Investigating Neurological Disease
Epidemiology for clinical neurology

In the clinical neurosciences, decision-making becomes ever more complicated because of rapidly emerging new diagnostic tests and treatments and increasing demands from patients to participate in their management. This concise but wide-ranging handbook reviews the epidemiology of neurological disease and the treatment and prognosis of major diseases of the nervous system. Part I offers essential guidance for clinicians to quantitative methods in research, including genetic epidemiology, decision analysis, meta-analysis, outcomes research and survival analysis, and thus provides a good understanding of the evidence underlying clinical management. The second part is devoted to individual neurological diseases, covering etiology, diagnosis, prognosis, interventions, and implications for clinical practice.

With contributions from leading international authorities, this book is an invaluable guide to clinical decision-making for neurologists and others involved in the management of neurological disease.

Albert Hofman is Professor in the Department of Epidemiology & Biostatistics at the Erasmus University Medical School, Rotterdam.

Richard Mayeux is Gertrude H. Sergievsky Professor of Neurology, Psychiatry and Public Health (Epidemiology) at the College of Physicians and Surgeons of Columbia University, New York.

Investigating Neurological Disease

Epidemiology for clinical neurology

Edited by

Albert Hofman

Erasmus University Medical School, Rotterdam

and

Richard Mayeux

College of Physicians and Sergievsky Center,
Columbia, New York

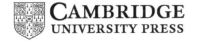

CAMBRIDGE
UNIVERSITY PRESS

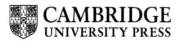

Shaftesbury Road, Cambridge CB2 8EA, United Kingdom

One Liberty Plaza, 20th Floor, New York, NY 10006, USA

477 Williamstown Road, Port Melbourne, VIC 3207, Australia

314–321, 3rd Floor, Plot 3, Splendor Forum, Jasola District Centre, New Delhi – 110025, India

103 Penang Road, #05–06/07, Visioncrest Commercial, Singapore 238467

Cambridge University Press is part of Cambridge University Press & Assessment, a department of the University of Cambridge.

We share the University's mission to contribute to society through the pursuit of education, learning and research at the highest international levels of excellence.

www.cambridge.org
Information on this title: www.cambridge.org/9780521000093

First published 2001

A catalogue record for this publication is available from the British Library

Library of Congress Cataloging-in-Publication data
Investigating neurological disease: epidemiology for clinical neurology / edited by Albert Hofman, Richard Mayeux.
    p. ; cm.
Includes bibliographical references and index.
ISBN 0 521 58065 X (hb) – ISBN 0 521 00009 2 (pb)
1. Nervous system – Diseases – Epidemiology.   I. Hofman, A.   II. Mayeux, Richard.
[DNLM: 1. Nervous System Diseases – Epidemiology.   2. Epidemiologic Methods.
WL 140 I62 2001]
RA645.N48 I56 2001
614.5'98 – dc21   2001025563

ISBN   978-0-521-00009-3   Paperback

....

Every effort has been made in preparing this book to provide accurate and up-to-date information which is in accord with accepted standards and practice at the time of publication. Although case histories are drawn from actual cases, every effort has been made to disguise the identities of the individuals involved. Nevertheless, the authors, editors and publishers can make no warranties that the information contained herein is totally free from error, not least because clinical standards are constantly changing through research and regulation. The authors, editors and publishers therefore disclaim all liability for direct or consequential damages resulting from the use of material contained in this book. Readers are strongly advised to pay careful attention to information provided by the manufacturer of any drugs or equipment that they plan to use.

Contents

Part I   Quantitative methods in clinical neurology

Part II   Neurological diseases

Contributors

A. Alpérovitch
INSERM U.360
Hôpital La Salpetrière
Paris Cedex 13 75651
France

John F. Annegers
Houston School of Public Health
University of Texas
PO Box 20186
Houston, Texas
USA

Ettore Beghi
Laboratory for Neurological Disorders
Istituto di Ricerche Farmacologiche Mario
Via Eritrea
Milano 20157
Italy

Kaj Blennow
Department of Psychiatry
Sahlgrenska University Hospital
S-413 45 Göteborg
Sweden

Monique M. B. Breteler
Department of Epidemiology & Biostatistics
Room Ee 2177
Erasmus University Medical School
PO Box 1738
3000 DR Rotterdam
The Netherlands

Richard K. Chan
Department of Clinical Neurological
Sciences
University of Western Ontario
Box 5339
339 Windermere Road
London
Canada N6A 5A5

Esther A. Croes
Department of Epidemiology & Biostatistics
Erasmus University Medical School
PO Box 1738
3000 DR Rotterdam
The Netherlands

Gerald J. Dal Pan
Food and Drug Administration
Division of Anesthetic, Critical Care and
Addiction Drug Products
5600 Fisheres Lane
Room 9B-45
Mail Stop HFD-170
Rockville, MD 20857
USA

Diederik W. J. Dippel
Department of Neurology
Room Ee 22-40A
Erasmus University Medical School
PO Box 1738
3000 DR Rotterdam
The Netherlands

Mitchell S. V. Elkind
Stroke Service, Neurological Institute
Columbia University
630 West 168th Street
New York, NY 10032
USA

Vladimir C. Hachinski
Department of Clinical Neuroscience
University of Western Ontario
Box 5339
339 Windermere Road
London N6A 5A5
Canada

Albert Hofman
Department of Epidemiology & Biostatistics
Erasmus University Medical School
PO Box 1738
3000 DR Rotterdam
The Netherlands

John F. Kurtzke
Dept of Veterans Affairs
Medical Center
50 Irving Street Horthvest
Washington DC 20422
USA

Richard B. Lipton
Neurology, Epidemiology & Social Medicine
Albert Einstein College of Medicine
Montefiore Medical Center
111 East 210th Street
Bronx, New York, NY 10467-2490
USA

Richard Mayeux
Sergievsky Center
Columbia University
630 West 168th Street
New York, NY 10032
USA

Justin C. McArthur
Johns Hopkins Hospital
Department of Neurology
Meyer 6-109
600 N. Wolfe Street
Baltimore, MD 21287
USA

Karin B. Nelson
Neuro-epidemiology Branch, ChP, DIR
Federal Building, Room 714
7550 Wisconsin Ave
Bethesda, MD 20892-9130
USA

Ruth Ottman
Sergievsky Center
Columbia University
630 West 168th Street
New York, NY 10032
USA

Maarten C. de Rijk
Dept of Epidemiology & Biostatistics
Erasmus University Medical School
PO Box 1738
3000 DR Rotterdam
The Netherlands

Walter A. Rocca
Department of Health Sciences Research
Mayo Clinic
200 First Street SW
Rochester, MN 55905
USA

Ralph L. Sacco
Columbia Presbyterian Medical Center
420 W 23rd Street
New York, NY 10011
USA

Ned C. Sacktor
Johns Hopkins Bayview Medical Center
Department of Neurology
B Building, Room 122
4940 Eastern Ave
Baltimore, MD 21224
USA

Ann I. Scher
Federal Building, Room 714
7550 Wisconsin Ave MSC
Bethesda, MD 20892-9130
USA

Ingmar Skoog
Department of Psychiatry
Sahlgrenska Hospital
University of Götenborg
Götenborg S-413 45
Sweden

Walter F. Stewart
Department of Epidemiology
Johns Hopkins Hospital
600 N. Wolfe Street Meyer 6-109
Baltimore, MD 21287-7609
USA

Therese A. Treves
Department of Neurology
Beilinson Hospital Rabin Medical Center
Petach Tikva 49100
Israel

Cornelia M. van Duijn
Department of Epidemiology & Biostatistics
Erasmus University Medical School
PO Box 1738
3000 DR Rotterdam
The Netherlands

Jan van Gijn
Afdeling Neurologie, Room G 03.228
Academisch Ziekenhuis Utrecht
Postbus 85500
3508 GA Utrecht
The Netherlands

W. A. van Gool
Divisie Neurozintuig Specialismen H2-214
Academisch Medisch Centrum
Postbus 22700
1105 AZ Amsterdam
The Netherlands

R. van Koningsveld
Department of Neurology
University Hospital Rotterdam
Dr Molewaterplein 40
3015 GD Rotterdam
The Netherlands

F. G. A. van der Meché
Department of Neurology
Dijkzigt Ziekenhuis
Dr Molewaterplein 50
3015 GD Rotterdam
The Netherlands

M. Vermeulen
Department of Neurology
Academic Medical Centre
University of Amsterdam
Meibergdreef 9
1105 AZ Amsterdam
The Netherlands

Mitchell T. Wallin
Neurology Service
VAMC
Washington, DC 20422
USA

Philip A. Wolf
Neurological Epidemiology and Genetics
Boston University School of Medicine
715 Albany Street B608
Boston, MA 92118-2526
USA

Preface

Neurological diseases are a major burden for patients and populations. There are few animal models in which human diseases can be easily studied making it mandatory to investigate these problems in humans. Many of these diseases have still largely unknown causes, but considerable progress has been made in recent years in diagnosis, prognosis and treatment. The quantitative approach to neurological diseases has contributed substantially to the increase in insight into the clinical aspects of these diseases and this book is a reflection of that. In this quantitative approach a key role in this is played by clinical epidemiology. Epidemiology addresses all major topics in medicine – etiology, diagnosis, prognosis and treatment. It also addresses, in principle, all diseases. More recently, epidemiology has combined the tools developed in molecular biology and genetics with large-scale epidemiological approaches to identify fundamental causes for some of these nervous system disorders with the long-term goal of successful intervention.

This book has two main sections. In the first part a general account of principles of quantitative research in clinical neurology is presented. This section addresses the design and analysis of clinical studies in neurology, the genetic approach to neurological diseases, diagnostic research and clinical decision analysis, prognosis research, in particular outcomes research and survival analysis, and the role of the clinical trial in efficacy studies.

In the second part most major neurological diseases are discussed in a systematic fashion with an emphasis on etiology, diagnosis, prognosis and intervention. For all diseases, implications of these findings for clinical practice are discussed.

We hope that this book will prove helpful for those interested in clinical neurology and the neurosciences, and in particular for those aiming at clinical research of the neurological diseases.

Albert Hofman and Richard Mayeux, editors

2001

Part I

Quantitative methods in clinical neurology

Clinical research design: analytical studies

Richard Mayeux

Analytic studies are used to define the relationship between a disease and its etiology or factors that may alter the course or manifestations of the disease. While these studies provide measures of the association between a risk factor, an exposure or a gene and a disease, Glynn (1) points out that the association may also be due to chance, the result of an inherent bias or confounding. Analytic studies usually take the form of observational investigations, but can also include randomized clinical trials. All aspects of the disease pathway may be investigated in this fashion.

Disease pathway

The model of the classical disease pathway (Figure 1.1) offers a way of conceptualizing how and when factors act in the process of disease. *Etiology* refers to a specific cause, while *pathogenesis* defines the mechanism by which the etiology results in disease. The period between exposure to the cause and the initiation of the disease process is referred to as the *induction period*. This period of time is dependent on the etiology or cause; no specific time period can be defined. The period between the induction of disease and its detection has been termed by Rothman (2) as the *latency period*.

In many neurologic disorders both the latency and induction periods may be lengthy. Associations between factors and disease may indicate where influences act in the disease pathway. For example, risk factors that act during the induction period will, most likely, have direct effects on risk. Traumatic head injury is an example of a risk factor that is considered by some to increase the risk of Alzheimer's disease by promoting the extracellular release of β-amyloid in the brain (3). Thus, by acting as an inducer of disease, head injury might be expected to increase the risk of Alzheimer's disease.

Queries concerning exposures during the latency period, however, might actually identify risk factors that modify (increase or decrease) the risk associated with the true etiology, or alternatively, factors that might result from the disease.

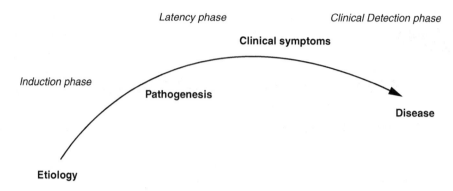

Figure 1.1   Causal pathway of disease.

For example, several case-control investigations had suggested that cigarette smoking is associated with a decreased risk of Alzheimer's disease (4,5). In some cross-sectional and case-control studies, a history of having smoked is less frequent among patients with Alzheimer's disease than among healthy controls. While it is possible that smoking decreases the risk of disease, it is also possible that smoking behavior diminishes as a result of the disease. That is, that smoking behavior changes during the latency period before the disease is diagnosed. Thus, a reduction in smoking during the latency period might actually reflect a manifestation of disease not a true modifier of disease risk.

Risk factors and causal inference

Risk factors are antecedents that are considered to be components of the disease pathway. Many are related to the etiology or cause of the disease (or outcome being investigated; the same principles may apply to clinical trials where the outcome is prevention or successful treatment of a disease and the risk factor is the therapy or intervention used). Cause and causal inference are the subject of great philosophical debate among clinical scientists (2,6–8). The investigator needs always to consider the possibility that the association might be due to chance or to some factor. The "cause" of a disease has been defined "as an event, condition or characteristic that plays an essential role in producing an occurrence of the disease." Rothman (2) argues that "cause" is a relative concept. For example, he cites that while smoking "causes" lung cancer, it does not do so in everyone. Smoking probably causes lung cancer only in those individuals susceptible to those effects of smoking. Nonetheless, risk factors, both genetic and environmental, may be considered "causal" by researchers if they are found in a higher proportion of individuals with, than without, the disease or if the risk of developing the disease over a specified time is greater for those individuals with, than those without, a particular risk factor. However, it is often very difficult to distinguish between a "causal" and "noncausal" association for any given factor and a disease.

Epidemiologists rely on the principles of causal inference first described by Hill (6), and further developed and refined over the last few decades by Susser (7,8) and Rothman (table 1) (2). In brief, associations should be strong on the argument that weak associations may be due to confounding or bias. Consistency and specificity of the relationship between the putative risk factor and disease are also important criteria. Temporal relationship is the most difficult to establish in cross-sectional or case-control studies. This criterion requires that the risk factor be present before the disease. Because ascertainment of cases and information regarding risk factors is often obtained at the same time it is often difficult to confirm the timing of the exposure with regard to disease onset. Biological gradient or "dose-response" implies that as the degree of exposure increased to a putative risk factor or as the number of alleles of a specific gene increases, the risk of disease will be greater. Biologic plausibility is also an important criterion, demanding a biological reason for any "causal" association.

Clearly, using these principles can help to establish the type of relationship between exposure and a disease. The use of appropriate statistical tests reduces, but does not eliminate, the possibility that chance alone accounts for the observed association. Appropriate study design and consideration to systematic bias and confounding also help to establish association between the exposure and disease. The purpose for maintaining the principles of causal inference and eliminating chance, bias, and confounding is to establish validity.

Types of analytic studies of risk factors

Typically, we investigate relationships between risk factors and disease using one of the approaches illustrated in Figure 1.2. The *case-control* study is essentially retrospective and estimates the "odds" of having *been* exposed to a risk factor, given case-control status. The advantage of a case-control study is its relatively low cost and efficiency in its design and conduct. Cases are selected by some a priori criteria and matched with healthy controls (those without the disease) from the same population. The investigator ascertains historical information regarding the type, duration, and means of exposure. The case-control design has limitations in that patient status and risk factors are determined at the same time. Therefore, the temporal sequence is often difficult to establish and one cannot measure incidence rates of disease in those exposed and unexposed to a risk factor. Thus, it is difficult to establish attributable risks (risk differences) between those exposed and unex-posed. Another problem is eliminating recall bias. Cases are more likely than

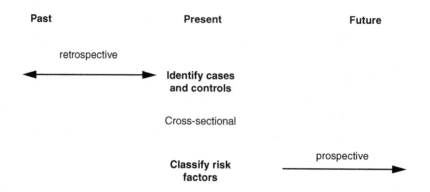

Figure 1.2   Types of analytic studies in epidemiology.

controls to have considered possible explanations for their illness (real or imagined). Given the structure of a case-control or cross-sectional study, the investigator is usually able to derive a testable hypothesis rather than firmly establish a cause–effect association.

The *cohort study* is prospective in design and generally allows the ascertainment of exposure before the occurrence of disease. This allows calculation of incidence rates in those exposed and unexposed to the risk factors, but requires follow-up of a large number of individuals because risk factor data are collected prior to disease onset. It is costly and investigators are not always able to control confounding variables and maintain high follow-up rates. Other outcomes may be expected. For example, a prospective study of Alzheimer's disease or Parkinson's disease would likely encounter heart disease and stroke at greater frequency. Another problem with longitudinal follow-up is that the risk factors under observation may become less important during the period of observation. For example, a study of smoking behavior and the risk of Alzheimer's disease may need to include the use of estrogen supplements by women. If the investigators did not include that information at the baseline interview, it will be difficult to add the study at a later date without biasing the results.

Occasionally, a cohort may have been gathered for a specific investigation and followed for a period. Later an investigator may want to reconstitute the cohort in order to investigate another disease entity. He or she may wish to study factors that were collected previously but will investigate new outcomes or disease which were not part of the original study goals. This "*retrospective cohort*" has the design of a prospective study but cases are determined in the present time. These types of study are more practical and less costly than prospective cohort studies, but it is often difficult to reconstruct the original cohort and identify other factors accounting for disease occurrence at follow-up. Thus, validity is a concern.

Table 1.1. Types of bias

Selection bias
Diagnosis bias (*Berkson's bias*)
Recall and information bias
Prevalent case bias (*Neyman's fallacy*)

An alternative, but less often used method, is the *case-base* method in which a random (stratified) sample of the base or referent population is interviewed for the putative risk factors. Then all incident cases are identified from the entire base population over a specified time period and the frequencies of risk factors in these cases are similarly determined. Because the sampled base yields essentially complete information on the base population, the investigator is able to estimate rates of disease in those exposed and unexposed to the risk factors of interest, assess attributable risk, and establish risk profiles with considerable economy over the cohort method. The problem of temporal direction is difficult to establish in this type of investigation because the same issues that limit the usefulness of case-control studies apply here as well: ascertainment of patient status and risk factors occurs at the same time.

Thus, while cross-sectional, case-control and case-base studies are economical and more pragmatic than longitudinal studies, they may only be useful for deriving hypotheses. In most instances, definitive analytic studies need to rely on prospective, cohort studies of risk factors.

Validity

The most serious concern in analytic studies is maintaining validity. To paraphrase Glynn (1), bias is usually minimized rather than eliminated and misclassification or exposure or diagnosis can have a major effect on the outcome of the study. Simply relying on the use of statistical significance or "p" values is insufficient.

Bias

In epidemiological studies two or more groups are usually compared for the frequency of exposure to a putative risk factor or factors. Procedures in the selection of either cases or controls can lead to a biased or invalid study (Table 1.1). Methods used for the selection of both cases and controls are the subject of intense discussion (9). In brief, case definitions must be considered in terms of sensitivity, specificity, and their effect on the validity, sample size, precision, and power. Overly restrictive case selection (lack of sensitivity) can lead to a loss of precision and power by reducing the sample size, and broad criteria (lack of specificity) produces misclassification that may bias the measure of any effect. Validity should always outweigh power and precision, and specificity (and the more restrictive case definitions) should outweigh sensitivity (and the more inclusive case definitions). The choice of a control implies some concept of the source population for both cases and controls. That is, controls should be selected to represent the population from which the cases were identified. Most importantly, controls should be from the same population at risk of the disease or condition being investigated.

Selection bias can result from any known or unknown influence motivating the way in which the selection of subjects for the study occurred. For example, if an individual is convinced that exposure to certain toxic fumes leads to Alzheimer's disease, then individuals with a history of such an exposure might seek to participate in a study of toxic fumes and Alzheimer's disease. The *self-selection* bias in this type of study might lead to the conclusion that toxic fumes are related to the cause of Alzheimer's disease.

Diagnostic bias can also be a problem. Berkson's bias refers to the probability of a hospitalization among patients with one or more conditions compared with that among patients with only one of the conditions. Thus, individuals drawn from hospital populations are likely to be different and most likely "sicker" than a group of cases drawn from a general population. This type of bias extends to the use of cases in tertiary centers or specialized centers. It is quite likely that the patients in a specialized center are also self-selected and the motivation for coming to the clinic is immeasurable. Thus, any set of risk factors, environmental or genetic, might be unique to such a group of individuals.

The use of prevalent versus incident cases in observational, correlative, or case-control studies can also be a source of bias. Because prevalence is the product of incidence × duration, prevalent cases may acknowledge factors that promote longer and better survival than incident cases. Thus, one is obtaining risk factors potentially related to survival rather than disease risk. As with the other forms of bias, *prevalent case* bias or Neyman's fallacy, promotes the underlying concern that the relationship between a risk factor and disease is different for those who participate (self-selected, specialty clinical hospital cases or prevalent cases) than for individuals who would have been eligible to participate but were otherwise aware of the study (9).

Information bias primarily concerns the collection of information from participants in a study. For case-control studies of risk factors the potential for one type of information bias, *recall* bias, is always present. Cases and controls differ in that one has the disease, the other does not. This difference, while obvious, may affect recall of exposure differently for cases than for controls. This is further complicated in studies of Alzheimer's disease where the individual is not capable of describing previous exposures. A spouse or family member may be called upon to provide such information. Alzheimer's disease may have affected the ability of a family member or spouse to remain objective in recalling past exposures in their affected family member. Differential misclassification (usually in cases) of exposure in a study has disastrous effects on validity. A highly motivated spouse as an informant for a patient with Alzheimer's disease might have strong opinions about a potential risk factor–disease relationship, whereas a control or his or her spouse may not have such opinions. This leads to differential misclassification of exposures, and could promote an association where none existed. Nondifferential misclassification of exposure is less severe, favoring a null effect of no association. Nondifferential exposure often occurs when the ability to remember an exposure (e.g., early life event) is equal for both cases and controls. Differential recall bias can be overcome by using a prospective cohort design in which exposure to risk factors is obtained before individuals develop disease.

Confounding

Confounders are, by definition, extraneous factors that are related to the disease and to a risk factor or exposure related to the disease (2). The confounder usually predicts disease in the absence of any risk factor. Perhaps the best known confounder is age. Advancing age is associated not only with Alzheimer's disease, but with a large number of disorders. Thus, age is not a "cause" but represents a confounder because it is involved in the relationship between any putative risk factor (environmental or genetic) and disease.

It is often difficult to be certain that a risk factor is not a confounder. Scientific judgement, experience, and investigation can help to clarify these relationships. In fact, the relationship between a confounder and disease may be stronger than that between a specific risk factor and disease. Finally, potential confounders must be accounted for by statistical adjustment or stratification in order to fully appreciate the relationship between a risk factor and disease. Nonetheless, the effects of strong confounders such as age, gender, or ethnic group may not be fully eliminated in any statistical association.

Conclusions

Analytic studies are increasingly important for understanding relationships between diseases and their causes. Each study design has its strengths and weaknesses. Exploratory studies should take the form of cross-sectional or case-control investigations with the goal of looking at many factors in order to derive general hypotheses. The more expensive cohort study can be used to test specific hypotheses. Investigators have to consider cost and efficiency in their design as well as the potential public health impact of any observed association.

Acknowledgements

This work is from the Gertrude H. Sergievsky Center, the Department of Neurology, Psychiatry, The Taub Center for Alzheimer's Disease Research Center and the Division of Epidemiology in the School of Public Health.

Support was provided by Federal Grants AG07232, AG10963, AG08702, NS15076 and RR00645, The Taub Foundation, the Charles S. Robertson Memorial Gift for Alzheimer's Disease Research from the Banbury Fund and the Blanchette Hooker Rockefeller Foundation.

REFERENCES

1. Glynn JR. A question of attribution. *Lancet* 1993;342:530–52.
2. Rothman KJ. *Modern Epidemiology.* Boston: Little, Brown and Company, 1986; 7–21.
3. Roberts GW, Gentleman SM, Lynch A, et al. β amyloid protein deposition in the brain after severe head injury. *J Neurol Neurosurg Psychiatry* 1994;57:419–25.
4. van Duijn CM, Hofman A. Relation between nicotine intake and Alzheimer's disease. *BMJ* 1991;302:1491–4.
5. Graves AB, White E, Koespell T, et al. A case-control study of Alzheimer's disease. *Ann Neurol* 1990;28:766–74.
6. Hill AB. The environment and disease: Association or causation? *Proc R Soc Med* 1965;58:295–300.
7. Susser M. *Causal Thinking in the Health Science. Concepts and Strategies in Epidemiology.* New York: Oxford University Press, 1973.
8. Susser M. What is a cause and how do we know one? A grammar for pragmatic epidemiology. *Am J Epidemiol* 1991;133:635–48.
9. Lasky T, Stolley PD. Selection of cases and controls. *Epidemiol Rev* 1994;16:6–17.

2

Genetic epidemiology in neurologic disease

Ruth Ottman

Rapid developments in molecular genetics in recent years have afforded tremendous growth in our understanding of the pathophysiology of many neurologic diseases. However, progress has been slower for common diseases of major public health impact (e.g., Alzheimer's disease, essential tremor, epilepsy) than for rare Mendelian disorders (e.g., Huntington disease, neurofibromatosis). The reason for this slow progress is that in most common neurologic disorders, the genetic contributions are exceedingly complex. The research tools of *genetic epidemiology* are uniquely suited to deal with this type of complexity (1). This multidisciplinary field, which has emerged over the last 15–20 years, combines concepts and methods from epidemiology, biostatistics, clinical genetics, molecular genetics, and population genetics, as well as new approaches developed specifically for study of the genetic contributions to complex diseases.

This brief introduction to genetic epidemiology in neurologic disease will address : (1) the basis of the complexity in the genetic contributions to common neurologic disorders, (2) gene–environment interaction, (3) the pathway for investigating the genetic contributions to disease risk, (4) methods for collection of accurate information on disease occurrence in families, and (5) research strategies commonly employed in genetic epidemiology.

Genetic epidemiologists frequently distinguish between "simple" and "complex" genetic diseases. Simple genetic diseases have inheritance patterns that conform to classical Mendelian laws, whereas complex diseases do not. Complex diseases tend to aggregate in families, but their familial distributions are inconsistent with straightforward Mendelian modes of inheritance (autosomal or X-linked, dominant or recessive). Moreover, with complex diseases both genetic and environmental factors generally contribute to susceptibility, and may interact in their influence on risk (2–4). Clinical presentation varies widely, and the role of genetic susceptibility may differ among subgroups defined by features such as age at onset or clinical severity. Within narrowly defined clinical subsets, the important genetic and nongenetic mechanisms may differ among families. Even within

Table 2.1. Sources of complexity in "complex" diseases

1. Reduced penetrance
2. Etiologic/genetic heterogeneity
      Genetic vs. nongenetic causes
      Locus heterogeneity
      Allelic heterogeneity
3. Pleiotropy
4. Epistasis
5. Gene–environment interaction

the same family, the effect of a specific genotype may differ among individuals because of the modifying effects of other genes or environmental factors.

Most simple genetic diseases are very rare. For example, the birth prevalence of von Recklinghausen neurofibromatosis, an autosomal dominant disease, is approximately 0.02% (i.e., 1/5000 births). Investigation of the genetic epidemiology of simple genetic diseases might include assessment of the efficacy of genetic screening programs (e.g., adult screening for Tay Sachs disease, neonatal screening for phenylketonuria), comparison of gene frequencies across different populations, and investigation of the causes of chromosomal abnormalities such as trisomy 21 (the cause of Down syndrome).

In general, complex diseases are much more common than simple genetic diseases. Some examples in neurology would include (among many others): epilepsy, Alzheimer's disease (AD), Parkinson's disease (PD), migraine, essential tremor, and amyotrophic lateral sclerosis (ALS). Lifetime cumulative incidence of epilepsy (to age 74) is approximately 3% (5), 150 times as high as the birth prevalence of von Recklinghausen neurofibromatosis.

The fundamental basis for the complexity in these diseases is that there is an imperfect correspondence between the genotype (i.e., the actual genes) and phenotype (i.e., the anatomic or functional manifestation of the genotype). Five reasons for this imperfect correspondence are listed in Table 2.1. First, the genotypes raising risk for complex diseases may have *reduced penetrance*. Penetrance is the probability that a person with a specific genotype will manifest the disease. If penetrance of a disease susceptibility genotype is reduced, some persons with the high risk genotype will be unaffected, suggesting that nongenetic factors may be required for phenotypic expression. The implication is that in studying complex diseases in families, one cannot assume that unaffected individuals do not carry a susceptibility gene. A related concept is *variable expressivity*, in which disease manifestations vary across individuals in terms of age at onset, clinical severity, etc. Variable expressivity is sometimes observed even in so-called simple genetic diseases. With neurofibromatosis, for example, the severity of clinical symptoms may range from barely visible to dramatically abnormal, even within a single pedigree.

Second, *etiologic/genetic heterogeneity* is common in complex diseases. Disease risk is often influenced by different genetic and nongenetic factors in different families, or in different clinically defined subsets of the disease. Etiologic heterogeneity here refers to genetic or nongenetic mechanisms as alternative causes of the same phenotype. The genetic epidemiology of epilepsy provides a clear example of etiologic heterogeneity. There is strong evidence for a genetic contribution to idiopathic/cryptogenic epilepsy, where no specific environmental insult has been identified. However, recent studies indicate that the genetic contributions are minimal for epilepsy occurring in the context of an identified postnatal environmental insult to the central nervous system (6), and the same clinical form of epilepsy, in terms of seizure type, age at onset, etc., can occur either in the presence or the absence of an environmental insult.

Two types of genetic heterogeneity may be distinguished. With *locus* heterogeneity, mutations at different genetic loci may produce the same clinical phenotype. With *allelic* heterogeneity, alternative alleles at a single locus may produce the phenotype. Both locus and allelic heterogeneity have been demonstrated in AD. So far, four susceptibility genes have been found, on chromosomes 1, 14, 19, and 21 (7,8); and other, as yet unidentified, loci probably also contribute to susceptibility. For two of the mutations that have been identified, allelic heterogeneity is extensive. Multiple different disease-causing mutations have been found in the amyloid precursor protein gene (APP) on chromosome 21, and in the presenilin-1 gene on chromosome 14 (7).

Third, disease susceptibility genotypes often have *pleiotropic* effects, resulting in multiple phenotypic manifestations affecting several different disorders, or even different organ systems. The implication is that when we study a single complex disorder in families, we might be leaving out other disorders that result from the same genotypes. For example, in a recent study of the families of persons with ALS, risk was increased not only for ALS, but also for dementia, and possibly PD, suggesting an underlying genetic susceptibility may raise risk for all three disorders (9). Similarly, a gene localized to chromosome 17 apparently has multiple phenotypic effects, including dementia, parkinsonism, amyotrophy, and disinhibited behavior (10).

Fourth, some genetic influences on susceptibility to complex diseases may involve *genetic interaction (epistasis)*. With epistasis, the genotype that raises risk for the disorder involves the interacting effects of alleles at different loci. One possible example of epistasis was reported in a study of familial AD, where carriers of a mutation in the APP gene on chromosome 21 had younger age at onset of AD if they also carried APOE-ε4 alleles than if they did not (11).

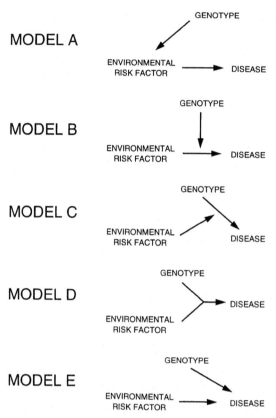

Figure 2.1   Five biologically plausible models of gene–environment interaction that may apply to diseases with complex genetic influences.

Fifth, disease risk may involve *gene–environment interaction,* defined as a different effect of a susceptibility genotype on disease risk in individuals with different environmental exposures (4). This can complicate study of both genetic and environmental factors in disease causation, because the effect of a genotype might be greater in exposed than in unexposed persons, or might be restricted to those exposed.

Figure 2.1 illustrates five biologically plausible models of gene–environment interaction that may apply to diseases with complex genetic influences (2,4). In Model A, the effect of the genotype is to produce, or increase expression of, a "risk factor" that can also be produced environmentally. In Model B, the genotype exacerbates the effect of the risk factor, but there is no effect of the genotype in unexposed persons. In Model C, the exposure exacerbates the effect of the genotype, but there is no effect of the exposure in persons with the low risk genotype. In Model D, both the exposure and the genotype are required to increase risk. Finally, in Model E, the exposure and the genotype each affect

Table 2.2. Pathway for studying the genetic contributions to disease risk

1. Is the disease familial?

2. What causes the familial aggregation?
   Shared behaviors/cultural factors (e.g., diet, smoking)
   Common environmental exposures (e.g., air or water pollution)
   Genetic susceptibility

3. What types of genetic effects are there?
   Single major genes (dominant or recessive, autosomal or X-linked)
   Epistatic effects
   Polygenic effects
   Chromosomal abnormalities

4. How do the gene(s) influence disease risk?
   Chromosomal localization
   Gene identification
   Functional studies

disease risk when they occur individually, and when they occur together risk may be higher or lower than predicted from their individual effects.

A recent study tested consistency with these models in an analysis of the relations between genetic susceptibility and head injury on the risk of AD (12). Risk of AD has consistently been found to be increased in individuals either heterozygous or homozygous for the ε4 allele of the apolipoprotein E (APOE) gene on chromosome 19 (13); thus APOE genotypes were used as a measure of genetic susceptibility to AD. When individuals with neither APOE-ε4 alleles nor head injuries were used as the reference group, risk of AD was not increased in head-injured individuals without APOE-ε4 alleles, but was increased two-fold in APOE-ε4 carriers without head injuries, and 10-fold in APOE-ε4 carriers with head injuries. These results are generally consistent with model C; they suggest that head injury has no effect on AD risk when acting by itself, but it exacerbates the effect of APOE-ε4 on AD risk.

The pathway for studying the genetic contributions to disease risk begins with investigation of the degree to which the disease aggregates in families (Table 2.2). If familial aggregation is observed, this does not necessarily imply a genetic etiology. Alternative explanations include behavioral risk factors shared by family members (e.g., diet, smoking, exercise habits), and common environmental exposures to family members who live together (e.g., air pollutants, water pollutants, radiation). Thus the second step in investigation of a complex disease involves disentangling genetic from environmental causes of familial aggregation. If genetic influences do appear to be important, the third step involves investigation of the types of genetic effects that are important, whether they involve single genes, combinations of genes (epistatic or polygenic effects), or chromosomal abnormalities. Finally, studies are designed to identify the susceptibility genes themselves, and to determine the mechanisms by which they influence disease risk.

Collection of accurate information about the disease status of family members is essential to all study designs in genetic epidemiology. There are two basic designs for collection of this type of information. In family *history* studies, information about disease in family members is obtained indirectly, from *family informants*. For many disorders, data obtained in this way have low sensitivity, i.e., many of the relatives who are truly affected are missed. For example, in a recent study of the validity of family history data on migraine headache, only 44% of the relatives who were diagnosed with migraine, based on self-reported symptoms, were reported by family informants to be affected (14). Sensitivity of family history data can be improved by restricting data collection to close relatives of the informants (generally *first-degree* relatives, i.e., parents, siblings, and offspring), selecting the informants likely to have the most complete information about the disease of interest, and interviewing multiple informants.

In *family studies*, on the other hand, data on the disease status of family members are obtained directly, through interviews or diagnostic testing of the relatives themselves. The data collected using this approach have higher sensitivity than those from family history studies. However, family studies are much more costly and time-consuming than family history studies. Also, data collection in family studies is necessarily incomplete because some relatives are always unavailable for direct testing (e.g., those who are deceased, cannot be located, or refuse to participate). Thus in practice, an intermediate approach between these two methods generally must be used (15).

Table 2.3 lists seven research strategies commonly used in genetic epidemiology. *Familial aggregation studies* focus on the first step in the pathway outlined in Table 2.2. The essential question posed in such studies is, "Does the disease occur more commonly in the families of affected individuals than in the families of unaffected individuals?" The data used to answer this question may be analyzed from two different perspectives (16). From the classical case-control perspective, a "positive family history" of disease is viewed as a risk factor, or "exposure," and disease status in cases and controls is viewed as the outcome. This can be problematic because the probability that a case or control has a family history of disease is influenced by the number of relatives at risk of disease in the family, and the age and other risk factors of the relatives. An alternative perspective, termed the "reconstructed cohort approach," treats the *relatives* of the cases and the *relatives* of controls as a cohort whose disease risk is to be evaluated. The "exposure" is

Table 2.3. Research strategies commonly used in genetic epidemiology

---

1. Familial aggregation studies

   Does the disease occur in some families more often than expected by chance?

2. Twin studies

   Is the concordance rate higher in monozygotic twins than in dizygotic twins?

3. Adoption studies

   Is the risk higher in biological relatives of affected adoptees than in biological relatives of unaffected adoptees?

4. Path analysis

   Are the similarities among relatives in the disease or trait explained by shared genes or shared environmental factors?

5. Seregation analysis

   Is the distribution of affected individuals in families consistent with a specific mode of inheritance?

6. Linkage analysis

   Is a disease susceptibility gene located on a chromosome, near a genetic marker?

7. Disease–genotype association studies

   Is the frequency of a marker allele higher in affected individuals than in unaffected individuals of the same ethnicity?

---

then defined by relatedness to the cases or controls. The hypothesis to be tested is that the disease risk is higher among relatives of cases than among relatives of controls. Control for the relatives' years-at-risk of disease (and any other information that might be available on the relatives' risk factors) can easily be accomplished through survival-based methods (e.g., life tables or Cox proportional hazards modeling) (17).

Twin studies, adoption studies, and *path analysis* are all designed to address the second stage of investigation in Table 2.2, namely distinction between genetic and nongenetic causes of familial aggregation. Twin studies can be used to advantage for investigating both genetic and environmental effects. In investigating genetic effects, the within-pair similarities of monozygotic and dizygotic twins are compared, on the assumption that genetic effects would produce greater similarity in the two cotwins of a monozygotic pair (who share 100% of their genes) than in the two cotwins of a dizygotic pair (who share on average 50% of their genes). To elucidate environmental influences on disease risk, discordant monozygotic twins can be compared with respect to their histories of environmental exposure.

Adoption studies can be designed in two ways. The first asks the question, "Is the disease risk higher in the biological than in the adopted relatives of affected adoptees?" This is potentially biased because of social differences between people who adopt children and those who put children up for adoption, which may be associated with risk for some diseases. The alternative, preferred approach asks the question, "Is the disease risk higher in biological relatives of affected adoptees than in biological relatives of unaffected adoptees?"

In path analysis, multiple regression-based statistical techniques are used to investigate the extent to which phenotypic similarities among relatives can be explained by shared environmental factors as opposed to genetic factors. This method is often used for analysis of data from twin and adoption studies, as well as for analysis of other types of familial data.

Segregation analysis is focused on the third stage of investigation in Table 2.2, namely elucidation of the types of genetic effects that underlie familial aggregation of the disease or trait. In this method, the observed familial distribution is compared with the distribution expected from various specific genetic models, to determine the most likely mode of inheritance.

Linkage analysis generally asks the question, "Is a disease susceptibility gene located on a chromosome near a genetic marker?" Chromosomal localization of a susceptibility gene is a first step in the final stage of investigation in Table 2.2, namely identification of the pathogenic mutation. The linkage approach involves statistical assessment of the evidence for cosegregation, within families, of a disease phenotype and a genetic marker. The analysis must be performed within families, because the specific marker allele associated with the disease generally varies from family to family, in accordance with the allelic distribution of the marker in the population. Such a within-family association is not likely to occur because of systematic bias, because most genetic markers have no clinical manifestations or social connotations, and marker information is collected by laboratory analysis of biological samples, independently of disease status. It provides strong evidence both that disease susceptibility is influenced by a gene (otherwise the disease would not be expected to cosegregate with a genetic marker), and the chromosomal location of the susceptibility gene is near that of the marker. The power of this method has been greatly expanded in recent years, due to developments in molecular biology, statistical genetics, and computer applications.

Finally, studies of *disease–genotype associations* ask, "Do affected individuals have a higher frequency of a specific marker allele than unaffected individuals (or the general population)?" This type of association is not expected in most cases of genetic linkage. If it is observed, then great care must be taken to rule out, as an explanation, confounding effects arising from different distributions of ethnicity in cases and controls. This problem can occur as a result of *population stratification*, where marker allele frequencies vary by ethnicity. If confounding effects can be ruled out, then the association could reflect either linkage disequilibrium (implying very tight linkage between a disease gene and the genetic marker), or a direct, causal effect of the associated allele on the disease. The consistent association of AD with APOE-ε4 provides an excellent example of this type of association. Since APOE plays an important role in amyloid deposition, the association may result from a causal effect of APOE-ε4 on AD risk (13). However, the APOE association appears to vary by ethnicity, suggesting that it may be due to linkage disequilibrium with another susceptibility locus on chromosome 19 (18).

In summary, many common neurologic disorders appear to aggregate in families in patterns that do not conform with simple Mendelian laws. For these disorders, the effects of genetic susceptibility on disease risk are unclear. Elucidation of these effects holds great promise for increasing understanding of basic pathophysiologic mechanisms. The research tools of genetic epidemiology, aimed at unraveling the genetic and environmental contributions to disease and their interactions, offer an exciting opportunity to resolve some of the most important current questions in neurologic research.

REFERENCES

1. Khoury MJ, Beaty TH, Cohen BH. *Fundamentals of Genetic Epidemiology.* New York: Oxford University Press, 1993.
2. Ottman R. An epidemiologic approach to gene–environment interaction. *Genet Epidemiol* 1990;7:177–85.
3. Ottman R, Susser E, Meisner M. Control for environmental risk factors in assessing genetic effects on disease familial aggregation. *Am J Epidemiol* 1991;134:298–309.
4. Ottman R. Gene–environment interaction: definitions and study designs. *Prev Med* 1996;25:764–70.
5. Hauser WA, Annegers JF, Kurland LT. Incidence of epilepsy and unprovoked seizures in Rochester, Minnesota: 1935–1984. *Epilepsia* 1993;34:453–68.
6. Ottman R, Annegers JF, Risch N, Hauser WA, Susser M. Relations of genetic and environmental factors in the etiology of epilepsy. *Ann Neurol* 1996;39:442–9.
7. Van Broeckhoven CL. Molecular genetics of Alzheimer's disease: identification of genes and gene mutations. *Eur Neurol* 1995;35:8–19.
8. Levy-Lahad E, Wasco W, Poorkaj P, et al. A candidate gene for the chromosome 1 familial Alzheimer's disease locus. *Science* 1995;269:973–7.
9. Majoor-Krakauer D, Ottman R, Johnson WG, Rowland LP. Familial aggregation of amyotrophic lateral sclerosis, dementia, and Parkinson's disease: evidence of a shared genetic susceptibility. *Neurology* 1994;44:1872–7.
10. Lynch T, Sano M, Marder KS, et al. Clinical characteristics of a family with chromosome 17-linked disinhibition-dementia-parkinsonism-amyotrophy complex. *Neurology* 1994;44:1878–84.

11. Sorbi S, Nacmias B, Forleo P, et al. Epistatic effect of APP717 mutation and apolipoprotein E genotype in familial Alzheimer's disease. *Ann Neurol* 1995;38:124–7.

12. Mayeux R, Ottman R, Maestre G, et al. Synergistic effects of traumatic head injury and apolipoprotein-ε4 in patients with Alzheimer's disease. *Neurology* 1995;45:555–7.

13. Strittmatter WJ, Roses AD. Apolipoprotein E and Alzheimer disease. *Proc Natl Acad Sci* (USA) 1995;92:4725–7.

14. Ottman R, Hong S, Lipton RB. Validity of family history data on severe headache and migraine. *Neurology* 1993;43:1954–60.

15. Ottman R, Susser M. Data collection strategies in genetic epidemiology: the Epilepsy Family Study of Columbia University. *J Clin Epidemiol* 1992;45:721–7.

16. Susser E, Susser M. Familial aggregation studies: a note on their epidemiologic properties. *Am J Epidemiol* 1989;129:23–30.

17. Chase GA, Folstein M, Breitner J, et al. The use of lifetables and survival analysis in testing genetic models, with an application to Alzheimer's disease. *Am J Epidemiol* 1983;117:590–7.

18. Maestre G, Ottman R, Stern Y, et al. Apolipoprotein E and Alzheimer's disease: ethnic variation in genotypic risks. *Ann Neurol* 1995;37:254–9.

3

Gene–environment interaction in neurologic disorders

Cornelia M. van Duijn

Introduction

In the past decade considerable progress has been made in unraveling the etiology of important major genetic diseases including neurogenetic disorders such as Huntington disease and autosomal dominant forms of Alzheimer's disease. At present, genetic research focuses on common neurologic diseases including Alzheimer's disease, Parkinson's disease, stroke and multiple sclerosis. Although it will be far more difficult to uncover the genetics of these complex disorders, as the Human Genome Project and molecular technology advances, the chances of success appear to be high. The pathogenesis of these disorders is more complex in that multiple genetic and environmental factors may interact. For the purpose of research as well as clinical practice, a key issue to resolve will be the interaction of genetic and environmental factors. In this chapter, the basic concept of gene–environment interaction will be discussed including the definition and principal mechanisms. Further, the evidence for gene–environment interaction will be addressed. Finally, some critical considerations for future research will be given.

Definition

Gene–environment interaction may be defined in several ways. From the perspective of a neurogenetic disorder, gene–environment interaction implies that the risk of disease associated with mutations or common genetic variations (i.e., polymorphisms) in genes is altered by a nongenetic risk factor. It is important to realize that in the case that an environmental factor causes a mutation, e.g., radiation leading to germ-line and/or somatic mutations, this does not imply there is evidence for interaction. In most cases it may be solely the mutation that determines the risk of disease without any interference of the environmental factors in the disease pathogenesis.

The environment may play a role at any level of the pathogenesis of a

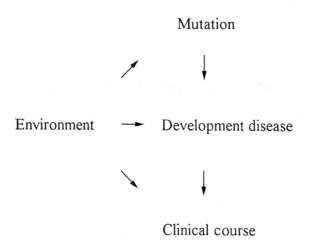

Figure 3.1 Gene–environment interaction in the disease pathogenesis.

neurogenetic disease (see Figure 3.1). At the stage of the etiology of the disease, genetic and environmental factors may interact and the risk of disease may be determined for a large part by the interplay between genetic and environment factors. However, the interaction between genetic and nongenetic factors is likely to determine also the course of disease after diagnosis. The most evident example from clinical practice is that genetic factors may determine in part the disease prognosis. If the course of disease is modified by therapeutic intervention, genetic factors may also interfere with their efficiency of drugs.

Mechanisms

Although gene–environment interaction is expected to be complex, Ottman (1) has shown that there are only a limited number of pathways through which a genetic and environmental factor may interact. If one considers the most simple case of the interaction between one genetic and one environmental factor, there are only four models possible (Figure 3.2). Under the first model, the genetic factor is the primary determinant of the disease, while the environmental factor has no effect by itself but merely modifies the risk associated with the genetic factor. *Vice versa*, model 2 specifies that the environmental factor is the primary determinant of the disease, while the genetic factor modifies only the risk associated with the environmental factor but the genetic factor does not have an effect by itself. In model 3, a mechanism is specified in which only subjects exposed to both the genetic and environmental factor are at increased or decreased risk of a certain outcome. Finally, in model 4, both the genetic and environmental factor may increase or decrease risk of a certain outcome by themselves, but the effect of each of these factors depends on the presence or absence of the other factor.

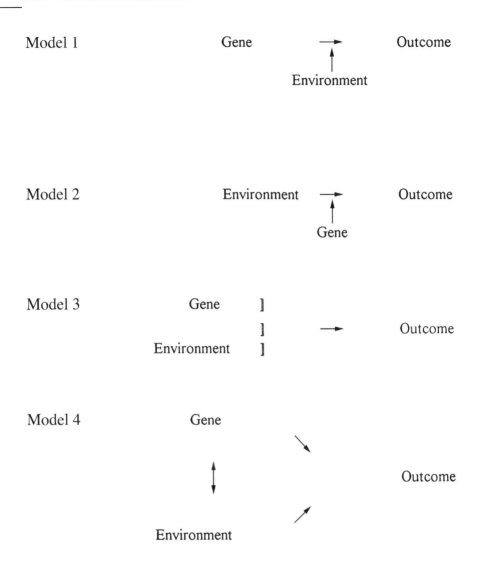

Figure 3.2   Models for gene–environment interaction according to Ottman (1990).

Since gene–environment interaction implies that the risk of disease associated with a certain factor is altered by another factor, it can be shown that the different models underlying the interaction may be disentangled simply by stratifying the data according to the presence or absence of the two factors under study (1). The hypothesis to be tested under model 1 specified in Figure 3.2 is that the risk of a certain outcome associated with the genetic factor differs significantly between those exposed and nonexposed to the environmental factor.

These models can be easily extrapolated to the interaction between multiple genetic and environmental factors. The number of possible mechanisms will grow tremendously when the interaction between multiple factors is addressed. This not only makes the interpretation of findings less straightforward, but also imposes a study design in which large numbers of subjects are to be studied, in order to have sufficient statistical power for the extensive subgroup analyses required.

Empirical evidence

Although gene–environment interaction may occur at any level of the pathogenic process, interactions may be particularly important from the point of disease prevention in neurodegenerative diseases with a late onset. Modifiable age-dependent environmental factors are likely to influence the risk and onset of disease. Genetic factors play an important role in the etiology of various neurodegenerative disorders such as Alzheimer's disease (AD), amyotrophic lateral sclerosis (ALS) and Parkinson's disease. For ALS and Parkinson's disease these concern Mendelian dominant or recessive mutations. Given the strength of familial aggregation and the variable disease expression, it is to be expected that also genetic factors with a more modest effect are implicated. The effect of these genetic risk factors may for a large part be determined by other, genetic and nongenetic factors. In particular, the findings of a high incidence of subclinical Parkinson's disease in genetically identical cotwins at positron emission tomography but major differences in clinical expression suggests that environmental factors modify the disease expression (2,3).

In recent years, remarkable progress has been made in the unraveling of the genetic basis of AD (4). Various mutations in three genes (Amyloid Precursor Protein gene, Presenilin-1 and -2 genes) have been identified which can lead to AD, but these are all extremely rare. The apolipoprotein E gene is a more common factor involved in Alzheimer's disease. As the risk associated with the polymorphisms known to date is highly variable, this gene has been a suitable candidate for studies of gene–environment interactions. There is evidence that the risk associated with the apolipoprotein E is modified by other genetic and nongenetic factors including head trauma, estrogen use, viral infections, smoking, and vascular disease and risk factors.

Considerations

It is becoming increasingly clear that a great number of common neurodegenerative disorders result from an interplay of genetic and environmental risk factors. The clinical and public health implications of genetic factors in terms of disease prevention and care are not straightforward if risks associated with these genetic factors are not properly quantified. Studies of gene interactions will be of growing import in etiological and clinical research.

For most neurologic disorders, little is known of gene–gene and gene–environment interactions. This is partly explained by the lack of knowledge of the genetic and environmental factors implicated in the disease pathogenesis. However, a major methodologic problem in studies of gene–environment interaction concerns the statistical power. To address the issue of gene–gene interactions and gene–environment interaction with sufficient statistical power, large numbers of patients and controls have to be studied (5). The most important issue to resolve is the low statistical power of studies of gene interactions. The statistical power decreases further when studying the interaction between three or more factors. Thus, to determine the relative contribution of various genetic factors to the occurrence and progression of disease in interaction with nongenetic factors and therapeutic interventions requires extensive studies of genetic and environmental factors in large study populations.

REFERENCES

1. Ottman R. An epidemiologic approach to gene–environment interaction. *Genet Epidemiol* 1990;7:177–85.
2. Smith PG, Day NE. The design of case-control studies: the influence of confounding and interaction effects. *Int J Epidemiol* 1984;13:356–65.
3. Burn DJ, et al. Parkinson's disease in twins studied with ^{18}F-DOPA and positron emission tomography. *Neurology* 1992;42:1894–1900.
4. Holthoff VA, et al. Discordant twins with Parkinson's disease: positron emission tomography and early signs of impaired cognitive circuits. *Ann Neurol* 1994;36:176–82.
5. Slooter AJC, Van Duijn CM. Genetic epidemiology of Alzheimer's disease. *Epidemiol Rev.* 1997;19:107–19.

4

Analysis, reanalysis, and meta-analysis in neurology

Walter A. Rocca

Introduction

The scope of this chapter is to illustrate the problems and the methodologic issues involved in collaborative reanalyses. The theoretical discussion and the definition of terms are kept to a minimum (1,2). Emphasis is given to factual examples derived from the neurologic literature and from the personal experience of the author.

The chapter covers an example of reanalysis of descriptive epidemiologic data (e.g., incidence and prevalence studies) and an example of reanalysis of analytic epidemiologic data (e.g., case-control and cohort studies). The much more prominent application of reanalysis to experimental epidemiology (e.g., clinical trials) is not covered here. The two examples used concern Alzheimer's disease (AD) and are derived from the extensive work of the European Community Concerted Action Epidemiology and Prevention of Dementia (EURODEM) (3–6). Some of the problems and methodologic issues illustrated may refer specifically to AD and may not be generalizable to other diseases; however, the two examples should conveniently illustrate some general aspects of reanalysis.

The next few paragraphs define the terms used and explain the disagreement on the definition of meta-analysis. *Analysis* is the application of statistical techniques to describe the data collected or to test hypotheses on the data collected in an individual epidemiologic study. *Reanalysis* is the subsequent analysis of a database from which primary analyses have been reported. Reanalyses are conducted when, for example, a new hypothesis has been proposed after the initial analyses had been completed. Data from an individual study may also be reanalyzed using a different statistical approach.

The term *collaborative reanalysis* is used when reanalyses involve more than one database, in general with the collaboration of several investigators who conducted the initial studies. A collaborative reanalysis is generally more sophisticated and powerful than a traditional *literature review*. An important limitation of literature reviews is that the reviewer(s) must rely upon published data. Almost always, the format of data reported varies across studies; for example, age classes for incidence or prevalence figures are aggregated according to the structure of the specific population or according to some conventional format. Another common problem is the use of open age classes, e.g., prevalence or incidence figures for the age class "85 +" or "90 +." In addition, journal editors often impose limits to the display of data; this policy may impede the reanalysis of published data. A common example is the publication of prevalence or incidence figures without displaying their denominator, or the report of an age- and sex-specific graph without a corresponding table with the numerator and denominator data. For case-control studies, it is common to report odds ratios, p values, and confidence intervals without displaying the actual numbers from which these measures were derived (7).

When reanalyses involve the *pooling* of data from randomized clinical trials, cohort studies, or case-control studies, the term *meta-analysis* has often been used in recent years (1). Meta-analysis has a qualitative component, namely the application of criteria of quality for the selection of studies to be included, and a quantitative component, namely the integration of numerical information (2). Meta-analysis includes aspects of an overview, and of pooling of data, but implies more than either of these processes (2).

Clayton suggests that the term meta-analysis should be restricted to the pooling of data from randomized clinical trials in which both bias and possible confounding are eliminated (or at least reduced) by the use of blindness and random allocation (8). In analytic epidemiology, pooled analyses may not add substantially to individual analyses because of the possibility of bias and confounding. An increase in the sample size of a study without an accompanying improvement in the quality of data will not necessarily yield benefit (9). The uncertainty regarding the interpretation of results from a case-control or cohort study is due primarily to the possibility of bias (10). The uncertainty caused by limitations in statistical power is only a small component of the overall uncertainty. Pooling of data may, at best, reduce statistical uncertainty, but it does not shed light on the quality of the data in the individual studies. Pooling of data and increasing the statistical power may actually be risky because it may give a "statistical blessing" to data that are fundamentally biased. These considerations apply more strongly to case-control studies than to cohort studies because case-control studies are particularly susceptible to various types of bias (7,8,10).

In this chapter, the term collaborative reanalysis is used for both descriptive and analytic data; this terminology is consistent with the publications from the EURODEM group (3–6). Figure 4.1 shows the steps common to most types of collaborative reanalyses. Each specific study may deviate to some extent from this general scheme; however, the fundamental steps remain constant.

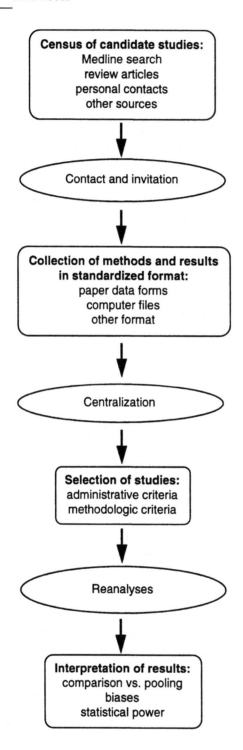

Figure 4.1   Steps involved in a collaborative reanalysis of descriptive or analytic epidemiologic data.

Reanalysis of descriptive epidemiologic data

An example of collaborative reanalysis of descriptive epidemiologic data is the comparison of prevalence data of AD by the EURODEM group (4). The objective of this study was to investigate geographic differences, age and sex patterns, and time trends in the prevalence of AD. Good quality data on the distribution of AD by place, time, and personal characteristics may be of extreme value in etiologic research (11,12).

Comparability of prevalence data on AD from various studies requires a homogeneous definition of the study population, common diagnostic criteria, equivalent case-finding strategies, and similar data analysis and reporting. Although comparability can be best achieved by the joint design and conduct of prevalence studies in several populations, collaborative reanalyses of existing data can be a step in that direction.

The study included the following steps: (i) census of existing prevalence surveys, (ii) contact and invitation of the investigator(s), (iii) collection of information on methods and results, (iv) centralization, (v) selection of methodologically comparable studies, (vi) study of AD distribution by time, place, and personal variables, and (vii) interpretation of results (Figure 4.1).

Census of studies, contact and invitation, data collection, and centralization

Current prevalence studies of dementia were identified from the following three sources: (i) Medline search and review papers, (ii) personal contacts of coordinating scientists and (iii) communication with dementia experts in each country. All the scientists identified were in turn asked for names of other investigators in their country who might have data of interest. Each potential co-investigator was then invited to participate in this collaborative study and to send suitable data sets to the coordinating SMID Center in Florence, Italy. Unpublished studies were included.

To report methods and findings in a standard format, each investigator completed a specifically designed data form including study title and investigators' information; time frame; characteristics of the study population or sample; diagnostic criteria for dementia and specific dementing disorders; case-finding procedures and their reliability and validity; response rate and sample attrition; tables of results; and publications from the study. Tables of results included number of patients, population at risk, and prevalence by 5-year age group, sex, and specific dementing disorder.

Selection of studies

The following eligibility criteria were applied to the recruited data sets: (i) studies conducted in Europe, (ii) conducted or published after 1979 (1980–1990), (iii) minimum sample of 300 subjects 65 years of age or older, (iv) case-finding through direct individual examination, (v) inclusion of institutionalized individuals, and (vi) clinical diagnosis of dementia based on the *Diagnostic and Statistical Manual for Mental Disorders, Third edition* (DSM–III), or equivalent criteria (13). The data sets fulfilling these criteria were used for a comparison of the prevalence of dementia in Europe reported elsewhere (3).

To be eligible for the comparison of AD prevalence, the following two additional criteria were used: (i) clinical diagnosis of AD based on the National Institute of Neurological and Communicative Disorders and Stroke-Alzheimer's disease and Related Disorders Association (NINCDS–ADRDA) or equivalent criteria (14), and (ii) sample yielding at least 10 patients with AD.

Reanalyses and results

Numerators, denominators, and prevalence figures were reported by 5-year age classes when the numerator included five or more patients with AD or when information within a decade was restricted to such an interval; otherwise, data were lumped into 10-year age classes coincident with decades. Prevalence from one study was reported by 5-year age classes because only two such classes were investigated. Prevalence estimates over the age of 89 years that were based on fewer than five patients were discarded. Because most studies to be compared were based on a complete enumeration of all individuals in a finite population, no sampling was involved, and confidence intervals for the prevalence estimates were not used (15).

Geographic differences were investigated through tables and graphs of age-specific prevalence for men and women separately; to enhance clarity of graphs, only prevalence figures over the age of 60 years were represented. Age and sex patterns within individual data sets were compared by graphing age- and sex-specific prevalence figures from cach study. Time trends were investigated by age and sex subgroups in the one suitable data set.

From an original roster of 23 data sets submitted to the project, 12 met the criteria for study of dementia prevalence in Europe (Figure 4.2). Eleven surveys were excluded for the following reasons: conducted and published before 1980 (one survey); insufficient sample size (two surveys); case-finding limited to existing medical documentation (one survey); institutionalized individuals excluded (four surveys); and only "cognitive impairment" investigated (two surveys). One study was excluded because it covered only institutionalized individuals; however, the results of this survey were combined with those from another study covering the household individuals of the same population.

Six of the 12 data sets were eligible for the comparison of AD prevalence and were included in the present study (Figure 4.2). In five of the six excluded surveys,

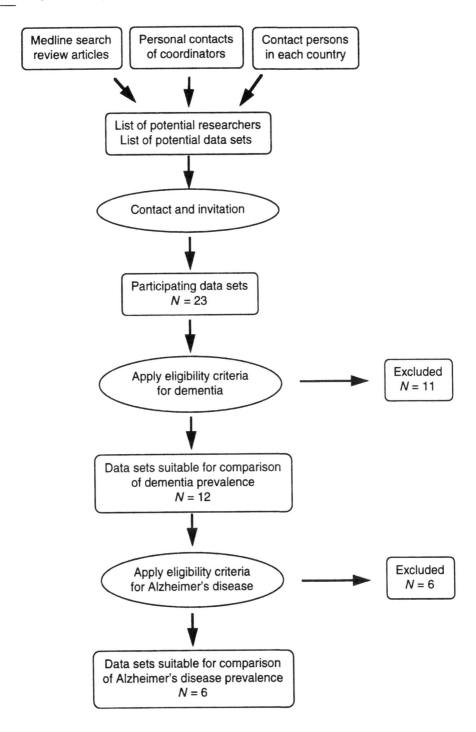

Figure 4.2 Steps involved in the EURODEM collaborative reanalysis of prevalence studies of Alzheimer's disease. Indicated also is the impact of individual steps on the number of studies involved.

AD was not separated from other dementing disorders; in one, the diagnosis of AD was not equivalent to the NINCDS–ADRDA criteria. The six eligible studies were from the following five European countries: Finland, Italy, Spain, Sweden, and the UK (two studies). Details on characteristics of the study population, case-finding procedures, and diagnostic criteria for dementia and specific dementing disorders were reported elsewhere (3,4).

When age and sex were considered, there were no major geographic differences in the prevalence of AD across European studies (Figure 4.3). Prevalence increased exponentially with advancing age in all studies and, in some populations, was consistently higher in women (4). Prevalence remained stable over 15 years in one study (4).

Interpretation

Rather than a traditional literature review, a collaborative reanalysis of results from existing surveys was undertaken. For this reason, access to the raw data was required. Some unpublished European studies, or studies reported in sources not easily retrieved, may have been overlooked. This fact might bias our results; however, none of the known data sets were withdrawn from consideration.

Suitable data sets were selected by qualitative judgement. Because of the rapid evolution of the diagnostic criteria for dementia and AD in recent years, we considered only studies conducted, or at least published, after 1979. We required the direct contact of study subjects for case-finding because many patients in the population do not come to medical attention for their dementia, and would be missed by searching only existing medical documentation. In addition, because in developed countries severely demented people are often institutionalized, we required the inclusion of institutionalized inhabitants of the study area (11,16).

The most important methodological issue in interpreting our findings is the comparability of various case-finding procedures. In surveys calling for the direct contact of each individual in the sample, the following two approaches can be used: (i) study subjects are directly examined by the specialist who makes the diagnosis of dementia (*single-phase study*), or (ii) study subjects undergo a screening procedure, and only individuals failing the screening are extensively evaluated (*two-phase study*). The first approach was used in one study; the remaining five studies followed a two-phase design. Unfortunately, different screening instruments were used. Two studies applied the Mini-Mental State examination, but the instrument was used in different languages and with some adaptations to the local culture (17). Distinct instruments, or different translations and cutoff levels of a common test, may have different sensitivity. This may introduce spurious variations in the observed prevalences.

The following are two common approaches to measuring the sensitivity of a

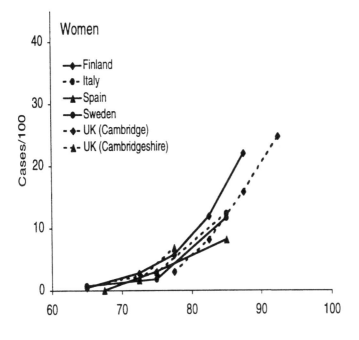

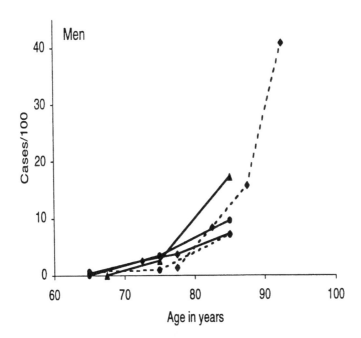

Figure 4.3   Age- and sex-specific prevalence of Alzheimer's disease from six European studies (data from (4)). In the Cambridgeshire, United Kingdom study, only women were surveyed.

screening instrument: (i) a validity study is conducted before beginning the survey, often on a different sample; or (ii) the validation is incorporated in the survey by submitting to clinical examination not only subjects who failed the screening, but also a sample of those who passed the screening. In both cases, results of the screening test are compared with the clinical diagnosis, which serves as the standard for comparison. In three of the five European surveys, the screening instrument was validated and sensitivity was found to be high. In another study, the investigators judged sensitivity to be high.

In the Finnish survey, mild dementia was explicitly excluded. In other studies, an effort was made to find all "detectable cases"; however, it is possible that some early or mild cases of dementia were missed by less sensitive screening procedures. On the other hand, neither the DSM–III nor the NINCDS–ADRDA criteria (13,14) define levels of severity, and terms such as "mild", "moderate", or "severe dementia" may not be comparable across studies.

Because DSM–III and NINCDS–ADRDA criteria are clinical diagnostic guidelines, and do not specify, for example, which laboratory tests are mandatory for a given diagnosis, different groups of researchers may disagree on their interpretation and use (13,14). Most problematic is the differential diagnosis of AD, vascular (including mixed), and secondary dementias. Also, the exclusion of cases of secondary dementia depends on the intensity and completeness of the search for specific causes. Most important for this search are imaging and hematological tests. In only two of the six European studies, imaging tests were conducted on some of the prevalent cases; therefore, greater weight was given to clinical criteria than to imaging findings in all studies. Similarly, a specific list of blood tests was performed routinely in only one study; however, in three others, blood tests were performed when suggested by medical history or physical examination. In two studies, hematological tests were not performed.

In some surveys, an effort was made to account either directly or indirectly for each individual originally included in the study sample; in others, information was missing on varying percentages of population. In four of the five two-phase studies, the response rate ranged between 89 and 97% for the screening phase; the response rate for phase 2 was between 82 and 98%. In the single-phase study, the response rate was 89%. In one study, response rates to both phase 1 and 2 were high but not quantified.

An effort was made in this study to select those European prevalence surveys that used more comparable methods. Unfortunately, the six studies selected may still be only partially comparable. The most important uncertainties relate to the sensitivity of case-finding procedures and the interpretation and use of allegedly common diagnostic criteria in various surveys. Even with these limitations, our findings suggest that the prevalence of AD is similar in various European countries, it increases exponentially with age, is higher in women, and has remained stable over time (4).

Reanalysis of analytic epidemiologic data

The example of collaborative reanalysis of analytic epidemiologic data is the comparison and pooling of case-control studies of AD by the EURODEM group. The objective of this study was to establish the consistency of findings across studies, to investigate rare exposures, and to conduct subgroup analyses (8). The most important objective was to establish consistency across studies. Although the same source of bias or confounding may be operating in all studies, consistency of findings across case-control studies conducted in various countries with different methodologies is crucial. Consistency of findings is one of the key criteria to establish a causal link in epidemiology (2). Consistency is more conveniently assessed within the frame of a collaborative reanalysis, because it is best assessed if comparable analyses are available. It is in general problematic to investigate consistency from published findings because investigators use different cutoff points for exposures, adjust for various confounders, and may report only summary results. For risk factors for which consistency of results across studies has been established, "pooling" may be useful to study confounders and to conduct subgroup analyses. Single studies are in general too small for multivariate or subgroup analyses. In addition, when an exposure is rare among controls (reflecting the general population), pooling may be indispensable to reach informative numbers even for the overall analysis.

A general discussion of the methods used in this EURODEM reanalysis is reported here; however, because methods varied slightly from risk factor to risk factor, the association between AD and family history of Down's syndrome is used as a specific example (18). For a complete report on the reanalyses, the reader is referred to the published monograph (6).

The study included the following steps: (i) census of existing case-control studies, (ii) contact and invitation of the investigator(s), (iii) collection of information on methods and results, (iv) centralization of the relevant segment of the database, (v) selection of methodologically comparable studies, (vi) reanalyses, and (vii) interpretation of results (Figure 4.1).

Census of studies, contact and invitation, data collection, and centralization

Case-control studies of AD were identified through the following three sources: (i) Medline search, (ii) review papers, and (iii) personal contacts of coordinating scientists. To obtain information regarding selection of cases, selection of controls, and collection of data on exposure in individual studies, each investigator completed a specifically designed data form. In addition, the risk factor question-naire of each study was translated into English.

The relevant segment of the database of each case-control study was centralized at the Department of Epidemiology and Biostatistics of the Erasmus University Medical School, in Rotterdam, The Netherlands. Data were transferred using magnetic tapes and were loaded on a central computing facility. Data format and coding were homogenized across studies. For example, the data on number of cigarettes per day and duration of smoking were transformed into a common analyzable format.

Selection of studies

The following preliminary inclusion criteria were applied early in the study, before inviting the investigators to participate: (i) studies conducted before January 1, 1990; (ii) studies using NINCDS–ADRDA, DSM–III, or equivalent criteria for AD (13,14); and (iii) studies that investigated a series of risk factors. Several small studies investigating a single risk factor for AD (e.g., maternal age) were not considered. On the other hand, non-European studies were included. The most important eligibility criterion was symmetrical data collection for cases and controls. Since data collection for cases was generally through a next-of-kin interview, the same procedure was also required for controls. In one study, however, data collection was through abstracting of medical records; in a second study, it was through a mailed questionnaire; and in a third, through a telephone interview. Other aspects of the study design, such as the type of controls, were considered in the analyses and in the interpretation of findings but were not used as eligibility criteria.

Reanalyses and results

For each specific risk factor, analyses were conducted on eligible studies with suitable exposure information. The strength of the association between AD and a given factor was measured by the odds ratio, that is an estimate of the relative risk. We obtained maximum likelihood estimates of the odds ratio and 95% confidence intervals based on asymptotic standard errors. Since all studies included were matched at least for age and sex, relative risks were estimated using conditional logistic regression models (7). When appropriate, potential confounding variables were entered into the models. For example, some analyses were adjusted for number of siblings, or for education (6).

Analyses were conducted on the individual data sets, on the pooled sample, and on subgroups of the pooled sample defined by sex, age at onset, or familial aggregation of AD cases. A case of AD was defined as "early onset" when the symptoms of the disease started before the age of 65 years, as "late onset" otherwise. A case of AD was defined as "sporadic" when the patient had no known first-degree relative affected by dementia, as "familial" when at least one first-degree relative was affected (6).

Applying the preliminary inclusion criteria, we were able to recruit 11 case-control studies of AD analyzing multiple risk factors (Figure 4.4). These studies are described in detail elsewhere (6). Two studies did not fulfill the criterion of symmetrical data collection and were subsequently excluded. In these two case-control studies, data regarding exposures of cases were collected through a next-of-kin interview, while data regarding exposures of controls were obtained by direct interview. Among the nine remaining case-control studies, only five investigated family history of Down's syndrome and were included in the specific reanalyses reported here (Figure 4.4). Family history of Down's syndrome was considered positive if at least one first-degree relative was affected.

In all five studies considered, the frequency of positive family history was higher in cases than in controls (Table 4.1). Overall, the odds ratio was 2.7 (95% CI: 1.2–5.7). The odds ratio was similar in men and women and for early onset and late onset AD patients. By contrast, the risk was suggestively higher for familial AD than for sporadic AD; however, the difference was not statistically significant (18).

Interpretation

In all five studies included in the reanalyses for family history of Down's syndrome, data on exposure were homogeneously collected through a next-of-kin interview for both cases and controls. None of the studies with alternative data collection strategies mentioned above were involved.

Some of the studies can be considered "quasi" population-based because an attempt was made to ascertain all cases of AD in a defined geographic area. However, since case-finding was invariably obtained through existing medical services in a defined geographic area, the actual exhaustiveness of case-ascertainment remains uncertain. Door-to-door studies of dementia have repeatedly shown that a high percentage of cases are not routinely recognized by the health services (11). In all events, these "quasi" population-based studies were probably less prone to *selection bias* than samples of other studies that were derived from hospitals or outpatient clinics (10).

Unfortunately, none of the case-control studies were based on incident cases, i.e., cases investigated at the time they developed the disease. By contrast, studies were based on prevalent cases, i.e., cases alive at a given point in time. Therefore, a second possible cause of selection bias is survival (*incidence-prevalence bias*) (10). The observed risk factors may be spurious because they may be determinants of survival rather than of risk.

In one study (Italy), two groups of controls were used. For comparability with

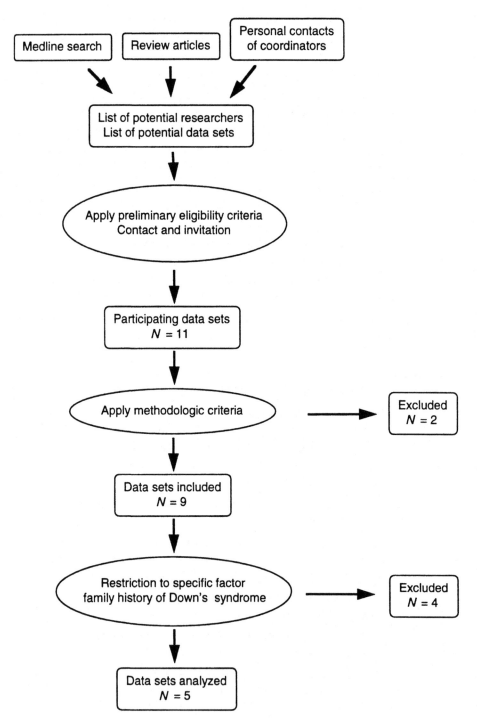

Figure 4.4   Steps involved in the EURODEM collaborative reanalysis of case-control studies of risk factors for Alzheimer's disease. Indicated also is the impact of individual steps on the number of studies involved.

Table 4.1. Results of case-control studies of the association between Alzheimer's disease and family history of Down's syndrome (data from (18))

Study or subgroup	Exposure frequency*			95% Confidence interval
	Cases	Controls	OR†	
Individual studies				
Australia	5/165	0/165	—	—
Italy	1/116	0/97	—	—
Netherlands	5/198	3/198	1.7	0.3–13.0
USA, Denver	2/64	0/64	—	—
USA, Durham	7/45	4/91	3.5	1.2–5.7
Overall analysis	20/588	7/615	2.7	1.2–5.7
Subgroups by sex‡				
Women	15/382	5/398	3.0	1.2–7.3
Men	5/206	2/216	2.6	0.6–10.5
Subgroups by family history of dementia‡				
With family history	12/227	3/248	4.0	1.3–12.5
Without family history	7/275	4/275	1.9	0.6–6.0
Subgroups by age at onset‡				
Before 65 years	9/327	3/348	2.8	1.1–7.5
65 years or over	9/243	4/241	2.6	0.7–10.0

*Subjects were considered exposed if they had at least one first-degree relative affected by Down's syndrome.

†OR, odds ratio; the estimate was adjusted for age, sex, number of siblings, and education.

‡Subgroups analyses were conducted on the overall sample obtained by pooling the five independent studies.

other studies, only the population controls were used in these reanalyses. In another study (Denver, USA) only hospital controls were used. However, since results from the Denver study regarding family history of Down's syndrome were consistent with those from other studies, data were pooled. A formal test of heterogeneity was performed before pooling.

In all five studies, the analysis was restricted to Down's syndrome among first-degree relatives, and the potential confounding effect of the number of siblings in the family was addressed by including the number of siblings in the regression models. Unfortunately, in the Denver and Durham studies (USA), no distinction was made between Down's syndrome and mental retardation. In the other three studies, the question regarding Down's syndrome was more specific;

Table 4.2. Advantages and disadvantages of collaborative reanalyses

Advantages	Disadvantages
Maximize the use of existing data bases	May be misinterpreted
Stimulate collaboration and exchange	May lead to dogmatic views
Improve individual research efforts	May lead to statistical abuses
Offer unique learning experiences	
May lead to new findings	
May lead to new concepts	

however, the ability of a next-of-kin to accurately report diagnoses of Down's syndrome among family members remains uncertain.

Our findings for family history of Down's syndrome are a good example of the advantages of pooled analyses. All studies were consistent in indicating a higher frequency of positive family history of Down's syndrome among cases; however, only the pooled sample showed a significantly increased risk. In addition, only in the pooled sample was it possible to conduct subgroup analyses. Down's syndrome is a relatively rare disease (the incidence rate is about 1.3 per 1000 live births) and large numbers of first-degree relatives are needed to establish an increased risk.

In interpreting the positive results of these reanalyses, we should consider the following limitations. Although the findings were consistent across studies and the pooled sample showed statistical significance, the numbers remained small and the relative risk estimate was relatively small. In addition, we cannot exclude the possibility of a *family information bias* occurring consistently in all studies (10). The association may be biased if relatives of AD patients serving as next-of-kin informants are more aware of the occurrence of other diseases in the family than relatives of controls. If a family information bias is present, it tends to occur in all case-control studies, and pooling will not cure but rather emphasize a biased finding.

Conclusions

Although reanalyses have a series of advantages, they also have disadvantages (Table 4.2). The most important disadvantage is that enthusiasm for statistical significance may distract the attention from the possibility of bias; therefore, reanalyses require more critical scrutiny than individual analyses. In addition, results from a collaborative reanalysis may be viewed as "dogmas," and they may discourage rather than encourage new testing of the hypothesis. Because many investigators from many countries may be co-authoring a reanalysis report, the weight of the conclusions may be perceived as greater than the weight of the conclusions from a single study. Unfortunately, consensus can be reached on wrong conclusions as well as on correct conclusions.

Acknowledgements

Part of the material in this chapter was used by the author for the American Academy of Neurology course entitled "Clinical Research Methods" held in Washington, DC, in May, 1994.

REFERENCES

1. Jenicek M. Meta-analysis in medicine: where we are and where we want to go. *J Clin Epidemiol* 1989;42:35–44.

2. Last JM. *A Dictionary of Epidemiology*, 2nd edn. New York: Oxford University Press, 1988.

3. Hofman A, Rocca WA, Brayne C, et al. The prevalence of dementia in Europe: a collaborative study of 1980–1990 findings. *Int J Epidemiol* 1991;20:736–48.

4. Rocca WA, Hofman A, Brayne C, et al. Frequency and distribution of Alzheimer's disease in Europe: a collaborative study of 1980–1990 prevalence findings. *Ann Neurol* 1991;30:381–90.

5. Rocca WA, Hofman A, Brayne C, et al. The prevalence of vascular dementia in Europe: facts and fragments from 1980–1990 studies. *Ann Neurol* 1991;30:817–24.

6. van Duijn CM, Hofman A, Kay DWK, eds. Risk factors for Alzheimer's disease: a collaborative re-analysis of case-control studies. *Int J Epidemiol* 1991;20(Suppl. 2):S1–73.

7. Schlesselman JJ. *Case-control Studies: Design, Conduct, Analysis.* New York: Oxford University Press, 1982.

8. Clayton D. The Eurodem collaborative re-analysis of case-control studies of Alzheimer's disease: some methodological considerations. *Int J Epidemiol* 1991;20(Suppl. 2):S62–4.

9. Felson DT. Bias in meta-analytic research. *J Clin Epidemiol* 1992;45:885–92.

10. Sackett DL. Bias in analytic epidemiology. *J Chron Dis* 1979;32:51–63.

11. Rocca WA, Amaducci L. Epidemiology of Alzheimer's disease. In: Anderson DW, ed. *Neuroepidemiology: A Tribute to Bruce Schoenberg.* Boca Raton, Florida: CRC Press, 1991:55–96.

12. Jorm AF. *The Epidemiology of Alzheimer's Disease and Related Disorders.* London: Chapman & Hall, 1990.

13. American Psychiatric Association. *Diagnostic and Statistical Manual of Mental Disorders*, 3rd edition (DSM–III). Washington, DC: American Psychiatric Association, 1980.

14. McKhann G, Drachman D, Folstein M, et al. Clinical diagnosis of Alzheimer's disease: report of the NINCDS–ADRDA Work Group under the auspices of Department of Health and Human Services Task Force on Alzheimer's disease. *Neurology* 1984;34:939–44.

15. Anderson DW, Mantel N. On epidemiologic surveys. *Am J Epidemiol* 1983;118:613–9.

16. Anderson DW, Schoenberg BS, Haerer AF. Prevalence surveys of neurologic disorders: methodologic implications of the Copiah County study. *J Clin Epidemiol* 1988;41:339–45.

17. Folstein MF, Folstein SE, McHugh PR. "Mini-mental state." A practical method for grading the cognitive state of patients for the clinician. *J Psychiatr Res* 1975;12:189–98.

18. van Duijn CM, Clayton D, Chandra V, et al. Familial aggregation of Alzheimer's disease and related disorders: a collaborative re-analysis of case-control studies. *Int J Epidemiol* 1991;20(Suppl. 2):S13–20.

5

Diagnostic research in clinical neurology

W. A. van Gool

Introduction

An accurate diagnosis is necessary, albeit not sufficient, for proper treatment and counseling of patients. According to Medline, the number of publications on the diagnosis of nervous system diseases has risen from almost 3500 in 1980 to more than 6000 in 1996. The proportion of papers on diagnostic innovations as measured by the percentage of papers containing adjectives such as "new," "novel" or "promising" rose from 3 to almost 7% in the same period. Thus, both in absolute as well as in relative terms clinicians are confronted with a continuing proliferation of reports on new diagnostic technologies.

New diagnostic tests may have important implications for everyday clinical practice, for research into pathogenic mechanisms, and sometimes even for classifications of diseases. In neurology, the advent of magnetic resonance imaging (MRI) has affected the diagnostic approach to a wide range of clinical problems in a fundamental way (1). Neuroreceptor imaging with radioactive tracers fuelled speculation on pathogenesis of several diseases and sequencing of the prion protein gene resulted in the definition of the new nosological entity of "prion diseases" encompassing various neurodegenerative syndromes with a distinct clinical phenotype (2,3). These different kinds of developments as a result of diagnostic innovations make diagnostic research ever more important.

Kent and Larson have proposed a standardized approach towards evaluations of new diagnostic technologies (4). They distinguish five levels of benefit attributable to diagnostic testing (Table 5.1), and the hierarchical nature of their framework implies that positive effects at higher levels of evaluation require good results at preceding levels. However, good performance at one of the lower levels of evaluation does not guarantee utility at the higher, clinically more relevant levels of evaluation. This chapter will be structured according to the Kent and Larson framework for a discussion of selected methodological issues relevant to research on diagnostic tests (4). The focus of this discussion is on diagnostic test research relevant for everyday neurological practice. Specific issues related to diagnostic testing for research purposes will be briefly mentioned only.

Table 5.1. Hierarchical framework for the evaluation of diagnostic test research, after Kent and Larson (4)

Study level	Examples of typical study result	Study frequency
1. Technical capacity	Test–retest variability	Common
2. Diagnostic accuracy	Sensitivity, specificity, receiver-operator characteristic curve	Common
3. Diagnostic impact	Diagnostic impact, test replacement	Rare
4. Therapeutic impact	Changes of management plan	Very rare
5. Health impact	Changes in functional status of patients, satisfaction of patients or caregivers	Almost absent

Technical capacity

A general and very basic requirement for any new diagnostic test is that it yields information that is valid and reliable. *Reliability* (or precision) of a measurement refers to the degree of variation in a series of observations of the same phenomenon. *Validity* (or unbiasedness) refers to the tendency to arrive at the correct value. The diagnostic procedure of measuring pupil size, for instance, is valid and unbiased if the average of different measurements corresponds to a true pupil size of 5 millimeters, but it is rather unreliable if these values range from 2 to 8 millimeters. If repeated exams of the same pupil give values varying from 2 to 3 millimeters, the measurement is very precise but biased.

Variations among observers, measuring instruments, laboratory conditions, or stability of reagents used may all affect the precision of a diagnostic test (4,5). A useful measure to specify agreement between observations on discrete or categorical data is the kappa statistic giving the ratio of the observed agreement beyond chance to the potential agreement beyond chance. For example, a kappa value of 1 indicating equivalence of the observed and potential agreement beyond chance, i.e., perfect agreement, was found in the identification of interacerebral hemorrhage on computed tomographic scans of stroke patients (6).

Technical capacity may refer to display of recognizable pictures in imaging studies or to stability of reagents in radioimmunoassay kits for determining levels of specific proteins in cerebrospinal fluid. Studies relevant to the technical capability of a new diagnostic method usually are performed in patients with a known disease status. Assessing test–retest variability in healthy subjects only may overestimate the precision of a diagnostic test. Specific disease characteristics such as, for example, severe dyskinesias or dementia may pose special technical problems in certain test situations, e.g., imaging studies.

Studies of technical capacity typically represent the first publications on a new diagnostic procedure. These studies tend to include few patients and they often lack control populations. As such, studies of technical capacity may identify high quality diagnostic tests which are not necessarily more accurate than the standard diagnostic approach in identifying subjects with a specific disease. MRI has a superior image quality but it is not more accurate than computed tomography (CT) in identifying meningiomas at the level of the hemispheres (1).

Diagnostic accuracy

Diagnostic accuracy refers to the capacity of a particular test to discriminate between presence and absence of a certain disease. Characteristically, studies of diagnostic accuracy are performed in populations of patients having the target disease and in a population of controls (7,8). These studies require a well-defined "gold" standard defining the disease under study and diagnostic test results should be interpreted independent of the patient's disease status. Patients with the disease should represent an appropriate spectrum of disease. An accurate test late in the course of a disease when the diagnosis is obvious may not be useful in the earlier stages of the diseases (8). Control populations including patients with conditions often confused with the target disorder allow for a more valid estimate of test characteristics than inclusion of healthy subjects as controls. The results of these kind of studies are usually presented in terms of sensitivity, specificity, likelihood ratio, or area under the receiver-operator characteristic (ROC) curve (7,8). The sensitivity of a test is the proportion of patients with the disease under study who have a positive test result and the specificity is the proportion of controls who test negative. The likelihood ratio of a positive test result is the probability of a positive test result given the presence of the disease, divided by the probability of the same finding given the absence of disease. In other words, the likelihood ratio can be calculated by dividing the true positive rate (equal to the sensitivity) by the false positive rate (equal to 1 minus the specificity). ROC curves plot the true positive rate (sensitivity) against the false positive rate (1 minus specificity) for a range of cutoff values of possible test results. Values of the area under the ROC curve range from 0.5 for a completely noninformative test to 1 for a test perfectly discriminating between presence or absence of a disease.

Even if a study avoids the pitfalls of spectrum bias in patients or controls, there may remain some problems in the interpretation of these test characteristics. The vast majority of diagnostic accuracy studies are retrospective by nature. They consist of descriptions of series of patients which were neither consecutive nor selected according to another explicit criterion. In most studies the only condition patients had to fulfill in order to be included in the typical study of test characteristics is that a final verification of their disease status, e.g., by follow-up, biopsy, or postmortem, has been possible. Selection of patients for diagnostic studies on the basis of their final diagnosis rather than on the symptoms or complaints which were the indication for performing the test under study, may result in verification bias and in spurious estimates for sensitivity and specificity (8). Patients in which the diagnosis of amyotrophic lateral sclerosis (ALS) is confirmed at autopsy are not representative for the population presenting complaints of limb weakness or dysphagia 1 to 3 years before that point in time. A new test for ALS which appears to have nearly perfect test characteristics in the former population may be useless in the latter. Ideally studies of test characteristics should be prospective and they should include consecutive patients presenting with a specific clinical problem rather than patients with a well-defined disease. Obtaining a final diagnosis as a "gold" standard in all patients of such a prospective cohort is essential but it can be very difficult if this requires a long follow-up.

Diagnostic impact

Currently there is no well established methodology for diagnostic impact studies. Studies of diagnostic impact are much less frequently performed than studies on diagnostic accuracy, which require only a relatively simple procedure. Assessments of the diagnostic impact of a new diagnostic test may focus on one of two different aspects of clinical impact. The emphasis may be on the replacement of existing diagnostic techniques or on measurement of changes in clinicians' diagnostic confidence (9). A study of Teasdale and colleagues may serve as an example of the first approach (10). Patients suspected for lesions of the posterior cranial fossa were randomly allocated to CT or MRI. The number of subsequent requests for the alternative imaging technique were recorded. It was found that the number of requests for MRI after CT increased, whereas referrals for CT after MRI decreased over the study period. These results suggested a greater impact of MRI than CT in patients presenting with this specific clinical problem (10). Observational studies in a real clinical environment of this kind have a greater external validity than methods relying on panel reviews of diagnostic test results. Meetings of a panel review committee may not adequately reflect the decision process of clinicians on wards or in outpatient clinics.

If two competing diagnostic strategies are compared in the same series of patients several methodological requirements have to be met (9). The order of testing should be random, both strategies or tests should be performed within a narrow window of time in each patient, diagnostic confidence should be quantified and the tests should be interpreted independently of each other. In an exemplary study of diagnostic impact, O'Connor and colleagues for the Rochester–Toronto study group (11) compared the impact of CT plus trimodal evoked potentials (EP) versus MRI on neurologists' diagnostic labeling of patients with suspected multiple sclerosis (MS). After clinical assessment two neurologists recorded a diagnostic categorization according to explicit criteria. Subsequently all patients underwent MRI and CT plus EP and all tests were interpreted by a reader who was unaware of clinical details. For each patient one neurologist received first the MRI result only and the other neurologist was provided initially with the CT–EP results. The neurologists categorized the diagnosis in each patient again and subsequently they received the remaining test results, before making a final diagnosis of possible, probable, or definite MS, or not MS. The sequence of receiving test results was randomized. As expected, diagnostic categorizations became more definitive in the course of the diagnostic workup, and the greatest change of diagnostic confidence occurred when the first test results were obtained after taking the history and clinical examination. However, this increase was irrespective of the nature of the first ancillary test: there was no difference in diagnostic effect between MRI and CT plus trimodal EPs in this study (11).

In this unique randomized trial of test result sequencing diagnostic classification consisted of an ordinal categorization. In other studies diagnostic confidence has been recorded using visual analogue 0 to 10 scales as a simple method to obtain a measure of the degree of certainty (9). In this way both changes of diagnostic category as well as actual changes in diagnostic confidence can be specified. However, an independent reference ("gold") standard also remains indispensable in studies of diagnostic confidence to control for the pitfall of increased confidence in the wrong diagnosis (4).

Therapeutic impact

The assumption that a better quality of diagnostic testing leads to improvements of patient care is implicit to most diagnostic test research. However, studies in which the impact of the diagnostic process on treatment of patients is measured directly are extremely rare. This holds even if "treatment" is taken in its broadest sense as to include not only initiation of a specific therapy but also counseling of patients, families or other caregivers serving as a basis for reassurance or more understanding of the illness (4). In their classification of studies of diagnostic neuroimaging Kent and Larson aptly epitomized the category of therapeutic impact studies with "no studies, many claims" (4).

Assessment of therapeutic impact requires recording of the diagnosis and treatment plan before the test under study is performed. Outcome measures in these kind of studies could be the effects on patient management in terms of the initiation, any change or withdrawal of planned therapy. Randomized rigorously controlled trials, analogous to drug trials, are best suited to assess therapeutic impact of diagnostic tests. However, if a diagnostic strategy is accepted as standard clinical routine, such as vitamin B12 determinations in patients presenting with dementia for instance, randomization of patients to trial arms including a specific test or not, may be considered unethical. Despite these ethical problems and many other problems with the complicated logistics of randomized trials in diagnostic research, this design has important advantages compared with the alternative of observational studies of therapeutic impact. Observational studies compare the management plan recorded before a diagnostic test is performed with the actual therapeutic strategy after obtaining diagnostic test results. For the interpretation of these kind of studies it is problematic that one factor in this comparison consists of a subjective impression of clinicians of what "would have been" the treatment without obtaining the results of the diagnostic test under study. Direct comparison of actual treatments in different arms of a randomized diagnostic study offers a much more straightforward interpretation. Kent and Larson (4) point out that appropriateness ratings of the observed differences of treatment are crucial in this kind of study. A new and extremely sensitive diagnostic test for incipient myasthenia gravis for instance, may result in treatment in much earlier stages of this disease to the benefit of patients. However, as a trade-off of improved sensitivity, the diagnostic innovation may also cause an increase of the number of (healthy) subjects treated on false-positive grounds. Weighing of beneficial and adverse therapeutic impacts is as essential in randomized diagnostic test research as it is in conventional drug trials.

Health impact

The technical capacity and diagnostic accuracy of a (new) test in clinical neurology should ultimately translate in health benefits for patients through its diagnostic or therapeutic impact. If a diagnostic test with negligible risks accurately identifies patients suffering from a fatal disorder for which an effective treatment is readily available, the value of a diagnostic test is beyond doubt. However, there are many neurological conditions which can be diagnosed by accurate tests but with an uncertain impact on patient outcome. Walstra and colleagues (12) assessed the value of routine investigations in large prospective series of first referrals of elderly people with (suspected) dementia. Using clinimetric methods measuring cognition, disability in daily functioning, behavioral changes, and caregiver burden, the authors found a low percentage of patients who benefitted in terms of reversal of dementia, as a result of the standard battery of diagnostic investigations.

Assessments at the level of health can be directed at longevity or improved health status as outcome, but also less obvious dimensions can be measured such as reduction of burden in patients (or caregivers) as a result of increased diagnostic confidence. Improved diagnostic certainty even with respect to a disease which can not be cured as many neurodegenerative conditions for instance, may translate in health impact by avoiding additional diagnostic testing (with potential discomfort) or inappropriate treatments (with potential side-effects) (4). This point is illustrated by a study of O'Connor and colleagues (13) of health perceptions before and after a diagnostic work-up for suspected MS, showing that distress over physical symptoms was more likely to decrease even in those with an increased certainty of having MS.

Concluding remarks

In terms of the Kent and Larson (4) framework (Table 5.1) the current status of diagnostic test research in neurology can best be summarized by stating that for most diagnostic tests there is abundant documentation of technical capacities and that there are usually reliable data on tests' diagnostic accuracy. In contrast, diagnostic impact is largely unknown for most tests, and evidence of therapeutic or health impact of diagnostic testing is virtually absent for all tests recently introduced in neurological practice. This may appear a sobering state of affairs but the suspicion that the same most probably holds for other disciplines of medicine as well may perhaps offer at least some consolation. The value of the hierarchical categorization of diagnostic test research as reviewed here, is that it clearly identifies the opportunities for future diagnostic research (Table 5.1) (4,14).

As long as studies of diagnostic, therapeutic, and health impact of new diagnostic technologies are very rare, the technique of meta-analysis may be a valuable tool to obtain an overall picture of available data on diagnostic accuracy of new tests. First used to create synthesis of results of different drug trials, Irwig and colleagues (15) recently published guidelines for meta-analysis of diagnostic studies. In addition to the obvious difficulty of publication bias these guidelines should protect against the pitfalls of pooling data on diagnostic accuracy. The authors review methods to estimate summary receiver-operator characteristic (ROC) curves taking into account possible differences in test thresholds between studies (15). In addition to differences in cutoff values, heterogeneity of primary studies may be due to different gold standards or (technical) differences of test quality, e.g., imaging quality.

The extreme focus on "lower" levels of test evaluation may explain the repetitive cultivation of high hopes in nonsystematic reviews on diagnostic tests for a wide range of neurological conditions. The design and actual performance of diagnostic studies with a focus on diagnostic, therapeutic, or health impact is more complicated than studies of technical capacity or diagnostic accuracy. In addition, the tremendous commercial pressure which can be behind the speed with which preliminary data are being turned into a diagnostic test (16) may also explain in part the extremely skewed frequency distribution among the levels of evaluation of diagnostic research (Table 5.1) (4.14). However, overly optimistic claims by researchers and biotechnology companies on the clinical utility of a new diagnostic method are inappropriate if they are based exclusively on research into its technical capacity or diagnostic accuracy.

Diagnostic tests based on genetic traits deserve a special word of caution. Unlike conventional diagnostic tests, this specific category of tests not only reveals a characteristic of patients seeking medical advice but there is also a risk that family members may receive (unsolicited) information about their disease risks. This specific characteristic of genetic testing can have unexpected and potentially serious implications for the psychological well-being, family relationships, and employability and insurability of those tested (16); issues which are all relevant to apolipoprotein E genotyping in suspected Alzheimer's disease for instance (17).

Methods are needed to increase the *ecological validity* of diagnostic studies for clinical medicine by measuring impact of testing at the level of diagnostic confidence in physicians, and ultimately, at the level of patient (or caregiver) health status, satisfaction, or burden. A great amount of resources for research could be saved if studies of new diagnostic technologies would include these kinds of assessments in earlier stages of test evaluation.

It is important to note that the focus of this chapter was on the evaluation of diagnostic technologies for current neurological practice. Entirely different considerations apply to the use of diagnostic instruments in research settings. Studies of pathogenic mechanisms for instance, require highly specific tests to avoid spurious classification of cases as affected, whereas false-negative classifications (occurring on low sensitivity tests) are not as harmful in this setting as they may be in clinical practice. It may be reasonable by all standards to use high sensitivity and low specificity diagnostic tests for selection of cases for trials of new drugs with minimal side-effects and a great therapeutic potential, whereas any test with such characteristics would certainly fail the standard of quality for current clinical use of new diagnostic technology as discussed in this chapter.

REFERENCES

1. Kent DL, Haynor DR, Longstreth WT, Jr., Larson EB. The clinical efficacy of magnetic resonance imaging in neuroimaging [Review.] *Ann Intern Med* 1994;120:856–71.
2. van Royen E, Verhoeff NF, Speelman JD, et al. Multiple system atrophy and progressive supranuclear palsy. Diminished striatal D2 dopamine receptor activity demonstrated by 123I-IBZM single photon emission computed tomography. *Arch Neurol* 1993;50:513–6.
3. Prusiner SB, Hsiao KK. Human prion diseases. [Review.] *Ann Neurol* 1994;35:385–95.

4. Kent DL, Larson EB. Disease, level of impact, and quality of research methods. Three dimensions of clinical efficacy assessment applied to magnetic resonance imaging. [Review.] *Invest Radiol* 1992;27:245–54.

5. Jaeschke R, Guyatt G, Sackett DL. Users' guides to the medical literature. III. How to use an article about a diagnostic test. A. Are the results of the study valid? Evidence-Based Medicine Working Group. *JAMA* 1994;271:389–91.

6. Shinar D, Gross CR, Hier DB, et al. Interobserver reliability in the interpretation of computed tomographic scans of stroke patients. *Arch Neurol* 1987;44:149–55.

7. Jaeschke R, Guyatt GH, Sackett DL. Users' guides to the medical literature. III. How to use an article about a diagnostic test. B. What are the results and will they help me in caring for my patients? The Evidence-Based Medicine Working Group. *JAMA* 1994;271:703–7.

8. Sox HC. The evaluation of diagnostic tests: principles, problems, and new developments. [Review.] *Annu Rev Med* 1996;47:463–71.

9. Mackenzie R, Dixon AK. Measuring the effects of imaging: an evaluative framework. [Review.] *Clin Radiol* 1995;50:513–8.

10. Teasdale GM, Hadley DM, Lawrence A, et al. Comparison of magnetic resonance imaging and computed tomography in suspected lesions in the posterior cranial fossa. *BMJ* 1989;299:349–55.

11. O'Connor P, Tansey C, Kucharczyk W, Detsky AS. A randomized trial of test result sequencing in patients with suspected multiple sclerosis. Rochester–Toronto MRI Study Group. *Arch Neurol* 1994;51:53–9.

12. Walstra GJM, Teunisse S, Van Gool WA, Van Crevel H. Reversible dementia in elderly patients referred to a memory clinic. *J Neurol* 1997;244:17–22.

13. O'Connor P, Detsky AS, Tansey C, Kucharczyk W. Effect of diagnostic testing for multiple sclerosis on patient health perceptions. Rochester–Toronto MRI Study Group. *Arch Neurol* 1994;51:46–51.

14. Van Gool WA, Van Crevel H. Impact on management of new diagnostic tests in Alzheimer's disease. *Lancet* 1996;348:961.

15. Irwig L, Macaskill P, Glasziou P, Fahey M. Meta-analytic methods for diagnostic test accuracy. [Review.] *J Clin Epidemiol* 1995;48:119–30.

16. Hubbard R, Lewontin RC. Pitfalls of genetic testing. *N Engl J Med* 1996;334:1192–4.

17. Anonymous. Apolipoprotein E genotyping in Alzheimer's disease. National Institute on Aging/Alzheimer's Association Working Group [Review.] *Lancet* 1996;347:1091–5.

6

Decision analysis in clinical neurology

Diederik W. J. Dippel

Introduction

Patient management comprises three key elements: arriving at a diagnosis, assessing prognosis, and making a treatment choice. Many decisions have to be made along the way. Almost every clinical decision carries an element of uncertainty: uncertainty about the occurrence of events and about the value of these events. Especially in the clinical neurosciences, decision making becomes more complicated every day, because of rapidly emerging new treatments and diagnostic tests, and because of increasing demands from patients to be informed and to participate in decision making. By its explicit nature and strictly logical approach, decision analysis can be a helpful tool in everyday patient management. It can form the necessary link between the results of a randomized clinical trial or diagnostic study, and their application in clinical practice. Since the mid-1970s, more than 60 decision analyses of neurological management problems have been published, and their number is now growing fast (1).

Decision analysis is a theory of decision making under conditions of uncertainty, used for normative, prescriptive purposes (2,3). In *clinical* decision analysis an intriguing mixture of medical (Bayesian) statistics, clinical epidemiology and clinical science is added (4–6). A clinical decision analysis explicitly addresses the inevitable uncertainties in a clinical problem and combines these with preferences for health outcomes in a consistent framework that obeys the laws of probability calculus and the theory of subjective expected utility. This should lead to management advice concerning an individual patient, or a group of similar patients. First the basic steps and assumptions in a decision analysis will be outlined. Four stages can be conveniently identified (7).

- Defining and structuring the clinical problem in a decision tree. This includes description of the patient, the possible diagnostic and therapeutic actions, and the possible outcomes of treatment.
- Assessing probabilities and utilities (relative value judgements) for diagnostic and therapeutic outcomes.

- Performing the necessary computations, in order to determine the preferred course of action. These computations include sensitivity analyses, to check how sensitive the preferred choice is to plausible changes in the assumptions.
- Presentation of the results and conclusions in a clinically useful way.

In a journal article that describes a decision analysis, these four stages should be readily identifiable. The process of performing an analysis, however, requires a lot of discussion between a decision expert and his clinical counterpart, and a lot of switching back and forth between these stages.

To be useful in practice, a decision analysis should focus on a clinical situation, and provide a clinically relevant case and context description. All possible strategies should be considered, although the final decision tree may be pruned from clinically irrelevant strategies. The results of the analysis should be extendable to other, slightly different patients, for example by taking into account age and severity of symptoms. Of course an analysis should be up to date, with regard to the evidence on which it is based, and with regard to the diagnostic and therapeutic strategies that are considered.

The best way to get acquainted with the methodology and to learn to appreciate its possibilities, is to follow an example closely. We will present two outlines of studies, to illustrate the basic elements of a decision analysis. The first example concerns a diagnostic problem, and will be used to illustrate the modeling of a decision tree, the calculation of expected utility, and sensitivity analyses. In the second example, a therapeutic problem, quality adjusted survival analysis will be introduced.

Diagnostic decision making: duplex or angiography?

Consider a 65-year-old right-handed man, with a history of a transient right hemiparesis and aphasia, one month ago. He was treated for hypertension, but was otherwise healthy. Should this patient undergo carotid angiography or duplex ultrasound examination of the carotid arteries, and should angiography be used to confirm the results of a positive duplex or not?

Decision tree

The decision tree of Figure 6.1 shows four strategies that will be considered: carotid angiography only, duplex ultrasound of the carotid arteries, followed by confirmative angiography if positive, and duplex only. No testing was also considered, although this may be counterintuitive to some readers. In all branches the patient receives "best medical treatment." The decision tree should be read from left to right, and starts with a description of the patient and the clinical problem. The square decision node depicts the decision that has to be made. Chance nodes

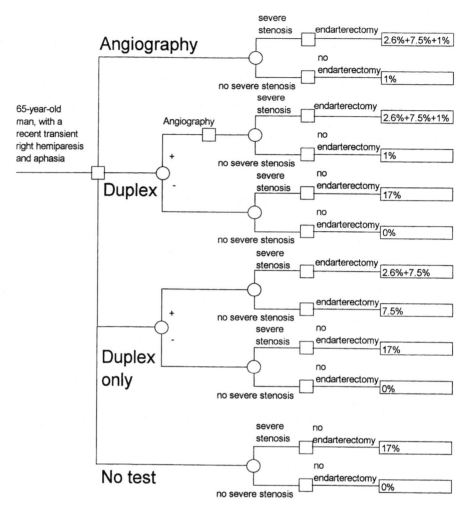

Figure 6.1   Duplex or angiography? Decision tree for the diagnostic management of a 65-year-old patient suspected of a severe symptomatic left carotid artery stenosis.

(circles) describe the occurrence of events that cannot be influenced by the decision maker. Outcome nodes (rectangles) describe the results of each action and event. When we proceed with carotid angiography directly, the patient will be exposed to a risk of stroke or death because of complications from this procedure. The angiogram may indicate a severe carotid stenosis, and the patient will be operated upon. When the angiogram does not reveal a severe carotid stenosis, no operation will follow. In the second strategy, duplex ultrasound may indicate a severe carotid stenosis. When this is confirmed by angiography, the patient will be operated on. When duplex does not indicate a severe carotid stenosis, the patient may in fact have one, although this will not be revealed to us. Thus, on the one

Table 6.1. Estimate for the decision analysis of the diagnostic management of a 65-year-old patient suspected of a symptomatic left carotid artery stenosis

	Point value (5)	95% Confidence interval
Three-year risk of ipsilateral stroke with a severe carotid stenosis	17	13–21%
Efficacy of endartererectomy	85	72–92%
Surgical mortality or stroke within 30 days	7.5	5–10%
Stroke or death risk after angiography	1	0.5–2%
Prior probability of a severe symptomatic carotid stenosis	22	16–29%
Sensitivity of duplex ultrasound	76	59–89%
Specificity of duplex ultrasound	85	78–91%

hand, duplex reduces the probability of unnecessarily undergoing carotid angiography, but on the other hand, there is a risk of missing an operable carotid stenosis. When angiography is not used to confirm a positive duplex result, as in the third strategy, the patient may be exposed to the risks of endarterectomy unnecessarily. When no diagnostic testing takes place, as in the fourth strategy, a severe carotid stenosis will remain undetected and the patient will not be treated.

Estimates

The decision tree helps in identifying the events and outcomes that have to be assigned a probability. Everyone involved in the management of this patient would have to admit that he could not predict with certainty what would happen to this patient after duplex ultrasound, angiography, and/or endarterectomy. That is the rationale for the use of probability calculus to assess the most reasonable management option. However, we are not even sure about the exact values of the probabilities that should be used, therefore 95% confidence intervals, or when the estimates are entirely subjective, plausible ranges of values will be suggested. The probability estimates (point values and 95% confidence intervals) were based on the literature, see Table 6.1. For the utilities a proxy of utility-loss was used, consisting of the combined risk of death (from stroke, surgery, or angiography) and nonfatal stroke. They are already inserted in the decision tree of Figure 6.1. Figure 6.2 shows how the proxies relate to an imaginary utility scale. Note that the risk of stroke from a moderate or mild carotid stenosis is not incorporated in the utility structure, because it is not influenced by the decision. The sensitivity and specificity of duplex ultrasound for severe carotid stenosis was estimated in a series

Table 6.2. Correlation of the results of duplex ultrasound and angiography for symptomatic carotid artery stenosis, in a series of 152 patients with transient ischemic attacks or non-disabling stroke from the Rotterdam Stroke Databank

	Angiography −	Angiography +	Totals	
				Se = 26/34 = 76%
Duplex −	100	8	108	Sp = 100/118 = 85%
Duplex +	18	26	44	PV + = 26/44 = 59%
Totals	118	34	152	PV = 100/108 = 93%

Se, sensitivity; Sp, specificity, PV +, positive predictive value; PV, negative predictive value.
Duplex −, negative duplex result, indicating a stenosis of less than 50%, or occlusion.

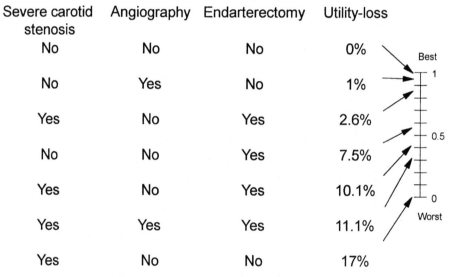

Severe carotid stenosis	Angiography	Endarterectomy	Utility-loss
No	No	No	0%
No	Yes	No	1%
Yes	No	Yes	2.6%
No	No	Yes	7.5%
Yes	No	Yes	10.1%
Yes	Yes	Yes	11.1%
Yes	No	No	17%

Figure 6.2 Duplex or angiography? Utility structure for the decision analysis of the diagnostic management of a 65-year-old patient suspected of a severe symptomatic left carotid artery stenosis.

of patients who were evaluated for transient ischemic attacks and were entered into the Rotterdam Stroke Databank. Table 6.2 is a simple contingency table of these data, that allows estimation of the sensitivity and specificity for a severe carotid stenosis. Note that although angiography is not infallible, it can be regarded as the gold standard diagnostic procedure in this case, because it was used to define the degree of carotid stenosis in the two clinical trials that proved the effectiveness of carotid endarterectomy (8,9). Actually, the duplex procedure yields a stenosis grading, from zero to occlusion, and a positivity criterion was determined by receiver-operater characteristic (ROC) analysis (10,11). Bayes' theorem could be used to compute the probability of duplex indicating a severe

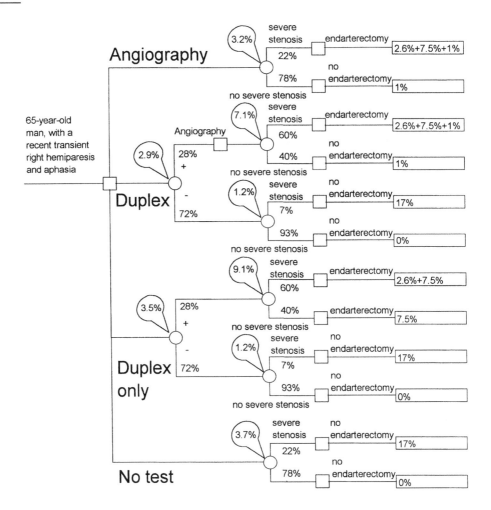

Figure 6.3   Duplex or angiography? Decision tree, folded back, for the diagnostic management of a 65-year-old patient suspected of a severe symptomatic left carotid artery stenosis.

carotid stenosis, and the probability of severe carotid stenosis, given a positive or negative duplex result (11).

Computations

Given the assumptions that were made, the best choice will be suggested by maximizing the expected utility, or minimizing the expected utility loss. This expectation can be simply computed by multiplying the probabilities of each branch of the tree with their associated utility losses. This has been done in Figure 6.3. This process is sometimes called *folding back*, because it is easier to start at the far end of the tree. In this case, the lowest risk of stroke or death is to be expected

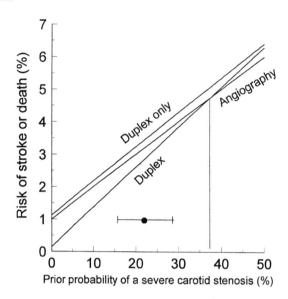

Figure 6.4   Duplex or angiography? Sensitivity analysis: dependency of the risk of fatal or nonfatal stroke attributable to the severe carotid stenosis, or death from surgery or angiography (y-axis) on the prior probability of a severe symptomatic carotid stenosis (x-axis), for three diagnostic strategies: angiography only, duplex followed by angiography if positive, or duplex only.

when the strategy "duplex, followed by angiography if positive" is adopted. Should we be satisfied with the analysis at this point? Clearly not, because the probability and utility estimates we made may not be as exact as they seem. How would plausible changes in these estimates affect the expected utility-loss of each management option? This question of secondary uncertainty can be addressed by sensitivity analyses. Another use of sensitivity analysis is to answer "what if" questions, such as, in this case, what if the patient had a cervical bruit, and his prior probability of a carotid stenosis would be approximately two-fold increased, or what if a CT scan had revealed a lacunar infarction, and the prior probability of a carotid stenosis would be much lower? A third reason for doing sensitivity analyses is to check the models' behavior, in order to find computational or conceptional errors (12).

Figure 6.4 shows the results of a one-way sensitivity analysis: low prior probabilities of a severe carotid stenosis result in lower expected risks of stroke and death for each strategy, but more so for "duplex followed by angiography if positive." High prior probabilities favor angiography. "Duplex only" is never the best option in this analysis. At some prior probability of severe carotid stenosis, the expected risk of death and stroke for angiography and duplex will be equal. This is called a threshold probability. It is indicated by a dotted vertical line in Figure 6.4. Below it, the threshold duplex is favored, and above it, angiography. The concept of a

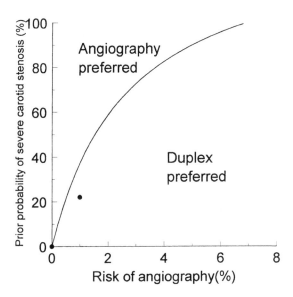

Figure 6.5   Duplex or angiography? Threshold analysis: combinations of the risk of stroke or death after angiography (x-axis) and prior probability of a severe symptomatic carotid stenosis (y-axis) that lead to equal expected utilities for two diagnostic strategies (i.e., duplex followed by angiography if positive, and angiography only.

threshold probability can be used in more extensive sensitivity analyses: the threshold analysis (sometimes wrongly called a two-way sensitivity analysis). Figure 6.4 gives an example. It shows how much the threshold probability for doing angiography only is increased when the risks of angiography itself are higher, and the other way around. Combinations of values of the prior probability and of the risks of angiography that favor one strategy are easy to find out. Note that the actual differences in expected utility loss are "concealed" in this graph; they can be quite small.

Sensitivity analyses of this kind can only consider a few variables at one time without becoming too complex. Moreover, plausible ranges of values are investigated, but the distribution of the values is not taken into account. Thus, an unequivocal conclusion cannot be reached. By doing a full Bayesian or probabilistic sensitivity analysis, this becomes possible. In Figure 6.5 the results of such an exercise are shown. The cumulative distribution of the difference in utility loss was estimated in a series of 1000 Monte Carlo simulations, where values of the probabilities and utilities were drawn from logistic approximations of their distributions, based on their 95% confidence intervals (12,13). The mean difference in utility loss between angiography and duplex followed by angiography if positive is 0.3% in favor of duplex, with a 95% confidence interval of −0.3% to 1.1%, indicated by two horizontal dotted lines in Figure 6.6. Note that even

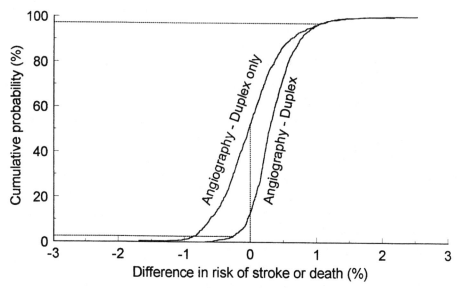

Figure 6.6   Duplex or angiography? Probability sensitivity analysis: cumulative distribution of the difference in risk of stroke or death between two diagnostic strategies.

though the 95% CI reaches beyond the boundary of no difference, for individual patient decision making this will not affect our choice, because the expected utility of each option will remain the same. A decision has to be made anyway, even though we are now aware that our knowledge is imperfect.

Conclusions

From this analysis, we concluded that duplex examination of the carotid arteries is a useful screening procedure for severe carotid artery stenosis, but it is not sufficiently accurate to serve as a single preoperative diagnostic procedure, without angiographic confirmation of positive results. The results of the Bayesian analysis may make us realize that when we want to make similar decisions in the future, more precise estimates, and therefore more studies, are needed.

Therapeutic decision making: asymptomatic carotid stenosis

Our patient, a 65-year-old right-handed man, has now undergone endarterectomy for a more than 70% symptomatic left carotid bifurcation stenosis. The operation was successful. His pre-operative angiogram however, had revealed a more than 70% stenosis of the right carotid artery as well. Should this patient now undergo endarterectomy for the asymptomatic stenosis?

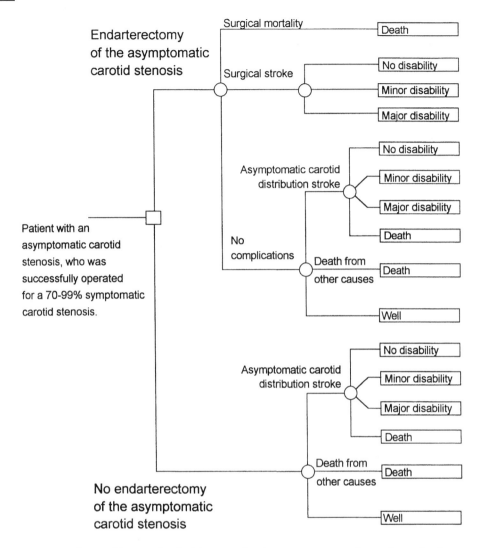

Figure 6.7   Asymptomatic carotid stenosis: decision tree for the management of a patient who has already been successfully operated for a left symptomatic carotid lesion (15).

Decision tree

This clinical problem is already well defined, and can be a basis for drawing a decision tree (Figure 6.7). The decision tree illustrates the trade-off that has to be made: reduction of the risk of stroke in the asymptomatic distribution against the risks of endarterectomy of the asymptomatic carotid artery. The upper part of the tree describes the chain of events after endarterectomy of the asymptomatic carotid artery, which may result in perioperative complications, e.g., stroke lasting more than seven days or death within 30 days of surgery. When the operation was uneventful, the patient may still suffer from a stroke, as with nonoperative treatment. The possibility of death from other causes than asymptomatic carotid distribution stroke (e.g., stroke in the symptomatic carotid distribution, myocardial infarction, etc.) is also included in the tree, because when this risk is high it will affect the benefit that is to be gained from the treatment under consideration.

The time horizon of the analysis is five years. The decision tree was analysed by computing the five-year risk of asymptomatic carotid distribution stroke lasting more than seven days, or surgical death. The tree structure seems simple but the tree is for illustrative purposes only. The actual computations are more complex: both main branches consist of subtrees denoting the chance of each outcome event at one, two, three, four, and five years from now.

Estimates

Two large, well-designed, randomized clinical trials of the management of patients with symptomatic carotid stenosis have been published, both suggesting that on average, these patients are better off with endarterectomy of the symptomatic carotid artery than without (8.9). Although these two studies answer the general question whether endarterectomy works as a treatment for patients with symptomatic carotid stenosis, their results definitely do not apply to our patient. In the American Carotid Atherosclerosis Study, a randomized trial of endarterectomy for asymptomatic carotid stenosis, less than one third of the patients had had endarterectomy for a contralateral *symptomatic* carotid stenosis (14). Moreover, the risks of endarterectomy in this study were very low. Its results may not be generalizable to the majority of patients with asymptomatic carotid stenosis, treated by vascular surgeons with less experience. We therefore estimated the risk of stroke in the asymptomatic carotid distribution in the subgroup of patients in the ECST who had a 30 to 99% asymptomatic contralateral carotid stenosis, and identified two prognostic factors by means of proportional hazards regression: severe carotid stenosis and hypertension (15). In Table 6.3 the probability estimates for our patient are listed. The assessment of quality adjusted life expectancy (QALE) will be described in the next section.

Computations

The estimated five-year risk of stroke in the asymptomatic carotid distribution in the key patient was 12.1% without, and 3.5% after endarterectomy of the asymptomatic stenosis. When the risk of death and stroke lasting more than seven days associated with endarterectomy itself was included, the risk after operation increased to 8.5%, still lower than after conservative management. The residual difference was largely due to differences in risk of minor disabling stoke, however. The five-year rate of death from any cause was also slightly in favor of endarterec-

Table 6.3. Probability estimates for a 65-year-old patient with an asymptomatic carotid stenosis who has been successfully operated for a symptomatic carotid lesion (15)

	Point estimate (5)	95% confidence interval
Data from ECST		
Five-year cumulative risk of asymptomatic carotid distribution stroke	12.1	8.3–17.5%
Death after stroke	22	9–35%
Major disability after stroke (Rankin 4 to 5)	24	10–38%
Minor disability after stroke (Rankin 1 to 3)	20	7–33%
No disability after stroke (Rankin 0)	34	20–52%
Five-year cumulative risk of death from causes other than asymptomatic carotid distribution stroke	27.1	21.6–33.7%
Surgical death	1	0.5–2%
Major disabling surgical stroke	1.5	1–3%
Minor disabling surgical stroke	1.5	1–3%
Nondisabling surgical stroke	1	0.5–2%
Efficacy	70	50–90%

tomy. Neither of these estimates make very good decision criteria, because surgical strokes and deaths occur early, and health status is not considered.

Therefore, the decision tree was used to compute the survival in different health states over the five-year period (Figure 6.8). These estimates were combined into time-restricted life expectancies, in order to compare the two treatment options. The time-restricted life expectancy was slightly in favor of endarterectomy, for a difference of 0.01 life years. When only survival in the normal healthy condition was considered, there was a slight difference in life expectancy in favor of no endarterectomy (0.02 life years). For the purpose of this analysis, the utility of intermediate health outcomes (minor and major disability from asymptomatic carotid distribution stroke or surgical stroke) was estimated (Table 6.4). It was decided to proceed with empirical validation of these estimates only if their exact values appeared crucial to the results and interpretation of the analysis.

Adjustment of the life years lived for preferences for health states was done by weighing each year spent in a certain health state with its utility value, and then computing the (time-restricted) quality adjusted life expectancy (QALE). The time-restricted QALEs for the two strategies were virtually equal. The estimated 95% confidence intervals for this difference (−0.16 to 0.10) indicated that the

Table 6.4. Utility estimates for a 65-year-old patient with an asymptomatic carotid stenosis who has been successfully operated for a symptomatic carotid lesion (15)

Utility of health outcomes	Point value	Plausible range
No disability (Rankin 0)	1	
Minor disability (Rankin 1 to 3)	0.90	0.80 to 0.99
Major disability (Rankin 4, 5)	0.50	0.25 to 0.75
Death	0	

Modified Rankin scale: Grade 0: no symptoms; Grade 1: minor symptoms not interfering with lifestyle; Grade 2: minor handicap, symptoms that lead to some restriction of lifestyle, but do not interfere with the capacity of the patient to look after himself; Grade 3: moderate handicap, symptoms that significantly restrict lifestyle and prevent totally independent existence; Grade 4: moderately severe handicap, symptoms that clearly prevent independent existence although not needing constant attention; Grade 5: severe handicap, totally dependent patient, requiring constant attention night and day.

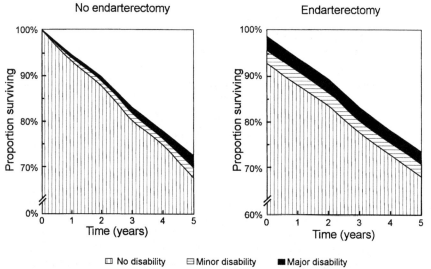

Figure 6.8   Asymptomatic carotid stenosis: partitioned survival curves, computed with the decision analysis model, showing the estimated cumulative proportions surviving with and without minor and major disability, as a function of time, for both treatment options; no endarterectomy (left) and endarterectomy (right). LE, time-restricted life expectancy; dfLE, diability-free life expectancy; QALE, time-restricted quality-adjusted life expectancy (15).

therapeutic yield will at best be small for this type of patient (Table 6.5).

Sensitivity analysis was used to examine the robustness of the analysis. We computed the effect of plausible changes in each estimate on the difference in time-restricted QALE between the two treatment options, when all other estimates

Table 6.5. Results of the decision analysis for a 65-year-old patient with an asymptomatic carotid stenosis who has been successfully operated for a symptomatic carotid lesion (15)

	No endarterectomy	Endarterectomy
Five-year risk of asymptomatic carotid distribution stroke, or surgical death	12.1%	8.5%
Five-year death rate	27.3%	25.9%
Life expectancy (years)	4.18	4.19
Disability-free life expectancy (years)	4.04	4.02
Quality-adjusted life expectancy (QALE)	4.14	4.14

were kept at their mean values. Only plausible changes in surgical risks changed the difference in time-restricted QALE in favor of endarterectomy. If the risks of surgical death and minor and major disabling surgical stroke were lower than the estimates that we used, there would be an advantage of endarterectomy over conservative management. If endarterectomy were completely without risk, this would amount to only 0.1 extra quality-adjusted life years, or five weeks per five years in the key patient. Plausible changes in the other estimates, and in the utility estimates, were of much less influence on the treatment recommendation.

There is some evidence that very severe stenosis of an asymptomatic carotid artery is associated with a particularly high risk of asymptomatic carotid distribution stroke, although this association could not be confirmed by the ACAS, probably due to small sample size (14). We used a separate regression model with the degree of asymptomatic carotid stenosis as a continuous variable to estimate the risk of stroke in the appropriate distribution. The subgroup of patients ($n = 27$, 3%) with a 80 to 99% stenosis and hypertension had a 25% five-year risk of asymptomatic carotid distribution stroke, sufficient to warrant endarterectomy according to the decision analysis (Figure 6.9). This figure also shows the difference in time-restricted QALE between the two treatments as a function of the degree of asymptomatic carotid stenosis. This turns in favor of endarterectomy at 75% stenosis (at least for patients with hypertension), but the gain is at most 0.12 quality-adjusted life years, even when surgical risks are low.

Conclusions

From this analysis we concluded that there is no good argument for performing endarterectomy in patients with an asymptomatic carotid stenosis who have been

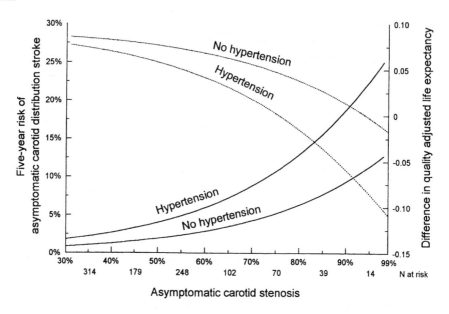

Figure 6.9   Asymptomatic carotid stenosis: five-year risk of asymptomatic carotid distribution stroke as a function of the degree of asymptomatic carotid stenosis (continued lines), and the difference in five-year-restricted quality-adjusted life expectancy (QALE) as determined with the decision analysis (dashed lines), for patients with and without hypertension. Positive values of the difference in QALE indicate an advantage of no endarterectomy, and negative values an advantage of endarterectomy for asymptomatic carotid stenosis (15).

successfully operated for symptomatic carotid stenosis, other than in the context of a randomized controlled trial.

Discussion

An analysis of diagnostic and one of therapeutic decision making have been used to illustrate the key elements and methodology of clinical decision analysis in neurology. This chapter is just meant to give a first impression, and therefore lengthy discussions of clinical or methodological topics have been avoided, but references for further reading have been provided.

It can be extremely difficult to formalize a decision-making process in a mathematical model, and not to violate the laws of logic and probability calculus on the one hand, or to lose contact with clinical reality on the other. Close collaboration between decision scientists with a feeling for the art of clinical decision making and clinicians with a background in clinical epidemiology and biostatistics is therefore indispensable. Several textbooks on clinical decision analysis exist (2–6,16–18), and some popular books on clinical epidemiology have merged the decision analysis approach with other quantitative methods (19–21).

Some medical textbooks already contain a chapter on decision analysis in general, although decision-oriented textbooks are still a rarity.

The most difficult part of a clinical decision analysis is the description of the clinical problem. The construction of a decision tree (graphically or mathematically) is a process that deserves care and time. Obviously, lack of case and context description poses a constraint on clinical applicability. The confusion about the application of a decision analysis can often be avoided with a descriptive branch that precedes the first node in the tree and provides a clinically relevant context and case description. This is important, because the basis for clinical applicability lies in the description of a typical patient, on which the assumptions are based. Only then will probability estimates be meaningful. In the stage where probability estimates are made, methodological problems do not often arise, although the lack of data that are readily applicable to the clinical situation may come as a surprise. The choice of a utility structure may be difficult. When utilities have to be estimated empirically, one will have to deal with several methodological and practical problems. Utilities are defined as relative value judgements based on substitution probabilities derived from standard reference gambles (3,6). Although theoretically correct, the standard gamble is an awkward measurement method in practice, because anxious and confused patients (but also volunteer medical students) are frequently not consistent in their preferences for health states, and their appreciation of risks (22). Alternative elicitation methods do not seem to measure what is needed, that is preferences for outcomes in risky choice situations (23). The use of quality adjusted life expectancy (QALE) seems to avoid some of these problems, but the estimation of parameters for the QALE model remains difficult (24). Fortunately, preferences for health states play a major role only in a minority of clinical problems, and many times, a suitable proxy is available. Sensitivity analyses of the impact of plausible alternative utility assumptions may many times obviate the need for exact estimates.

Although the results of a decision analysis can be helpful in clinical practice, the responsibility in clinical decision making will always remain with the clinician. He or she communicates with the patient, weighs the medical evidence, and determines how and whether decision analysis should play a role in the decision-making process, and where individual preferences come in. This process can never be replaced by any automated procedure.

Apart from being useful in individual patient management, decision analysis can help in identifying gaps in clinical knowledge that are important from a decision-making point of view. In this way, decision analysis can be used to direct future clinical research, and to evaluate the implications of the results of clinical trials for individual decision making. A step further along this path would be to integrate the decision analysis approach with the analysis of the results of clinical trials. This would imply first of all doing away with meaningless compound outcome measures such as "death or major morbidity." These should make way for survival estimates in different, well-defined health states (25–27). Moreover, decision analysis can be useful in (para)medical education and as a guide for protocol development (7).

Several circumstances have increased the need for decision support in the clinical neurosciences; they have been mentioned in the introduction. The availability of powerful personal computers, the growing familiarity with clinical epidemiology, and the emergence of centers for clinical decision science have facilitated the application of decision analysis to real clinical problems (1). However, decision-analytic applications have not found their way into the clinic as easily as was once predicted (7). Perhaps the main obstacle remains the reluctance of doctors to think in terms of probability, in spite of omnipresent uncertainty (17,28). Framing effects (overestimation of the likelihood of rare events, anchoring, etc.) may lead intuitively to other choices than a decision analysis recommends, which makes it sometimes difficult to accept the explicit advice (29). The quality of a single decision cannot be measured just by its result (30). Good choices can lead to bad outcomes, and the other way around. As a consequence, it will be difficult to prove that decision analysis indeed improves the quality of clinical decision making. Nevertheless, we owe it to ourselves, to our patients, and to the community that provides the resources for our health care system, that we adopt an explicit, consistent, rational, scientific, and communicative attitude in clinical decision making.

REFERENCES

1. Dippel DWJ, Habbema JDF. Decision analysis in the clinical neurosciences: a systematic review of the literature. *Eur J Neurol* 1005;2:523–39.

2. Raiffa H. *Decision Analysis. Introductory Lectures on Choices under Uncertainty*. Reading: Addison-Wesley, 1968.

3. Von Winterfeldt D, Edwards W. *Decision Analysis and Behavioral Research*. Cambridge: Cambridge University Press, 1986.

4. Dowie J, Elstein AS. *Professional Judgment, a Reader in Clinical Decision Making*. New York: Cambridge University Press, 1988.

5. Lusted LB. *Introduction to Medical Decision Making*. Illinois: Thomas Springfield, 1968.

6. Weinstein MC, Fineberg HV. *Clinical Decision Analysis*. Philadelphia: Saunders, 1980.

7. Habbema JDF, Van der Maas PJ, Dippel DWJ. A perspective on the role of decision analysis in clinical practice. *Ann Med Intern* 1986;137:267–73.

8. European Carotid Surgery Trialists' Collaborative Group. MRC European Carotid Surgery Trial: Interim results for symptomatic patients with severe (70 to 99%) or with mild (0 to 29%) carotid stenosis. *Lancet* 1991;337:1235–43.

9. North American Symptomatic Carotid Endarterectomy Trial Collaborators. Beneficial effect of carotid endarterectomy in symptomatic patients with high grade stenosis. *N Engl J Med* 1991;325:445–53.

10. Centor RM. Signal detectability: the use of ROC curves and their analyses. *Med Decis Making* 1991;11:102–6.

11. McNeil BJ, Keeler E, Adelstein SJ. Primer on certain elements of medical decision making. *N Engl J Med* 1975;293:211–15.

12. Habbema JDF, Bossuyt PMM, Dippel DWJ, Marshall S, Hilden J. Analysing clinical decision analyses. *Stat Med* 1990;9:1229–42.

13. Doubilet P, Begg CB, Weinstein MC, Braun P, McNeil BJ. Probabilistic sensitivity analysis using Monte Carlo Simulation: a practical approach. *Med Decis Making* 1985;5:157–77.

14. Executive Committee for the Asymptomatic Carotid Atherosclerosis Study. Endarterectomy for asymptomatic carotid artery stenosis. *JAMA* 1995;273:1421–8.

15. Dippel DWJ, Koudstaal PJ, Van Urk H, et al. After successful endarterectomy for symptomatic carotid stenosis, should a contralateral, but asymptomatic carotid stenosis be operated on as well? *Cerebrovasc Dis* 1997;7:34–42.

16. Llewelyn H, Hopkins A. *Analysing how we Reach Clinical Decisions*. London: Royal College of Phycisians, 1993.

17. Sox HC, Blatt MA, Higgins MC, Marton KI. *Medical Decision Making*. Stoneham: Butterworths, 1988.

18. Bradley GW. *Disease Diagnosis and Decisions*. Chichester: John Wiley, 1993.

19. Weiss NS. *Clinical Epidemiology. The Study of the Outcome of Illness*. New York: Oxford University Press, 1986.

20. Sackett DJ, Haynes RB, Guyatt GH, Tugwell P. *Clinical Epidemiology. A Basic Science for Clinical Medicine*, 2nd edn. Boston: Little, Brown & Co., 1991.

21. Ingelfinger JA. *Biostatistics in Clinical Medicine*, 2nd edn. New York: MacMillan, 1987.

22. Redelmeier DA, Rozin P, Kahnemann D. Understanding patients' decisions. Cognitive and emotional perspectives. *JAMA* 1993;270:72–6.

23. Stalmeier PFM, Bezembinder TGG, Unic IJ. Proportional heuristics in time tradeoff and conjoint measurement. *Med Decis Making* 1996;16:36–45.

24. Bleichrodt H, Gafni A. Time preference, the discounted utility model and health. *J Health Economics* 1996;15:49–66.

25. Glasziou P, Simes RJ, Gelber RD. Quality adjusted survival analysis. *Stat Med* 1990;9:1259–76.

26. Hilden J. Reporting clinical trials from the viewpoint of a patient's choice of treatment. *Stat Med* 1987;6:745–52.

27. Simes RJ. An application of statistical decision theory to treatment choices: implications for the design and analysis of clinical trials. *Stat Med* 1986;5:335–54.

28. Young DW. Numerical methods for decision making in clinical care: where to now? *J Roy Soc Med* 1988;81:128–9.

29. Balla JI, Elstein AS, Christensen C. Obstacles to the acceptance of clinical decision analysis. *BMJ* 1988;298:579–82.

30. Wulff HR. How to make the best decision. *Med Decis Making* 1981;1:277–83.

7

Outcomes research in clinical neurology

Mitchell S. V. Elkind and Ralph L. Sacco

Introduction

Outcomes research may be defined as the systematic collection and analysis of data regarding the results of medical care. In a broad sense, all clinical medical research, ranging from observational epidemiologic studies to randomized clinical trials, could be considered outcomes research since it is concerned with the results of the presence of disease or its treatment. Outcomes research in the present discussion, however, refers more specifically to several overlapping areas of research within the broader field of health services research which are directed at analyzing the results of medical care in real patients in real health care systems with the goal of improving their care. There is nothing fundamentally or conceptually novel about outcomes research, but in the current understanding of the term it is represented by a multidisciplinary field reliant upon contributions from physicians, health services researchers, economists, epidemiologists, statisticians, and others. Although it enjoys a strong commitment from national and private funding agencies, it is a young field whose benefits may only become apparent and generally accepted several years from now.

This chapter will provide an overview of the historical roots of outcomes research, describe the different types of studies which fall under the rubric of outcomes research, and discuss some of the major methodological issues which face the investigator interested in this area. The role of outcomes research in clinical neurology will be stressed, and examples from the neurologic literature, particularly from the authors' specialty field of stroke, will be used to illustrate our points.

Historical perspective

Historically, in the United States, outcomes research as it is currently conceived originated in the growing sense of a health care crisis that came about in the 1980s. Arnold Relman, the former editor of the influential *New England Journal of*

Medicine and an outspoken analyst of American health care, has described the 1980s as a period of great upheaval in our health care system following upon a period of great expansion (1). During the post-World War II period the United States experienced a dramatic increase in health care services provided to its citizens. The number of hospitals and physicians increased rapidly, and the amount of money expended both for clinical care and medical research grew tremendously, such that from 1960 to 1990 the proportion of the gross national product devoted to health care nearly tripled from 4.4% to 12%. The realization that continued unchecked growth of this sort would bankrupt the country led in the early 1980s to a policy of cost-containment, led by a Federal government initiative to decrease Medicare spending. This resulted initially in the institution of diagnostic-related groups, or DRGs, as a means of prospectively controlling government payments for hospital services, and more recently in the proposed Resource-Based Relative Value Scale as a means of controlling physicians' fees (2). Industry, concerned about its own loss of profits due to health care expenditures, has similarly reacted to the growth in costs, resulting in the growth of managed care plans of several varieties.

In Relman's view, the present climate of assessment and accountability is a reaction to the interest in cost containment. Part of this reaction led to the Federal Medical Treatment Effectiveness Program (MEDTEP) and in 1989 the establishment by Congress of the Agency for Health Care Policy and Research (AHCPR). This agency has awarded funding to several groups, or Patient Outcomes Research Teams (PORTs), to both study and to develop *methodologies* for studying effectiveness and economics of many common diseases and their treatment. PORTs so far have focused on common medical and surgical conditions including ischemic heart disease and hip fracture, but also two neurologic conditions: low back pain and stroke. The goals of these research projects are to assess the health care benefits and their costs of interventions for these conditions as they are treated in general medical practice, information which is of growing importance to the public.

While economic forces are crucial to understanding the interest in outcomes research, several other forces also operated to generate this interest (3). First, despite the remarkable technological and scientific discoveries which have contributed to the advance of modern medicine in the twentieth century, it has become increasingly apparent that there is a discrepancy between scientific knowledge and medical practice. In many cases, physicians lack an accepted scientific rationale for much of their medical practice. Variations in practice patterns between different geographic regions, for instance, have been frequently cited as evidence that nonscientific factors frequently influence medical decision making (4). Moreover, studies by the Rand group (5) and others have shown that physicians frequently make decisions that run counter to guidelines developed by professional consensus panels. One study (6) suggested that as many as 32% of carotid endarterectomies performed in 1981 were done for inappropriate indications. Even when clinical trials and other studies are able to show a benefit for a particular therapy, physicians in practice do not necessarily incorporate this knowledge into their practice. Outcomes research investigates the gap between scientific knowledge and expert opinion and its transition into medical practice. Third, the availability of computer capability to store and analyze huge quantities of data regarding health care (insurance claims, discharge diagnoses, and mortality, for example) has allowed a fundamental change in the ability of investigators to study outcomes in different environments. Physician decisions, at least in aggregate, have therefore become less private and more subject to investigation, analysis, and criticism than ever before. Fourth, because of the new and competitive health care payment systems manifested by the rise in health maintenance organizations, there is an increased interest in ensuring that health care is responsive to the needs and desires of patients as perceived by patients, not physicians. Outcomes research frequently incorporates in its analyses measures of patient quality of well-being or satisfaction in addition to those which may reflect physiologic or functional results.

Outcomes research and clinical neurology

Neurology has several features which render it especially amenable to outcomes research. First, neurologic conditions are highly prevalent. Stroke is the third leading cause of death in the United States, and the leading cause of disability (7). Headache and back pain, other common neurologic complaints, are among the most frequent reasons patients seek medical attention. Second, while tremendous progress has been made in identifying the etiology and pathophysiology of neurologic disease, substantial therapeutic progress has lagged behind, and is only now beginning to become a real possibility. Many neurologic diseases, such as Alzheimer's disease, Parkinson's disease, multiple sclerosis, and amyotrophic lateral sclerosis (ALS) are chronic conditions which are incurable but for which therapies in use and under development may lessen disability and offer symptomatic benefit. Outcomes research has a role to play in determining the benefits and costs of therapy for patients when standard objective indices such as mortality or incident clinical events are impractical. In such situations, analyses of functional status, cognitive test scores, or quality of life may better reflect therapeutic benefit.

Table 7.1. Types of outcome studies

Natural history studies
Efficacy studies
Effectiveness studies
Cost-effectiveness studies

Types of outcome studies

Natural history studies

Outcomes studies may be conducted in several different ways, and their designs often reflect their intended uses (Table 7.1). Observational studies of the natural history of disease over time provide an example of outcome studies in their simplest sense. Patients are enrolled in a study at the time of diagnosis or some particular clinical event and then followed to see what happens. Such studies may be either case series from a particular clinic or population-based studies which attempt to identify all the patients with a particular disease in a given population. They may be conducted retrospectively, by identifying a cohort based on a diagnosis made earlier in time, or prospective, in which the diagnosis is made in the present and the patient is followed into the future. Such studies have long been an important part of clinical neurologic epidemiologic research and may play an exploratory role in planning further analytic research. For example, studies of the natural history of patients with carotid stenosis with transient ischemic attacks (TIAs) (8,9) or without TIAs (10) showed that such patients had a several-fold increased risk of stroke compared to those without, thereby accelerating interest in the use of carotid endarterectomy to decrease the risk of stroke. Well-recognized limitations of such studies include the biases intrinsic to patient selection, and the variation among the ways in which different physicians may treat patients and assess their outcomes.

Efficacy studies

Outcome studies intended to provide more scientifically valid and potentially more useful results include efficacy and effectiveness studies. Efficacy analyses are studies which attempt to determine the benefit of a drug or other medical or surgical therapy in a scientifically rigorous and objective fashion. These studies are exemplified by the randomized controlled trial (RCT), in which patients with certain characteristics are selected and randomly assigned to an active treatment or placebo, or perhaps one active treatment versus another. Outcomes are then measured by observers blinded to the treatment status of the study subject, and outcomes are compared among treatment groups.

The recent NIH-sponsored study of the use of recombinant tissue plasminogen activator (rt-PA) in acute ischemic stroke is an example of a well-conducted randomized trial relevant to neurology (11). In this study, 333 patients with acute ischemic stroke within 3 hours of presentation were randomized to receive either rt-PA or placebo. The primary outcome measure of efficacy was a composite score measured at 3 months combining four different ranking scales measuring different aspects of functional status and neurologic deficit (Barthel index, modified Rankin scale, Glasgow outcome scale, and NIH stroke scale). The rt-PA treated group was 30% more likely to show minimal or no disability at 3 months.

The factors which make an efficacy study scientifically valid, however, are the very same factors which conspire to make it less generalizable to everyday clinical practice. Efficacy studies, for example, typically exclude patients with coexistent diseases which might either influence the prognosis or otherwise confuse the measurement of outcomes. The patients treated by clinicians every day, however, often have coexistent diseases which would cause them to be excluded from trials. Are therapies deemed efficacious in studies of highly selected patients necessarily beneficial for the potentially more complicated patients clinicians face in their offices? Similarly, physicians in the real world may behave very differently from those actively involved in enrolling patients in a clinical trial. A recent trial of thrombolysis (12) in acute stroke conducted in Europe makes this point nicely. In this study, which used a 6 hour time window, physicians were instructed to exclude patients with early evidence of infarction on CT. Despite this intended exclusion criterion, however, 66 patients were enrolled and treated despite what was later read by a review committee as evidence of either early infarction or hemorrhage on CT. The investigators provided analyses for two groups, an intention-to-treat group including the patients with abnormal scans, and a target group, which excluded those patients with abnormal scans. The target group analysis showed a benefit for rt-PA treated patients but the primary analysis – the intention-to-treat analysis – did not. It is unlikely, however, that neurologists in the community, without any special training in interpreting these films, would fare better in selecting patients than those physicians involved in the study itself.

Effectiveness studies

Studies which attempt to determine the outcome of therapies administered by physicians practicing in the community are termed effectiveness studies to distinguish them from studies in the more artificial and controlled atmosphere of efficacy analysis. In the above example, although rt-PA may be considered efficacious if administered appropriately within 6 hours based on the data from the European study, it is unlikely to be effective when used on a population-wide basis. In many clinical situations, moreover, there are no RCTs to guide treatment

Table 7.2. Characteristics of efficacy and effectiveness studies*

	Efficacy study	Effectiveness study
Study design	Randomized, controlled trial	Observational
Patient population	Well-defined, homogeneous	Heterogeneous
Provider	Academic investigator or experienced, expert clinician	"Usual" caregivers or physicians
Treatment	Comparison to placebo or standard therapy	Comparison of types of care ordinarily rendered
Sources of data	Primary data collected for purpose of study using specific instruments	Secondary data using administrative databases, literature review
Outcomes	Clinical events or measures	Clinical events, patient-related outcomes
Informed consent	Always	Not necessarily
Generalizability	Limited	Broad

*Adapted from (14).

decisions, and effectiveness studies are all clinicians may have to guide management.

The design and conduct of effectiveness studies is necessarily different from that of efficacy analyses since they attempt to assess actual practice (Table 7.2). Most importantly, the patients and clinical environments studied will be as unselected as possible in order to closely represent clinical practice. Because human factors are as important to the understanding of the results of the effectiveness analysis as medical or biologic principles, investigators attempt to use subjects from a variety of different types of practice settings and geographic locales to assess whether such factors influence outcomes. For example, a recent effectiveness study of the benefits of rehabilitation for patients with stroke or hip fracture (13) first selected a random sample of 92 rehabilitation facilities and skilled nursing facilities from 17 states. Patients who had been admitted to these facilities in a nonrandom fashion by their physicians, who are presumed to be exercising standard clinical judgement, were then selected at random for data collection and analysis. Data were collected on a range of different factors including functional and cognitive status at admission and after discharge, health care resource utilization, and location to which the patient was ultimately discharged. The study found that facilities which provide intensive inpatient rehabilitation result in better outcomes for stroke patients, but not for hip fracture patients, even after controlling for status on admission.

Effectiveness studies, moreover, may be used for purposes quite distinct from those of efficacy analyses. Such purposes include decision analysis, quality assessment, and disease management programs. Decision analysis is an attempt to formalize the process of decision making which occurs in clinical situations in which there are uncertain outcomes. This method relies on breaking down complex decisions into their component parts in order to make explicit the reasons governing choices of one option over another, thereby substituting a rational foundation for decision making where before there was only opinion. Effectiveness studies may provide data about the results of care which can be useful to the decision analyst in assigning the likelihood of certain outcomes to various decision points. Such analyses may be used by clinicians at the bedside or by administrators determining standards of care or clinical pathways. In similar fashion, one measure of quality of care offered by a provider is how effective it is in actual practice. Disease management programs are organizational structures which allow an institution to continually monitor the way in which it manages medical conditions and costs such that it can continually provide optimal care. It differs from the traditional paradigm of the individual physician encountering patients in the office and emphasizes instead a population-based approach in which persons at risk are identified, interventions are made, outcomes are measured, and care is continually adjusted to optimize outcomes based on new available data. Such systems of disease management are just in the early stages of their development and have yet to be proven effective themselves.

Effectiveness studies have important limitations. Because they are by definition aimed at uncovering actual unconstrained physician and patient behavior, they are likely to be conducted as observational studies rather than as interventional ones. It therefore becomes important in the analysis of the data to account for selection biases which may lead to differential case mixture and disease severity. Because of their noninterventional nature, they also tend to provide information about what is *done* rather than about what *might* be done. Some investigators, however, are designing effectiveness trials which would require patient recruitment, informed consent, randomization, and data collection similar to that used in efficacy studies, but would enroll a heterogeneous patient population more like those to whom the study is intended to generalize, use physicians like those in the community, and impose fewer protocol-related restrictions (14). The Cholesterol Reduction Intervention Study (15), for example, will randomize patients with hypercholesterolemia to receive either niacin and ordinary stepped-care according to the treating physician's preferences or to an HMG CoA reductase inhibitor (lovostatin).

Cost-effectiveness studies

While effectiveness studies have the advantage of offering clinicians assistance in

Table 7.3. Types of health economic evaluations

Type of analysis	Feature
Cost-minimization	Assumes that measure of health effectiveness for two alternatives is equal, and seeks to identify minimum cost strategy
Cost-effectiveness analysis	Determines cost in dollars to obtain a unit of health care outcome, in which the measure of outcome may be defined in any of several different ways
Cost–utility analysis	Determines cost in dollars to obtain a unit of health care outcome, in which the measure of outcome is universal and patient-centred (quality-adjusted life years)
Cost–benefit analysis	Places dollar value on the health care outcome itself, such that both costs and outcomes may be compared in monetary terms

choosing a particular mode of therapy, they do not provide policy-makers or third party payers information regarding the efficiency or costs of given interventions. Even effective treatments may still be too expensive, in society's opinion, to warrant their use. Health economic studies, an important and growing division of outcomes research, are a more specific type of analysis which attempts to relate a given increment in effectiveness to a dollar cost. Such analyses may be used to determine whether the spending of a given amount of money on a particular therapy results in a greater or lesser net effect on overall health outcome than spending the same amount of money on a different therapy.

The cost-effectiveness ratio is the central measure used in cost-effectiveness analyses. This is a measure of the incremental cost of obtaining a unit of health outcome from a particular intervention when compared with an alternative intervention (16). The ratio is obtained by dividing the difference between the two interventions in terms of their costs by the difference in their health outcomes (Equation 1).

$$C/E \text{ ratio} = \frac{(\text{Cost of intervention} - \text{Cost of alternative intervention})}{(\text{Effect of intervention} - \text{Effect of alternative intervention})}$$

$$= \frac{\text{Net cost}}{\text{Net effects}} = \frac{\text{Cost}}{\text{Unit of health}} \tag{1}$$

Several types of health economic evaluations exist (Table 7.3). In a cost-minimization analysis the health outcomes of the two interventions being compared are assumed to be equal, and the study seeks to determine the least expensive strategy. A cost-effectiveness analysis may use as its measure of effectiveness any index of health outcome, including lives saved, hospital days, or a change in a functional rating scale such as the Barthel index or Karnofsky score. A cost–benefit analysis is one in which the health outcomes themselves are converted into dollar amounts, for example by determining how much productivity is lost due to a given state of ill health. The dollar value of a health outcome may therefore be compared with the cost of obtaining that health outcome to determine an overall net value in dollars of an intervention. The advantage to such an analysis is that it allows the analysis of outcomes and costs to be conducted entirely in monetary units, but its disadvantage is that it requires assumptions to be made to determine monetary values of health states, and also reduces health states to monetary terms.

Cost–utility analyses: quality-adjusted life years

In many cases, the cost-effectiveness ratio must function as a comparator of different health care interventions with potentially different fundamental types of outcomes. For example, policy-makers using the results of the analysis may wish to choose between different interventions such as acute stroke therapies or treatments of chronic diseases such as ALS, the outcomes of which will likely need to be measured in very different ways. Because of this, the unit of health in the denominator of Equation 1 must be comparable across all types of study outcomes. A universal indicator of benefit, or outcome, which has been developed for this purpose is the quality-adjusted life-year, or QALY. A cost-effectiveness study which uses as a measure of effectiveness the QALY is more correctly labelled a cost–utility analysis, but the label cost-effectiveness is commonly used for this specific type of analysis, as well. The QALY allows investigators to determine the effects of an intervention on both quantity and quality of life. It is calculated by multiplying the number of years a person is expected to survive by a factor which represents the relative value of life in that state of health as compared to the state of perfect health. This factor is referred to as the "preference," "value," or "utility" of a given health state, and is represented by a number between 0 (dead, the minimal reference state) and 1 (normal healthy state).

Various methods exist for determining utilities of given states, and they usually require posing questions to subjects about their preferences for living in various states. Some common neurological conditions and the utilities assigned to them are given in Table 7.4. One example of the method involved in such utilities analysis in the neurologic literature comes from a study of patient preferences for stroke outcomes (17). Patients at risk for stroke were interviewed using case scenarios about possible stroke syndromes and outcomes, and asked to rate the relative outcome of each scenario. Not surprisingly, patients found increasingly unacceptable strokes of increasing severity. More notably, however, patients

Table 7.4. Utilities for selected health states*

Health state	Utility
Healthy (reference state)	1.0
Taking aspirin[†]	0.999
Taking warfarin[†]	0.990
Migraine[‡]	0.82
Depression[‡]	0.70
Moderate motor stroke[§]	0.43
Constant severe pain[**]	0.28
Dead (reference state)	0.00
Dementia[**]	<0.00
Coma[**]	<0.00
Severe hemiplegia[§]	<0.00

*Adapted from (23); [†]From (24); [‡]From (25); [§]From (17); [**]From (26).

valued states of severe hemiplegia less than those involving confusion, global aphasia, and death. Utilities for such states would thus appear as negative numbers on the 0 to 1 scale.

Although the advantage of using QALYs as a measure of health outcome is applicability across disease states, this universality creates limitations, as well. A gain in QALYs may be achieved in any one of several different ways. Lengthening a subject's life by 10 years in a state of severe disability with a utility of 0.10 (QALY = 10 × 0.1 = 1.0) is in this analysis equivalent to lengthening the life of a healthy person by one year (QALY = 1 × 1.0 = 1.0). This may not represent our true belief about how we would prefer health care decisions to be made, however. An extensive literature in utility analysis is undergoing development for the purposes of assessing this methodology.

Sources of data

The design of cost-effectiveness studies can take many different forms depending upon the type of intervention to be analyzed and the resources available to the investigator. The source of the data to be analyzed may come from either data collected as part of a study conducted at least in part as a cost-effectiveness analysis, or data obtained by a review of previously conducted research related to the intervention of interest. The former may be a cost-effectiveness trial, in which data regarding costs and effects are collected in subjects in the real world, randomized to one treatment or another, as in the effectiveness trials described above. Such studies are generally hard to conduct, however, because the length of follow-up needed to capture the relevant health outcomes and economic costs is generally longer than the time period of clinical trials and the sample sizes are very large due to the increased variance in economic as compared to clinical data. More reasonably, a cost-effectiveness trial may be "piggybacked" onto an existing randomized clinical trial which is in fact being conducted as an efficacy analysis. Economic data and health outcomes data incorporating results other than morbidity and mortality may be collected as part of the trial. Such studies may be limited, however, by their obvious focus on efficacy rather than effectiveness, and their need for larger sample sizes than the RCT itself. Additionally, the time period relevant to the cost data may be longer than that of the trial. A patient may reach a clinical endpoint in a trial at the time he suffers a disabling stroke, for instance, and so data collection may cease, but the costs which will be generated by his care from that point on are important for the economic analysis.

Because of these methodologic limitations, many CEAs utilize secondary data sources. These may include administrative databases such as HCFA records on hospital discharge diagnoses, published retrospective and prospective observational studies, RCTs, and meta-analyses. Statistical modeling may also be used as part of either type of study, and frequently allows some extrapolation from the available data.

Estimating costs

Once an investigator has chosen a means of evaluating a health outcome (to be discussed more fully below), a method of determining costs of an intervention and its alternative must be given. This process involves estimating the costs of each of the possible short- and long-term consequences of the intervention. These costs include direct and indirect costs. *Direct* costs may be medical, such as the value of all health-related goods and services consumed as a result of each of the consequences of the intervention, or nonmedical, such as the cost of transportation of the patient or the cost of time away from work to participate in the intervention. *Indirect* costs are those which accrue due to morbidity and mortality associated with an intervention and represent future lost productivity. Because such costs are actually reflected in the QALY determination related to the intervention, however, it may be more appropriate not to include these indirect costs in the numerator as a dollar cost of the intervention.

Various methods exist for determining the costs associated with the resources used for each intervention. Costs may be determined by a detailed itemization, accounting for the specific number of pills administered to a patient, or the number of bandages used. So-called microcosting, however, is generally too time-consuming, and so most investigators use gross costing techniques, which ascribe a certain value to a given procedure or therapy based upon its average cost, perhaps weighted by regional factors.

In assessing both costs and patient preferences for given outcomes, one important concept which may be taken into account is discounting, which simply reflects the fact that people value more highly resources which are available to them in the present than in the future. In addition, though it is somewhat controversial, they also appear to value more highly health states which occur in the present to those in the future. For these reasons, most investigators discount future costs and health care outcomes by about 3–6%, which is thought to reflect their present value.

The cost-effectiveness model: an example

A cost-effectiveness analysis, like a decision analysis, may be constructed using as a schematic model a branching tree in which each of the branch points represents alternative possible pathways with different probabilities and independent outcomes. The first branch point reflects the decision between choosing the intervention and the alternative with which it is to be compared. Subsequent branches will arise whenever there are different possible alternatives which may arise, either because of random variation or physician and patient choice. Each branch of the tree is associated with a given set of costs and health outcomes. Depending upon the relative probabilities of the different outcomes and the preferences for the resulting health states, different cost-effectiveness ratios will be generated. Construction of the schematic model is extremely important to the ultimate validity of the cost-effectiveness analysis, and great care must be used to ensure that it accurately and completely reflects clinical reality and decision making.

Figure 7.1 shows a model that was used in a recent cost-effectiveness analysis of anterior temporal lobectomy for intractable epilepsy (18). The first two major branches, or trunks, of the model represent the intervention and the alternative with which it is compared. In this example, a choice is made for each patient whether to continue with medical management or to proceed to further evaluation for potential surgical resection of an epileptogenic focus. Once the decision to proceed to further evaluation is made, the patient undergoes noninvasive electroencephalography. Depending upon the results of that test, the patient may (1) be deemed an unsuitable candidate for further evaluation, (2) undergo invasive monitoring, or (3) undergo anterior temporal lobectomy. The probability of each of these branches was determined in this case by a review of the available literature. Each alternative is associated with several possible outcomes, the probabilities of which were again determined by literature review: seizure control off medications, seizure control on medications, persistent seizures, morbidity of one of the procedures if performed, or death. The costs of each of the pathways and the

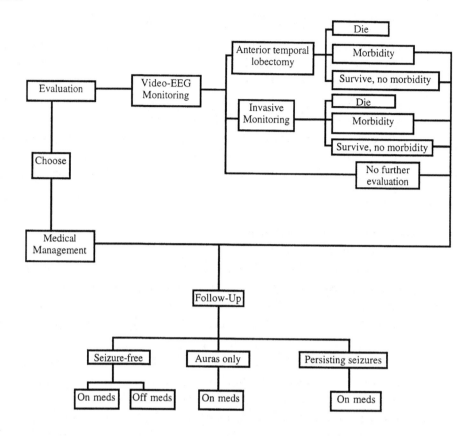

Figure 7.1   An example of a model for a cost-effectiveness analysis: anterior temporal lobectomy. Adapted from (18).

probability of its occurrence may then be multiplied to determine an overall cost of the intervention and its alternative. The utility (in QALYs) of each of the possible resultant health states is also determined and multiplied by the probability of its occurrence. In this case, the utility was based upon a quality-of-life instrument developed for use in epilepsy research, the ESI-55 (19), administered to epilepsy patients.

Because a cost-effectiveness analysis always involves some degree of artificiality in its model and assumptions, the robustness of its findings are assessed by conducting sensitivity analyses. This is simply a way of varying the assumptions, for example, about the relative probabilities of various outcomes and patient preferences which are important to the model in order to determine the effect such variations have on the final result. Ideally, for a cost-effectiveness ratio to be considered valid, one would like to see it change very little over a wide range of assumptions about a given parameter. Sensitivity analysis, moreover, should allow one to determine the threshold for a given parameter at which the cost-effectiveness changes significantly.

In the above example regarding temporal lobe resection (18), for instance, sensitivity analyses were conducted to determine what effect changing each of the important probabilities, costs, and outcomes through a range of plausible possibilities would have on the cost-effectiveness ratio. It was found, for instance, that using in the model increased probabilities of being selected for further evaluation after noninvasive electroencephalographic monitoring and of being seizure-free after surgery increased the cost-effectiveness of surgery. Alternatively, assuming a minimally improved quality-of-life with seizure control led to a lower estimate of cost-effectiveness. By performing computations using variations in different parameters simultaneously (multiway sensitivity analysis), the author was able to come up with "best" and "worst" case scenarios, or situations in which the cost-effectiveness is either minimized or maximized. For example, it appeared that under most ordinary clinical circumstances, evaluation for surgical resection was likely to be more costly, but also more effective, than medical management alone, and only under the most optimistic assumptions was surgery likely to provide long-term cost savings. Such information may be of use to both clinicians and organizations responsible for determining how to allocate scarce medical resources.

Outcome measures

Common to all of the above types of analyses, whether efficacy, effectiveness, or cost-effectiveness, is the need to measure outcomes in an appropriate, accurate, and valid fashion. Outcomes are essentially measures of the result of medical care, and they may be assessed in several different ways. One way of classifying outcomes is in terms of either specific events or repeated measures of some parameter. Certain neurological diseases, for example, lend themselves to the measurement of specific events: strokes, seizures, or mortality from glioblastoma, for example. The outcomes of other neurological diseases, however, may be better assessed by measuring some parameter representative of the patient's condition. Such parameters may be laboratory parameters, which may take a continuous range of values with some range of possibilities. Clinical trials of interferon-beta in multiple sclerosis, for example, have relied on evidence that there is a decrease in burden of disease as manifested by lesion volume on MRI in addition to clinical parameters of efficacy (20). It has been suggested, for example, that the outcome of an intervention in Alzheimer's disease may best be studied by a measure of the patient's cognitive or functional status repeated serially over time. Numerous rating scales have been developed for the purpose of measuring function over time

Table 7.5. Neurologic rating scales

Disease-specific scales
    The Unified Parkinson's Disease Rating Scale (UPDRS)
    Abnormal Involuntary Movement Scale (AIMS)
    National Institutes of Health Stroke Scale (NIHSS)
    Orgogozo Scale for Middle Cerebral Artery Infarction

Cognitive status scales
    Blessed Dementia Test
    Mini-Mental State Examination

Functional outcome scales
    Glasgow Outcome Scale
    Modified Rankin Scale
    Barthel Index
    Functional Independence Measure (FIM)

Quality-of-life measures
    Quality of Well-being (QWB)
    Quality of Life in Epilepsy (QOLIE) Instruments
    Epilepsy Surgery Inventory (ESI–55)

in Alzheimer's and other neurological conditions (Table 7.5). Some of these are disease-specific, such as the Unified Parkinson's Disease Rating Scale (UPDRS), which assesses motor function in that disease, or the NIH stroke scale, which is designed to measure the severity of neurological deficit after stroke. Other measures are more general measures of functional status, such as the Index of Independence in Activities of Daily Living or the Barthel Index.

Certain measures are particularly suited to outcomes research in its commitment to assessing overall patient well-being. Outcomes research seeks to expand beyond the confines of medical research as it has traditionally been conceived in terms of narrowly defined physiologic parameters or counts of mortality and morbidity. It thus uses as measures of outcome markers of overall well-being of the person in his or her social, as well as medical or health, context. As noted above, it is only in this way that measures of effectiveness can be compared across diseases and treatments. The Medical Outcomes Study (MOS) Short-form General Health Survey was developed specifically as a comprehensive, valid, but easy to administer general health survey. It utilizes 20 items designed to capture six health concepts: physical functioning, role functioning, social functioning, mental health, health perceptions, and pain. A measure which can incorporate weights reflecting individual's preferences for given health states, which is essential for cost-utility analysis, is the Quality of Well-Being (QWB) scale.

The choice of an appropriate measurement scale cannot be overstated. A recent clinical trial of the calcium-channel antagonist nimodipine in acute stroke demonstrates this point. In the American Nimodipine trial, analyses of the efficacy of the drug were performed using seven different stroke scales. It was found that the results of the study were statistically significant for two of the scales (the Matthew and Toronto scales), marginal for a third (NIH stroke scale), and not significant for four others (Canadian, Frithz–Werner, Orgogozo, and Scandinavian) (21). The scales which did show benefit, moreover, were most heavily weighted towards higher cerebral functions rather than sensorimotor function, suggesting that the choice of outcome and its measurement instrument may strongly influence the results of a study.

A recent study of selegeline and vitamin E in Alzheimer's disease used both event measures and repeated measures over time as outcomes. The primary outcome measure was a complex composite "event": the occurrence of any one of: death, institutionalization, loss of ability to perform at least two of three activities of daily living, or severe dementia, as determined by a Clinical Dementia Rating of 3. The secondary outcome utilized repeated measures at 3-month intervals on several different scales of dementia, behavior, functional status, and extrapyramidal motor symptoms. The investigators found a statistically significant benefit for each of the medications compared with placebo on the primary outcome measure, and a benefit of treatment on scales that involved assessment of activities of daily living, but not on cognitive scales. The authors speculated that ". . . functional and occupational measures of cognitive capacity are better indicators of disease progression than psychometric measures" (22). The composite primary outcome measure used in this study demonstrates, moreover, that event measures may be constructed to fit clinical scenarios other than events such as death or traditional clinical events. Whether outcomes in other neurological diseases with chronic, debilitating courses are best studied using event measures or repeated measures remains an open question.

Conclusions

Outcomes research is a new and growing field, particularly with respect to its role in neurology. The premises upon which the need for outcomes research has been based are strong. Financial resources are limited, and the public requires a rational basis for choosing and paying for various diagnostic and therapeutic interventions. Clinical practice often deviates from what has been determined the most efficacious care for various reasons, including differences in patient population and physician experience. Outcomes research, though imperfect, attempts to provide a way of addressing these issues in as scientifically valid a fashion as possible. Investigators are only beginning to grapple with the different methodologies required to perform analyses of effectiveness and cost-effectiveness. Constructing valid models for analyses that reflect clinical practice, determining appropriate measures of outcome for different diseases, and assessing patient preferences for various health states are all important areas for further development. The ability of neurologists to apply the increasingly exciting discoveries in neuroscience to patient care will likely depend on the ability of clinical scientists and health services researchers with an interest in neurology to perform outcomes research with the same expertise as investigators have traditionally performed basic and clinical science.

REFERENCES

1. Relman AS. Assessment and accountability: the third revolution in medical care. *NEJM* 1988;319:1220–2.
2. Hsiao WC, Braun P, Yntema D, Becker ER. Estimating physicians' work for a Resource-Based Relative Value Scale. *N Engl J Med* 1988;319:835–41.
3. Mulley AG. Outcomes research: implications for policy and practice. In Smith R, Delamothe T. (eds.) *Outcomes into Clinical Practice.* London: BMJ Publishing Group, 1995:13–27.
4. Wennberg JE. Dealing with medical practice variations: a proposal for action. *Health Affairs* 1984;3:6–32.
5. Chassin MR, Kosecoff J, Solomon DH, Brook RH. How coronary angiography is used – Clinical determinants of appropriateness. *JAMA* 1987;258:2543–7.
6. Chassin MR, Kosecoff J, Park RE. Does inappropriate use explain geographic variations in the use of health care services? *JAMA* 1987;258:2533–7.
7. Sacco RL. Stroke epidemiology and stroke risk factors. In Sacco RL (Ed.) *New Approaches to the Treatment of Ischemic Stroke.* The American Journal of Medicine Continuing Medical Education Curriculum Series 1996.
8. Heyman A, Leviton A, Millikan CH. Transient focal cerebral ischemia: epidemiological and clinical aspects. *Stroke* 1974;5:277–84.
9. Mohr JP. Asymptomatic carotid artery disease. *Stroke* 1982;13:431–3.
10. Wolf PA, Kannel MB, Surlie P, McNamara P. Asymptomatic carotid bruit and the risk of stroke. The Framingham study. *JAMA* 1981;245:1442–5.
11. National Institute of Neurological Disorders and Stroke rt-PA Stroke Study Group. Tissue plasminogen activator for acute ischemic stroke. *N Engl J. Med* 1995;333:1581–7.
12. Hacke W, Kaste M, Fieschi C, et al. Intravenous thrombolysis with recombinant tissue plasminogen activator for acute hemispheric stroke. *JAMA* 1995;274:1017–25.
13. Kramer AM, Steiner JF, Schlenker RE, et al. Outcomes and costs after hip fracture and stroke. A comparison of rehabilitation settings. *JAMA* 1997;277:396–404.
14. Epstein RS, Sherwood LM. From outcomes research to disease management: a guide for the perplexed. *Ann Intern Med* 1996;124:832–7.

15. Oster G, Borok GM, Menzin JJ, et al. A randomized trial to assess effectiveness and cost in clinical practice: rationale and design of the Cholesterol Reduction Intervention Study (CRIS). *Control Clin Trials* 1995;16:3–16.

16. Garber AM, Weinstein MC, Torrance GW, Kamlet MS. Theoretical foundations of cost-effectiveness analysis. In Gold MR, Siegel JE, Russell LB, Weinstein MC (Eds.) *Cost-effectiveness in Health and Medicine.* New York: Oxford University Press, 1996:25–53.

17. Solomon NA, Glick HA, Russo CJ, Lee J, Schulman KA. Patient preferences for stroke outcomes. *Stroke* 1994;25:1721–5.

18. Langfitt JT. Cost-effectiveness of anterotemporal lobectomyin medically intractable complex partial epilepsy. *Epilepsia* 1997;38:154–63.

19. Vickrey BG, Hays RD, Graber J, Rausch R, Engel J Jr., Brook RH. A health-related quality of life instrument for patients evaluated for epilepsy surgery. *Med Care* 1992;30:299–319.

20. Paty DW, Li DK. Interferon Beta-1b is effective in relapsing-remitting multiple sclerosis. *Neurology* 1993;43:662–7.

21. Mohr JP, Mast H, Thompson JLP, Sacco RL. Are more complex study designs needed for future acute stroke trials? *Cerebrovasc Dis* 1998;8(suppl.1):17–22.

22. Sano M, Ernesto C, Thomas RG, et al. A controlled trial of selegeline, alpha-tocopherol, or both as treatment for Alzheimer's disease. *N Engl J Med* 1997;336:1216–22.

23. Holloway RG. Economic outcomes research: in pursuit of cost-effective care. Course syllabus, American Academy of Neurology meeting, Boston 1997.

24. Naglie IG, Detsky AS. Treatment of chronic nonvalvular atrial fibrillation in the elderly: a decision analysis. *Med Decis Making* 1992;12:239–49.

25. Fryback DG, Dusbach EJ, Klein R, et al. The Beaver Dam Health Outcomes Study. Initial catalog of health-state quality factors. *Med Decis Making* 1993;13:89–102.

26. Patrick DL, Starks HE, Cain KC, Uhlmann RF, Pearlman RA. Measuring preferences for health states worse than death. *Med Decis Making* 1994;14:9–18.

8

Survival analysis in neurological diseases

John F. Kurtzke and Mitchell T. Wallin

Introduction to survival analysis

Survival analysis can be defined as the statistical processing of survival data. It allows one to examine the time interval from a given starting point (e.g., diagnosis of disease) to a discrete outcome (e.g., death) for a specified group. If this group is a random sample of the population, then the survival experience of the group will reflect that of the general population. It is the goal of this chapter to provide an overview of survival analysis as it relates to the major disorders within neurology. Death will be the predominant outcome measure in discussions. The field of survival analysis has had many recent advances and for a more technical discussion, the reader is referred to more exhaustive sources (1–4).

The ideal survival study would follow all members of a cohort from a specified time to a predetermined outcome. Unfortunately, the reality of assembling a survival cohort must allow for different outcomes. This is illustrated in Figure 8.1 where seven subjects were followed for variable lengths of time after an acute ischemic stroke. The outcome in this example was death. The subjects were recruited during a 2-year period and followed for 4 years. Subjects four, five, six, and seven reached the endpoint in the study prior to the end of the observation period. Subjects one, two, and three were censored. Censoring occurred in subjects two and three because they reached the end of the study before dying. This is called right censoring (5). Subject one was lost to follow-up prior to the end of the closing date and was thereby censored. On the other extreme, one must take into account different starting points. The goal is to summarize the probability of survival of a particular group over time in a table or survival curve (with the x-axis representing time and the y-axis representing the proportion surviving). Two commonly used methods to handle censoring and variable starting times include life table analysis and the Kaplan–Meier approach.

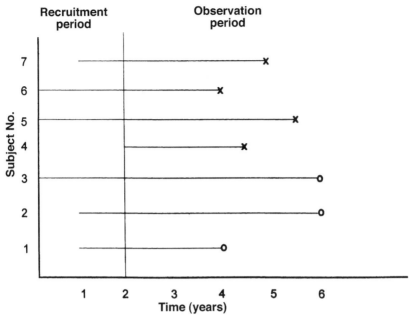

Figure 8.1   Patients with ischemic stroke that enter a study at different times with known (x) and censored (o) survival times (x, death; o, censored).

Life table method

The life table method (also called the actuarial approach) is often applied when survival data are grouped into regular time intervals (6). We will add some more data to the original stroke survival example to illustrate the technique. Suppose the goal is to define survival after acute ischemic stroke. In the community under study, 100 such patients at the time of the ictus and another 20 who had their strokes 1 year previously have been ascertained (Table 8.1). In the first year of follow-up, there are 20 deaths, but 10 patients have been lost from observation. The first line of Table 8.1 describes that year.

In this life table, the interval is years. While we know which year subjects were lost to follow-up (censored), we do not know exactly when they were lost. By custom, losses are considered equally distributed throughout the interval, so they contribute half their number to the cases at risk of death in that interval. The number at risk in the first year, then, is the number seen from onset (100) minus half the losses, or 95 cases. Twenty deaths in 95 give a ratio of 0.211, and thus 0.789 of the series are alive, giving a survival for the first year after stroke of 78.9%.

In the second year, the 70 survivors of year 1 (100 – 20 deaths – 10 losses) are added to the 20 cases first ascertained 1 year after the ictus. By adding subjects with different starting points at the proper observation year, the problem of a staggered entry into the follow-up period is solved. Note that it would have been improper

Table 8.1. Survival after ischemic stroke (hypothetical data)

Year	Number at risk	Deaths	Losses	Annual ratio		Percentage survival
				Dead	Alive	
1	$(100 - 5) = 95$	20	10	0.211	0.789	78.9
2	$(70 + 20 - 5) = 85$	15	10	0.176	0.824	65.0
3	$(65 - 3) = 62$	10	6	0.161	0.839	54.5
4	$(49 - 3) = 46$	5	6	0.109	0.891	48.6

to add these 20 before this point, as by definition they already had survived one-year post stroke. They can be included only from the time of ascertainment (5). These 90 minus one-half the losses result in 85 at risk, among whom 15 deaths occurred for a ratio of 0.176. The balance surviving (0.824) is multiplied by the previous year's balance surviving (0.789) to give a survival of 65.0% for 2 years after the stroke. This is an example of conditional probability where the probability of surviving from the beginning of the study until the end of year 2 is the probability of surviving year 2, conditional on having survived year 1. In this example, the median (50%) survival time is reached in the fourth year after ictus. A typical survival curve using the life table approach for a multiple sclerosis cohort is illustrated in Figure 8.2.

Kaplan–Meier method

In 1958, Kaplan and Meier first proposed a survival analysis method based on the precise survival time (7). As opposed to an arbitrary interval (i.e., life table method), the Kaplan–Meier method uses the exact time of an outcome in calculating survival. This leads to the characteristic irregular steps of the survival curve. Only subjects with exactly the same survival time are in each interval. This small interval essentially eliminates the need for the assumption of uniform withdrawals over the interval discussed above for life tables. Rather than using a correction equation for the interval, censored subjects are considered to be at risk until the time that they drop out. Between events, the proportion surviving remains unchanged, even if there are intermediate censored observations. With a small sample, the Kaplan–Meier method is more efficient than the life table method as exact times for the outcome of interest are used rather than an approximation (i.e., life table method).

The technique can be illustrated using the ischemic stroke sample data shown in Figure 8.1. The first step is to rank order the data based on the length of time (in years) in the trial. Censored items are marked with an asterisk:

2.5* 3 3.5 4 5* 5.5 6.0*

Table 8.2. Kaplan–Meier life table analysis (data in Figure 8.1)

Time (years)	Number at risk	Number of deaths	Death rate	Survival rate	Cumulative survival rate
3	6	1	0.17	0.83	0.83
3.5	5	1	0.20	0.80	0.66
4	4	1	0.25	0.75	0.50
5.5	2	1	0.50	0.50	0.25

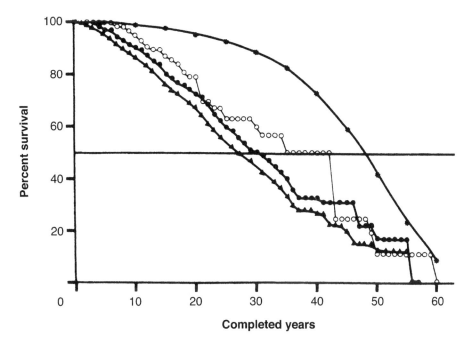

Figure 8.2   Percentage survival in multiple sclerosis by years after onset from: epidemiologic series of Lower Saxony (○–○); FRG original hospital series from 11 neurologic centres (▲–▲); revised FRG hospital series (cases with 2 + years under observation) (●–●); contrasted with expected survival from age 30 from FRG life tables 1976–78 weighted 1 : 2; M : F (*–*). From (16) with permission.

The next step is to put the data into a Kaplan–Meier survival table (Table 8.2). As opposed to the regular yearly intervals seen in the life table method (the far left-hand column of Table 8.1), the yearly intervals in the Kaplan–Meier table correspond to the exact year each subject dies. In the first line, there are six persons at risk because one person was censored at 2.5 years. The survival rate at 3 years is equal to 1 – death rate or $1 - 1/6 = 0.83$. At 5.5 years, three persons have died and one was censored leaving two persons at risk. The cumulative survival at year 5.5 is the probability of surviving 5.5 years for all subjects who started the study. It can be calculated by multiplying the cumulative survival rate at 4 years (0.50) times the survival rate (probability of survival for those starting the interval) at year 5.5 (0.50), which is 0.25. The median survival for this cohort occurs during the fourth year. A Kaplan–Meier curve showing the survival experience of two stroke cohorts is illustrated in Figure 8.7.

In most cases, both the life table method and the Kaplan–Meier method give similar survival probabilities. Some general assumptions must be emphasized with both methods:

(1) *A clear starting point.* This must be defined by the investigators with some possibilities including time of diagnosis, time of first symptom, or time of a particular procedure (e.g., carotid endarterectomy). Each possibility will have concerns regarding accuracy and reliability. A uniform, reproducible starting point must be applied to all subjects.

(2) *A clear end point.* While death is often used in studies and is very concrete, other measures (e.g., disability scales, quality of life indexes) that involve individual examinations and questionnaires are often applied. These carry the potential for bias because of variation in reporting. This variation can occur within reports generated by one investigator or reports generated between several investigators in a particular study.

(3) *Loss to follow-up should not be related to the end point.* One assumes that the reason a subject is censored before the end of the study is not related to the end point. In our example of stroke survival, if persons withdrew due to recurrent pneumonia from stroke-related swallowing disorder, they likely would have had a greater probability of dying than those remaining in the study. If these subjects are excluded, then the survival rate will be over-estimated and the death rate underestimated.

(4) *No secular changes.* Changes in diagnosis, treatment, and data collection techniques can often produce misleading results in a cohort assembled over a long period of time. Feinstein et al. showed how lung cancer survival rates falsely increased in more recent cohorts of patients (8). What actually happened was that the more recent cohorts of lung cancer patients demonstrated less severe disease due to improved imaging and diagnostic data. This resulted in a "stage migration." Because the prognosis of those who migrated, although worse than that for other members of the good-stage group, was better than that of the bad-stage group, survival rates rose in each group without any change in individual outcomes. This effect must be taken into account in studies that follow cohorts for long periods of time.

There are a number of ways to summarize survival data. The median survival time is a commonly used statistic. This is defined as the time at which 50% of the study population has reached the defined endpoint. Another frequently used term is the survival rate at a particular time, e.g., 5- or 10-year survival. The main problem with both of these statistics is that they do not describe the whole survival curve. The survival experience of subjects beyond the particular time interval (i.e., 10 years) may be very different than an earlier summary statistic (i.e., 5-year survival) would indicate. To avoid this problem, a survival table or curve is often the best way to evaluate trends in survival for a particular group or groups. Comparing survival between two or more groups requires significance testing.

Logrank test

The logrank test is a common statistic to compare groups in life tables and Kaplan–Meier curves. Despite the use of "log" in the title, the test does not incorporate logarithms. The test is nonparametric and is based on a modification of the Mantel–Haenszel chi-square test. The major advantage of this approach is that all the data are used and one avoids the problem of choosing a single point in the two survival curves as a basis for comparison.

As with the chi-square test, the logrank test for two groups can be written as:

$$\chi^2 = (O_1 - E_1)^2/E_1 + (O_2 - E_2)^2/E_2, \text{ with 1 df} \tag{1}$$

For each group (k), an observed (O) and an expected (E) number of events can be calculated. The results produce the familiar chi-square statistic with k − 1 degrees of freedom (df). The logrank test can also be expanded to include several groups or strata.

Cox proportional hazards model

The Cox proportional hazards model allows one to simultaneously predict the impact of several variables on the survival of a given group (9). It is a semi-parametric approach, meaning there is no assumption of a specific underlying distribution for survival times. The major assumption is that there can be no change in the effect of the prognostic variables over time. This can be stated as a constant risk-multiple over time for the prognostic variable. Besides the advantage of handling multiple factors (covariates) at one time, the technique treats continuous data as continuous and gives an estimate of the magnitude of the differences between factors in the form of relative risk. The actual method is very complex and this section only serves as an introduction to the methodology.

A hazard can be defined as the probability of occurrence of an outcome (e.g., death) for individuals who began a specified interval where:

$$q_i = D_i/R_i \tag{2}$$

Here q_i = probability of death in year i, D_i = the number of persons who died in year i, and R_i = the number of subjects at risk in year i. The proportional hazards model extends the definition to the probability of an event at time t, given survival up to time t, for a specific value of variable, x. The hazard function can be rewritten for several independent variables of interest (e.g., X_1 to X_m) so we can express the hazard at time t, $h(t)$, as:

$$h(t) = h_0(t) \times \exp(b_1 X_1 + b_2 X_2 + \ldots + b_m X_m) \tag{3}$$

The value $h_0(t)$ is equivalent to the hazard when all the variables are zero and must be estimated from the data. The value of the regression coefficients, b_1 to b_m, also must be estimated from the data.

The Cox model is fitted with the help of a computer software program. The interpretation of proportional hazards regression coefficients is analogous to logistic regression coefficients. A positive sign means the hazard is higher, and thus, if survival is being assessed, the prognosis is worse with higher values of the given variable. In the case where a binary variable is coded 0 or 1, the hazard ratio is equal to e^{b_1}.

Let us propose a model from a clinical trial comparing "drug A" to a placebo (0 = drug A and 1 = placebo) on survival of patients with brain stem gliomas. Suppose we find a value of $0.50 = b_{\text{drug A}}$ with other variables in the model including albumin (g/liter) and hepatitis B (0 = no; 1 = yes). Thus, the estimated hazard for the placebo is 1.65 ($\exp(0.50) = 1.65$) times that of drug A, adjusting for all other variables in the model. In other words, drug A reduced the hazard to $\exp(-0.50) = 0.61$ or 61% compared with the placebo and adjusted for the other variables in the model.

Continuous covariates (e.g., albumin) can be interpreted as an increase in log hazard for an increase of 1 unit (g/liter) in the value of the covariate. One can compare the relative risk at two different values of a specified covariate, h_1 and h_2 by:

$$h_1(t)/h_2(t) = h_0(t) \times \exp(bx_1))/h_0(t) \times \exp(bx_2) \tag{4}$$

This equation is equivalent to the relative risk of h_1 compared to h_2. For more discussion on the Cox proportional hazards model, the reader is referred to standard texts (1,2).

Multiple sclerosis

There have been a number of studies to elucidate the survival characteristics of individuals with multiple sclerosis (MS) (10–21). It is not clear, however, whether the risk factors that influence the diagnosis of MS might play a significant role in survival subsequent to MS onset. Because MS is a relatively rare disease (prevalence even in high-risk areas is some 30–200 per 100 000 population) with its peak incidence in young adults, assembling and following a survival cohort is often difficult (22). Country-wide data bases (e.g., Denmark), small population clusters (e.g., Olmsted County, Minnesota) and specialized population groups (e.g., United States (US) veteran population) have provided resources for long-term follow-up studies. Known risk factors for the diagnosis of MS that have been previously reported from cohort studies include (13–18):

- Female sex
- White race
- Northern latitude
- Higher education
- Urban residence
- Higher socioeconomic class
- Scandinavian ancestry
- Poor visual acuity at induction

Cohorts that utilize prospective analyses of incident cases provide the most unbiased assessment of risk factors. Unfortunately, due to the time and expense involved, there are only a handful of these studies available describing the survival in MS (11,15,17,20). We will highlight a few of these studies and then summarize MS survival characteristics.

Poser et al. reported the survival characteristics of a German population-based epidemiologic MS series and a hospital-based MS series and compared both to the standard survival of the German population (16). The population-based epidemiologic series included 224 persons, and the hospital-based series included 1429 persons, with deaths for both recorded between 1973 and 1981. Subjects were followed from disease onset to death. Figure 8.2 shows the percentage of survival in MS by years after onset for the two series and expected survival for the German population. A revision was made in the hospital series due to the high number of deaths in the first 3 years. In order not to delete too many cases, patients with at least 2 years of follow-up after ascertainment were included. The median survival for the population-based epidemiologic series was 35–42 years. The median survival for the revised hospital-based series was 30 years. While there were no significant differences between male and female survival, patients with onset greater than age 35 years had a significantly shorter survival than those with onset at ages under 35 years. The survival curves agreed with data from two other population-based estimates in Rochester, Minnesota (12) and in US World War II veterans (11).

Brønnum-Hansen et al. reported on the survival characteristics of a 6727 Danish population cohort followed for 39 years (20), the largest population-based cohort to date. There were minimal losses to follow-up, and Danish population statistics were used to calculate excess death rates between the MS cohort and the general population. A standard life table approach was used in the study. Median survival time from onset of the disease was 28 years in men and 33 years in women. Ten-year

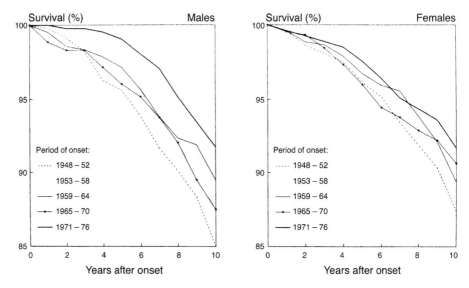

Figure 8.3   Ten-year survival in five cohorts of Danish patients with multiple sclerosis ascertained within 10 years of onset. From (20) with permission.

survival cohorts have been followed since 1948 (Figure 8.3), with more recent cohorts showing improved survival. Disease onset, as opposed to diagnosis, was used as the starting point. The survival for males improved to that of females in the period between 1971 and 1976. A significant decrease in the 10-year excess death rate helped to show that this trend was not due to a lower mortality trend versus that of the general population. Improved care and prevention of complications in MS patients is probably responsible for a large part of this change in mortality. Riise et al. found similar trends of improved survival with more recent cohorts (15).

In summary, the population-based incident cohorts (11,15,17,20) give a median survival range from disease onset of 28 to 35 years for both sexes. Considered separately, men have shorter median survival compared to women. Other risk factors that significantly worsen survival in MS include (4–7,10,11,15,17,20):

- Older age of onset
- Progressive disease course
- Severe MS disability
- Motor symptoms at onset
- Cerebellar symptoms at onset
- Short interval to first relapse of MS
- High socioeconomic status

With more knowledge about the risk factors for survival in MS, more realistic prognostic and treatment advice can be given to patients and hopefully more light can be shed on the etiology of the disease itself.

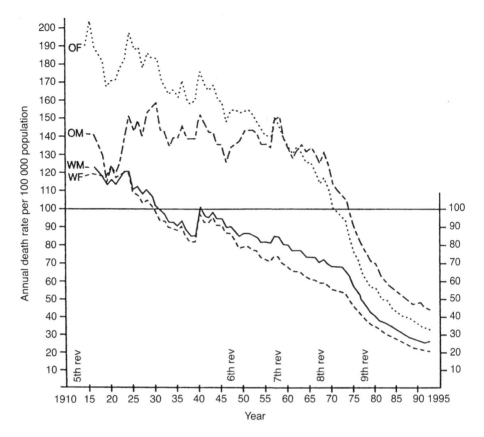

Figure 8.4   Cerebrovascular disease. Annual age-adjusted (USA 1940) death rates per 100 000 population by sex and colour, USA, 1915–93. Source: Adapted with permission from (102). OM,
other male; OF, other female; WM, white male; WF, white female.

Stroke

Cerebrovascular disease (CVD) or stroke is the third leading cause of death and a
significant cause of long-term disability in most industrialized nations (23). The
World Health Organization (WHO) defines stroke as "rapidly developing clinical
signs of focal (or global) disturbance of cerebral function, with symptoms lasting
24 hours or longer or leading to death, with no apparent cause other than of
vascular origin" (24). Because the definition of stroke is so broad, it has been
difficult to categorize uniformly its different etiologies and characterize its course.
In this section, we will highlight some of the recent trends in stroke mortality and
survival.

Stroke mortality in the United States has declined steadily from 1900 through
the mid-1970s, with possibly a more rapid decline through the 1980s. The decline
seems to have plateaued in the early 1990s. Figure 8.4 illustrates this trend. Stroke

data were collected from the US National Vital Statistics System. Since the 1950s, the age adjusted (to 1940 US population) death rate from cerebrovascular disease has declined by more than two-thirds (from 88.6 deaths/100 000 population to 28.0/100 000), twice the rate of decline of other causes of mortality. The decline is seen for both sex and race categories.

The decline in stroke mortality since the early 1900s in the US can be attributed to a number of different factors, including: changes in International Classification of Diseases (ICD) coding, increased diagnostic capabilities (e.g., magnetic resonance imaging), increased utilization of neurologists in the diagnosis of stroke, decreased stroke incidence and decreased case fatality rates (no. stroke deaths in a given interval/no. stroke cases in the same interval). Prior to the mid-1970s, there had been a true decrease in the incidence of stroke in addition to a decrease in the case fatality rate (25). This is at least in part due to improved treatment of comorbidities.

When looking at the type of stroke, there appears to be a large difference in the case fatality rate. Thirty-day case fatality rates by stroke type from the Framingham cohort are illustrated in Figure 8.5 (26). These data were obtained prospectively from 5184 subjects followed biennially for 26 years starting in 1949. Overall case fatality at 30 days was 22%. Subarachnoid hemorrhage rates were higher for men than women, but brain infarction rates were similar at around 15%. As age increased, so did the 30-day case fatality in brain infarctions for both men and women. For a similar period in a Rochester, Minnesota cohort, the 30-day case fatality rates for cerebral infarction, intracerebral hemorrhage and subarachnoid hemorrhage were 28, 84, and 52%, respectively (27).

The current evidence gives a mixed picture in regard to time trends. A small number of studies have shown a decrease in incidence and case fatality in the US (28–30), Finland (31), and Japan (32). Other studies have shown stable or increasing stroke incidence rates and decreasing case mortality (33–39). Two Minnesota groups reported a shift toward increasing incidence and stable to decreasing case fatality rates in stroke cohorts from the late 1980s (40,41). In Rochester, Minnesota, a population followed since 1955 showed a rather notable increase in incidence of stroke to levels higher than those of the 1970s (1985–1989 annual age and sex-adjusted stroke incidence rate was 145 per 100 000 population, 13% higher than the rate during 1975–1979). Overall survival after first stroke (measured at 30 days and 1 year) was not significantly different during 1985–1989 compared to 1980–1984 (1985–1989 30-day/1-year survival for all strokes: for men 86%/77%; for women 75%/61%). A Cox proportional hazards model revealed that age and calendar year were significant risk factors for 30-day and 1-year survival after first ischemic stroke. Short- and long-term survival improved for intracranial hemorrhages over the last 15 years (41).

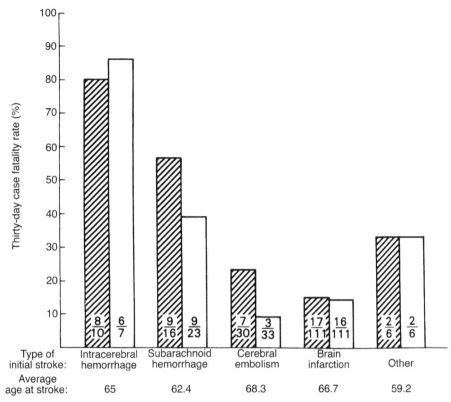

Figure 8.5 Thirty-day case fatality rates by stroke type from the Framingham cohort (from (26) with permission). ▨, men; ☐, women.

Most industrialized countries have shared similar time trends in stroke mortality. Intercountry comparisons, however, bring concerns regarding accuracy and validity of data. The World Health Organization (WHO) initiated the first integrated international study of stroke, called MONICA (Monitoring Trends and Determinants in Cardiovascular Disease) (42). From 1982–1986, age standardized stroke mortality rates were calculated from 18 collaborating countries (16 European and two Asian) and weighted to a derived standard. The average case-fatality rate at 28 days was 30%, but ranged between 15% and 57%. The lowest case fatality rates were reported from Scandinavian countries (Denmark, Finland, and Sweden), West Germany, Lithuania, Novosibirsk, and the Russian Federation. The highest rates were found in Eastern Europe and Italy. Men had higher case fatality rates in all populations except Lithuania and Novosibirsk.

Survival after an initial ischemic stroke is shown in Figure 8.6. The life table method was used to obtain the curves. These data are from a 26-year follow-up of the Framingham cohort (starting in 1949) described above (26). Overall 10-year

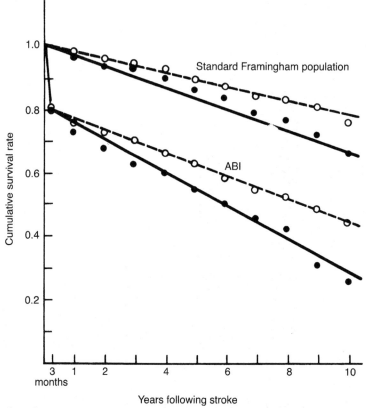

Figure 8.6   Survival after an ischemic stroke, using the life table method. Data are from the Framingham cohort (from (26), with permission). ABI, acute brain infarction. ●—●, males, $n = 111$ (average age 66.6); ○—○, females, $n = 111$ (average age 66.8).

survival for all strokes combined was 35%, with women showing improved survival compared to men. Because the ages of both sexes were similar, age cannot explain this disparity in survival. The survival rate for acute brain infarction was similar to the rate for all strokes combined. Five-year survival rates for acute brain infarction for men and women were 56% and 64%, respectively. This compares to a five-year survival rate for the standard population of 89%.

As health care resources become more restricted in most countries, there has been increasing concern about the type of care received for life-threatening disorders such as stroke. The reduction of services to decrease costs has been documented in health maintenance organizations (HMOs), especially in terms of home health care (43,44). Retchin et al. reported the outcomes of elderly stroke patients managed in fee-for-service (FFS) and managed care (HMO) settings in 12 states in the US (45). Figure 8.7 shows that both the FFS and the HMO group experienced similar survival during the follow-up period after a stroke. However,

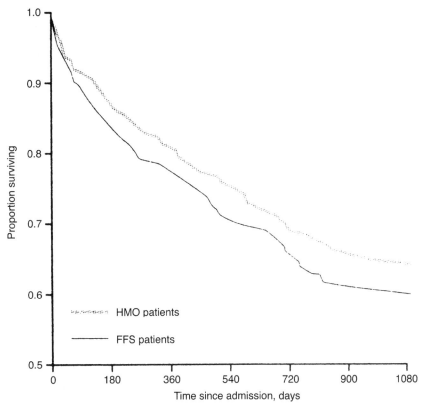

Figure 8.7   Kaplan–Meier survival function estimates comparing the proportion of patients surviving after stroke who were enrolled in health maintenance organizations (HMOs) vs. fee for service (FFS). From (45) with permission.

in a regression model controlling for age, marital status, and characteristics of dependency at discharge, HMO patients were more likely than FFS patients to be sent to nursing homes (HMO, 41.8%; FFS, 27.9%) and less likely to be discharged to rehabilitation hospitals or units (HMO, 16.2%; FFS, 23.4%). While scales of morbidity and quality of life were not taken after hospitalization in this study, identification of therapeutic endeavors that alter functioning after stroke will be of utmost importance in the economic management of this disorder.

HIV-related neurologic disease

As of December 1994, the Centers for Disease Control (CDC) had reported 426 978 cases of AIDS have been diagnosed in the US and 267 479 of these patients have died (46). The WHO has estimated that since the early 1980s through 1994, approximately 18 million people had been infected with the HIV virus and 4.5 million of these had developed AIDS (47). This pervasive disease is caused by a retrovirus and spread by body fluids. After acute infection, most persons enter an asymptomatic period for approximately 8 to 10 years. Most nervous system complications of HIV appear late in the course (48). Despite a poor long-term prognosis, short-term survival time from diagnosis of AIDS for all cases has improved during the 1980s (49–52). In a New York State cohort, median survival increased from 5.3 months pre-1984 to 13.2 months in 1987–1989 (51). This trend is in part related to improved treatments for HIV (zidovudine), better detection of secondary diseases (e.g., *Pneumocystis carinii* pneumonia), and changes in the definition of AIDS in 1985 (53) and 1987 (54).

The classification system for staging HIV-1 infection has been developed by the CDC and most recently modified in 1993 (55). The current system uses illness categories (A–Asymptomatic, B–Symptomatic, C–AIDS defining illness) and CD4+ cell counts to help define the course of HIV disease. The biggest change in the 1993 modification was the inclusion of patients infected with HIV-1 having a CD4+ lymphocyte count less than 200/uL, irrespective of their clinical status. Vella et al. evaluated the impact of this new CDC definition on the survival of AIDS patients in an Italian cohort (56). Compared to the 1987 CDC case definition, the study population with the 1993 case definition increased by 188%, and the median survival more than doubled (median survival 1987 definition: 24 months; 1993 definition: 57 months). The presence of an AIDS-defining illness was a powerful independent predictor of death. This modification in the diagnostic classification of AIDS is a secular trend with obvious implications on survival analysis. Time trend analyses in HIV/AIDS must take the changing definition into account. In the remaining discussion, we turn to survival issues in some of the major HIV-associated neurologic diseases.

HIV-dementia

HIV-dementia is largely a subcortical disorder involving deficits in cognition, behavior, and the motor system. The prognosis for HIV-dementia is dismal with an average survival of 6 months from onset of symptoms to death. In examining four separate Kaplan–Meier survival curves from patients diagnosed with HIV-dementia (pre-1987, 1989/90, 1987/88, 1991/92), a median survival of 4.3 months was calculated without change over the time periods (48).

Ellis et al. recently showed that HIV-infected individuals with neuropsychological (NP) impairment had a higher risk of dying than those who were neuropsychologically normal (57). NP impairment was defined by the operational criteria for HIV-associated minor cognitive motor disorders (MCMD), and as having two or more NP test domains that were impaired (NP-I). The median survival for the MCMD group was 2.2 years and for the NP-I group, 3.8 years.

Cryptoccocal meningitis

Cryptoccocus neoformans causes meningitis in approximately 10% of AIDS patients (58). It is the most common CNS opportunistic infection in AIDS patients. Chuck and Sande (59) showed in a Cox regression analysis that the growth of cryptococcus from an extrameningeal site (median survival 147 days if positive vs. 265 days if negative) and the presence of hyponatremia (median survival of 113 days if present vs. 214 days if absent) were independent predictors of shorter survival. In a study of 131 patients receiving fluconazole (200 mg per day) or amphotericin B (0.4 mg/kg/day), early mortality in the first 2 weeks was higher in the fluconazole group (15%) compared with the amphotericin group (8%) (60). This rather high mortality was in part due to low doses of that antifungal therapy. The most important predictors of death were abnormal mental status (lethargy, somnolence, or obtundation), CSF cryptococcal antigen titer $> 1:1024$, and CSF WBC < 20 cells/mm^3.

CNS toxoplasmosis

CNS toxoplasmosis results from the reactivation of latent infection of the obligate intracellular protozoan, *Toxoplasma gondii*. The disease causes multifocal cerebral abscesses and usually develops when the CD4 cell count is fewer than 200 cells/mm^3. In a treatment trial consisting of pyrimethamine, sulphadiazine and leucovorin in 114 AIDS patients with CNS toxoplasmosis (1981–1990), 95% of patients responded with improved follow-up MRI scans at 2 weeks (61). Mean survival of patients who died after their first episode of CNS toxoplasmosis was 265 days ± 212 days. Multivariate analysis showed that a history of PCP and a blood lymphocyte count of $< 24\%$ were independent predictors of decreased survival. A more recent cohort of HIV-infected patients followed and treated in Baltimore, Maryland from 1989–1995 had a median survival of 180 days after a diagnosis of *Toxoplasmosis gondii* encephalitis (62).

Progressive multifocal leukoencephalopathy

Progressive multifocal leukoencephalopathy (PML) is caused by a papovavirus that infects oligodendrocytes and astrocytes. The disease causes progressive focal demyelination of the CNS. The mean survival with PML and AIDS is 4 months from the onset of neurological symptoms (63). Fong et al. reported on the survival of 28 AIDS patients with a history of PML from Canada (64). The overall mean survival time after presentation of neurological symptoms was 5.6 months. A Cox regression analysis showed that patients with CD4 + cell counts of < 90/mm^3 were nearly 3.4 times more likely to die earlier than were patients with CD4 + cell counts of ≥ 90/mm^3. Moreover, patients diagnosed with AIDS prior to developing PML had a 2.8 times higher risk of dying compared to patients for whom AIDS was not previously diagnosed.

Primary CNS lymphoma

Upwards of 2% of AIDS patients develop primary CNS lymphoma, and in 0.6% of patients it will be the AIDS-defining illness (65). Typically the presentation is one of progressive deterioration of neurologic function with death in 3 months. CNS lymphoma usually develops in the late stages of HIV disease with CD4+ cell counts of less than 100 cells/mm³ (66). If untreated, the median survival after diagnosis of primary CNS lymphoma is less than one month (67,68). Radiation therapy may prolong median survival to 4–6 months (67–71).

Dementia

Within the past two decades, Alzheimer's disease (AD) has been confirmed to be responsible for the majority of primary degenerative dementias (72,73). AD is largely a diagnosis of exclusion and many studies have utilized the guidelines developed by the National Institute of Neurological and Communicative Disorders and Stroke and the Alzheimer's Disease and Related Disorders Association (NINDS/ADRDA) to identify cases (74). Newer criteria for diagnosis have been defined in the Tenth Revision of the International Classification of Diseases (75) and in DSM–IV (76). Clinicopathologic correlation is relatively high with these clinical criteria. Vascular dementia remains the second most common cause of dementia, responsible for 10–20% of cases (77). The Hachinski score (78) and the more restrictive American–European criteria (79) have been used to more accurately define cases of vascular dementia. This discussion on survival will be limited to AD and multi-infarct dementia (MID).

The survival of patients with dementia has been reviewed by van Dijk et al. (80). Forty-one papers representing 38 dementia survival studies were reviewed. These studies were selected out of a total of 90 papers based on dementia diagnosis, a well-defined cohort population and use of the life table or Kaplan–Meier methods in the survival analysis.

Figure 8.8 lists the calculated 2-year survival rate for the 38 studies. Broad differences can be appreciated based on the reference cohort of interest. Two-year survival rates for patients in community based studies range from 37–86%. Patients with dementia in the outpatient clinic setting have a 2-year survival rate of 75% (range 60–95%) and those in nursing homes, 50% (range 30–65%). Those patients admitted to mental and psychiatric hospitals had a 2-year survival rate of about 40% (range 20–60%). Some general conclusions about patients with dementia were made from the review:

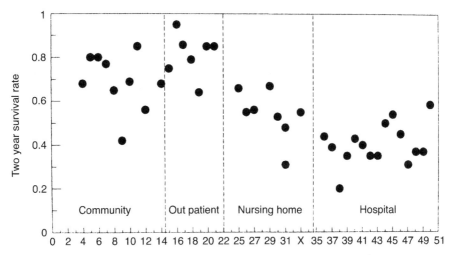

Figure 8.8   Two-year survival rates for 38 follow-up studies of demented patients. Numbers on x-axis are reference numbers, ordered according to calendar time to each type of study population. x represents results of van Dijk PTM, et al. From (80) with permission.

- Women seem to have longer survival than men
- Mortality increases with increasing age
- There is substantial excess mortality compared to the general population

Differences in survival between patients with AD and MID were small and more recent studies have shown a more favorable prognosis for AD. McGonigal et al. described survival in patients who had died of both pre-senile AD and pre-senile MID (81). The duration of survival was greater from symptom onset to death in AD (mean 7.4 years) compared with MID (mean 5.8 years). Most of the difference was accounted for by the longer duration between symptom onset and presentation to the hospital in the AD group (mean 3.2 years) and the MID group (mean 2.4 years). Other studies have shown that in AD, early-onset patients live longer on average (median 6.7–8.1 years) (82,83) than those with late-onset disease (median 4.8–9.7) (84,85). Life expectancy in AD is shorter for those with more severe cognitive impairments (86,87). More quantitative studies are needed concerning the rate of progression of dementia and risk factors for survival.

Primary CNS neoplasms

Over 17 000 primary brain tumors were newly diagnosed in the US during 1995. Only about half of these patients were expected to be alive 1 year after diagnosis (88). Primary brain tumors are classified by site and histologic type as given by the International Classification of Diseases for Oncology (ICD–O). The three most common primary brain tumors in adults are glioblastoma, meningioma, and low-grade astrocytoma, respectively.

The most recent cancer survival statistics (1988–1992) show an increased 5-year survival for all primary nervous system tumors (White 29% and Black 32%) compared with rates from 1960–1963 (White 18% and Black 19%) (89). Five-year survival for primary brain tumors in an Australian cohort was 52% for females and 37% for males (90). Five-year survival for nerve sheath tumors, meningiomas, and "other" (mostly nonmalignant) was 100%, 92%, and 96%, respectively. Patients with ependymomas and oligodendrogliomas had survival rates at 5 years of 65% and 61%, respectively. This is in contrast to medulloblastomas at 43% and astrocytomas at 44%. Overall 5-year survival was worst for glioblastoma multiforme at 5%; even after treatment, 2-year survival is reported to be only 5–10% (91,92).

A study of malignant cerebral gliomas (grade 3 or 4) from the UK evaluated survival and disability using Kaplan–Meier techniques and a Cox proportional hazards model (93). Median survival for those receiving radiotherapy was 10.3 months. Multivariate analysis revealed that the initial WHO clinical performance status was the most important component in predicting survival. Other variables that were significantly related to survival in the Cox analysis were history of seizures and extent of surgery. Disability-free survival rate (as judged by a Barthel score <20) by initial WHO performance status criteria (0 – normal activity to 4 – no self care/confined to bed or chair) was assessed by Kaplan–Meier analysis. Seventy-four percent of those with the highest clinical performance (Grade 0–1) maintained disability free living for 6 months in contrast to less than 10% of the lowest grade (3–4) at 6 months. Sixty-five percent of those on the lowest clinical performance scale also spent at least a month in the hospital for treatment as compared to 20% of all others.

Status epilepticus

Status epilepticus (SE) is often defined as "an epileptic seizure which is so frequently repeated or so prolonged as to create a fixed and lasting condition" (94). Hauser has estimated that 12% of patients with a first diagnosis of epilepsy present in status epilepticus (95). In regard to the etiology, two broad groups have been defined: those without a new structural CNS lesion and those with an acute CNS injury (96). The latter group has a much higher mortality than the former (96,97). Mortality figures in SE range between 14% and 59% in adults, with much lower figures for children (98).

Most epidemiologic studies that deal with SE have not been population-based. DeLorenzo et al. recently published a review of SE in the Richmond, Virginia metropolitan area (99). The absolute incidence rate was 41 cases/100 000 residents/year. The overall mortality rate was 22%, with individual rates in pediatric, adult and elderly populations of 2.5, 14, and 38%, respectively. The top etiologies for mortality from SE in adults were anoxia, hypoxia, and cerebrovascular accident, respectively. Mortality from SE tended to increase with age. The number of deaths expected per year from SE in the US population were estimated to be between 22 000 and 42 000.

Comments

The study of survival within populations has greatly improved our understanding of the natural history of many neurologic disorders. Dramatic improvements in stroke mortality have occurred over the last 50 years. Hopefully, advances in understanding CNS neoplasms, dementia, and AIDS will further improve outcomes in these diseases as well. Developments with protease-inhibitor combinations and HIV disease have been particularly encouraging (100). By further defining risk factors for morbidity and mortality, we will hopefully come closer to understanding the etiology of disease and thereby make prevention and treatment more realistic. As our population ages, understanding the time trends of major neurologic diseases becomes paramount as two of the four leading causes of death in the elderly are stroke and dementia. Currently, those 85 years and older in the US represent the fastest growing segment of our population with a projected increase to 15 million persons by 2050 (101). Making decisions regarding prevention, education, research, and treatment in these times of limited resources can be aided through our knowledge of the time trends of disease.

REFERENCES

1. Altman, AG. *Practical Statistics for Medical Research.* London: Chapman and Hall, 1991:365–94.
2. Kahn HA, Sempos CT. *Statistical Methods in Epidemiology.* Oxford: Oxford University Press, 1989.
3. Peto R, Pike MC, Armitage P, et al. Design and analysis of randomized clinical trials requiring prolonged observation of each patient. I. Introduction and design. *Br J Cancer* 1976;34:585–612.
4. Peto R, Pike MC, Armitage P, et al. Design and analysis of randomized clinical trials requiring prolonged observations of each patient. II. Analysis and examples. *Br J Cancer* 1977;351:1–39.
5. Kurtzke JF. On estimating survival: a tale of two censors. *J Clin Epidemiol* 1989;42:169–75.
6. Kurtzke JF. Clinical manifestations of multiple sclerosis. In Vinken PJ, Bruyn GW (Eds), *Multiple Sclerosis and Other Demyelinating Diseases. Handbook of Clinical Neurology*, vol 9. Amsterdam: North-Holland, 1970:161–216.

7. Kaplan EL, Meier P. Nonparametric estimation from incomplete observations. *J Am Stat Assoc* 1958;53:457–85.

8. Feinstein AR, Sosin DM, Wells CK. The Will Rogers phenomenon. Stage migration and new diagnostic techniques as a source of misleading statistics for survival in cancer. *N Engl J Med* 1985;312:1604–8.

9. Cox DR. Regression models and life tables. *J Royal Stat Soc B* 1972;34:187–220.

10. Leibowitz U, Kahana E, Alter M. Survival and death in multiple sclerosis. *Brain* 1969;92:115–30.

11. Kurtzke JF, Beebe GW, Nagler B, Nefzger MD, Auth TL, Kurland LT. Studies on the natural history of multiple sclerosis. V. Long-term survival in young men. *Arch Neurol* 1970;22:215–25.

12. Percy AK, Nobrega FT, Okazaki H, Glattre E, Kurland LT. Multiple sclerosis in Rochester, Minnesota; a 60-year appraisal. *Arch Neurol* 1971;25:105–11.

13. Visscher BR, Liu K-S, Clark VA, Detels R, Malmgren RM, Dudley JP. Onset symptoms as predictors of mortality and disability in multiple sclerosis. *Acta Neurol Scand* 1984;70:321–8.

14. Phadke JG. Survival pattern and cause of death in patients with multiple sclerosis: results from an epidemiological survey in north east Scotland. *J Neurol Neurosurg Psychiatry* 1987;50:523–31.

15. Riise T, Gronning M, Aarli JA, Nyland H, Larsen JP, Edland A. Prognostic factors for life expectancy in multiple sclerosis analyzed by Cox-models. *J Clin Epidemiol* 1988;41:1031–6.

16. Poser S, Kurtzke JF, Poser W, Schlaf G. Survival in multiple sclerosis. J Clin Epidemiol 1989;42:159–68.

17. Wynn DR, Rodriguez M, O'Fallon WM, Kurland LT. A reappraisal of the epidemiology of multiple sclerosis in Olmsted County, Minnesota. *Neurology* 1990;40:780–6.

18. Miller DH, Hornabrook RW, Purdie G. The natural history of multiple sclerosis: a regional study with some longitudinal data. *J Neurol Neurosurg Psychiatry* 1992;55:341–6.

19. Sadovnick AD, Ebers GC, Wilson RW, Paty DW. Life expectancy in patients attending multiple sclerosis clinics. *Neurology* 1992;42:991–4.

20. Brønnum-Hansen H, Koch-Henriksen N, Hyllested K. Survival of patients with multiple sclerosis in Denmark: a nationwide, long-term epidemiologic survey. *Neurology* 1994;44:1901–7.

21. Midgard R, Albrektsen G, Riise T, Kvåle G, Nyland H. Prognostic factors for survival in multiple sclerosis: a longitudinal, population based study in Møre and Romsdal, Norway. *J Neurol Neurosurg Psychiatry* 1995;58:417–21.

22. Kurtzke JF, Beebe GW, Norman JE. Epidemiology of multiple sclerosis in US veterans:1. Race, sex and geographic variation. *Neurology* 1979;29:1228–35.

23. Bonita R. Epidemiology of stroke. *Lancet* 1992;339:342–4.

24. Thorvaldsen P, Asplund K, Kuulasmaa K, et al. Stroke incidence, case fatality, and mortality in the WHO MONICA Project. *Stroke* 1995;26:361–7.

25. McGovern PG, Shahar E, Sprafka JM, et al. The role of stroke attack rate and case fatality in the decline of stroke mortality: The Minnesota Heart Survey. *Ann Epidemiol* 1993;3:483–7.

26. Sacco RL, Wolf PA, Kannel WB, McNamara PM. Survival and recurrence following stroke – The Framingham Study. *Stroke* 1982;13:290–5.

27. Matsumoto N, Whisnant JP, Kurland LT, Okazaki H. Natural history of stroke in Rochester, Minnesota, 1955 through 1969: an extension of a previous study, 1945 through 1954. *Stroke* 1973;4:20–9.

28. Brown RD, Whisnant JP, Sicks JD, O'Fallon WM, Wiebers DO. Stroke incidence, prevalence, and survival: secular trends in Rochester, Minnesota, through 1989. *Stroke* 1996;27:373–80.

29. Garraway WM, Whisnant JP, Furlan AJ, Phillips AH, Kurland LT, O'Fallon WM. The declining incidence of stroke. *N Engl J Med* 1979;300:449–52.

30. Kagan A, Popper J, Reed D, McLean CJ, Grove TS. Trends in stroke incidence and mortality in Hawaiian Japanese men. *Stroke* 1994;25:1170–5.

31. Tuomilehto J, Bonita R, Stewart AW, Salonen JT. Hypertension, cigarette smoking, and the decline in stroke incidence in eastern Finland. *Stroke* 1991;22:7–11.

32. Ueda K, Omae T, Hirota Y, et al. Decreasing trend in incidence and mortality from stroke in Hisayama residents, Japan. *Stroke* 1981;12:154–60.

33. Kramer S, Keamond EL, Lilienfeld AM. Patterns of incidence and trends in diagnostic classification of cerebrovascular disease in Washington County, Maryland, 1967–1971 to 1974–1976. *Am J Epidemiol* 1982;115:398–411.

34. Howard G, Toole JF, Becker C, et al. Changes in survival following stroke in five North Carolina counties observed during two different periods. *Stroke* 1989;20:345–50.

35. Ahmed OI, Orchard TJ, Sharma R, Mitchell H, Tallot E. Declining mortality from stroke in Allegheny County, Pennsylvania: trends in case fatality and severity of disease, 1971–1980. *Stroke* 1988;19:181–4.

36. McGovern PG, Burke GL, Sprafka JM, Xue S, Folsom AR, Blackburn H. Trends in mortality, morbidity, and risk factor levels for stroke from 1960 through 1990: The Minnesota Heart Survey. *JAMA* 1992;268:753–9.

37. Wolf PA, Agostino RB, O'Neal A, et al. Secular trends in stroke incidence and mortality: the Framingham Study. *Stroke* 1992;23:1551–5.

38. Modan B, Wagener DK. Some epidemiological aspects of stroke: mortality/morbidity trends, age, sex, race, socioeconomic status. *Stroke* 1992;23:1230–6.

39. Bonita R, Broad JB, Beaglehole R. Changes in stroke incidence and case-fatality in Auckland, New Zealand, 1981–1991. *Lancet* 1993;342:1470–3.

40. Shahar E, McGovern, Pankow JS, et al. Stroke rates during the 1980s. The Minnesota Stroke Survey. *Stroke* 1997;28;275–9.

41. Brown RD, Whisnant JP, Sicks JD, O'Fallon WM, Wiebers DO. Stroke incidence, prevalence, and survival. Secular trends in Rochester, Minnesota, through 1989. *Stroke* 1996;27:373–80.

42. Thorvaldsen P, Asplund K, Kuulasman K, et al. Stroke incidence, case fatality, and mortality in the WHO MONICA Project. *Stroke* 1995;26:361–7.

43. Miller RH, Luft HS. Managed care plan performance since 1980: a literature analysis. *JAMA* 1994;271:1512–19.

44. Shaugnessy P, Schlenker RE, Hittle DF. Home health care outcomes under capitated and fee-for-service payment. *Health Care Financing Rev* 1994;16:187–222.

45. Retchin SM, Brown RS, Yeh SCJ, Chu D, Moreno L. Outcomes of stroke patients in Medicare fee for service and managed care. *JAMA* 1997:278:119–24.

46. Centers for Disease Control and Prevention: US HIV and AIDS cases reported through December 1994. *HIV/AIDS Surveillance Report* 1994;6:1–39.

47. *World Health Organization: The HIV/AIDS Pandemic: 1993 Overview.* Geneva: World Health Organization, 1993:1–17.

48. Harrison MJ, McArthur JC. *AIDS and Neurology.* Churchill Livingstone, 1995.

49. Blum S, Singh TP, Gibbons J, et al. Trends in survival among persons with acquired immunodeficiency syndrome in New York City. The experience of the first decade of the epidemic. *Am J Epidemiol* 1994;139:351–61.

50. Seage GR, Oddleifson S, Carr E, et al. Survival with AIDS in Massachusetts 1979 to 1989. *Am J Public Health* 1993;83:72–8.

51. Chang HH, Morese DL, Noonan C, et al. Survival and mortality patterns of an Acquired Immunodeficiency Syndrome (AIDS) cohort in New York State. *Am J Epidemiol* 1993;138:341–9.

52. Lemp GF, Payne SF, Neal D, Temelso T, Rutherford GW. Survival trends for patients with AIDS. *JAMA* 1990;263:402–6.

53. Centers for Disease Control. Revision of the case definition of acquired immunodeficiency syndrome for national reporting – United States. *MMWR Morb Mortal Wkly Rep* 1985;34:373–5.

54. Centers for Disease Control. Revision of the CDC surveillance case definition for acquired immunodeficiency syndrome. *MMWR Morb Mortal Wkly Rep* 1987;36:3S–14S.

55. Centers for Disease Control and Prevention. 1993 revised classification system for HIV infection and expanded surveillance case definition for AIDS among adolescents and adults. *MMWR Morb Mortal Wkly Rep* 1992;41(RR-I7):1–19

56. Vella S, Chiesi A, Volpi A, et al. Differential survival of patients with AIDS according to the 1987 and 1993 CDC case definitions. *JAMA* 1994;271:1197–9.

57. Ellis RJ, Deutsch R, Heaton RK, et al. Neurocognitive impairment is an independent risk factor for death in HIV infection. *Arch Neurol* 1997;54:416–24.

58. Larsen RA, Leal MA, Chan LS. Fluconazole compared with amphotericin B plus flucytosine for cryptococcal meningitis in AIDS: a randomized trial. *Ann Intern Med* 1990;113:183–97.

59. Chuck SL, Sande MA. Infections with *Cryptococcus neoformans* in acquired immuno-deficiency syndrome. *N Engl J Med* 1989;321:794–9.

60. Saag MS, Powderly WG, Cloud GA, et al. Comparison of amphotericin B with fluconazole in the treatment of acute AIDS-associated cryptococcal meningitis. *New Engl J Med* 1992;326:83–9.

61. Porter SB, Sande MA. Toxoplasmosis of the central nervous system in acquired immuno-deficiency syndrome. *N Engl J Med* 1992;327:1643–8.

62. Moore RD, Chaisson RE. Natural history of opportunistic disease in an HIV-infected urban clinical cohort. *Ann Intern Med* 1996;124:633–42.

63. Berger JR, Kaszovitz B, Post MJD, Dickinson G. Progressive multifocal leuko-encephalopathy associated with human immunodeficiency virus infection. *Ann Intern Med* 1987;107:78–87.

64. Fong IW, Toma E and the Canadian PML Study Group. The natural history of progressive multifocal leukoencephalopathy in patients with AIDS. *Clin Infect Dis* 1995;20:1305–10.

65. Berger JR, McArthur JC. The neurological manifestations of Human Immunodeficiency

Virus infection. In Bradley WG, Daroff RB, Fenichel GM, Marsden GD (eds.) *Neurology in Clinical Practice*, 2nd Edition. Butterworth-Heinemann, 1996:1276–92.

66. Simpson DM, Tagliati M. Neurologic manifestations of HIV infection. *Ann Intern Med* 1994;121:769–85.

67. Gill PS, Levine AM, Meyer PR, et al. Primary central nervous system lymphoma in homosexual men. Clinical, immunologic, and pathologic features. *Am J Med* 1985;78:742–8.

68. Baumgartner JE, Rachlin JR, Beckstead JH, et al. Primary central nervous system lymphomas: natural history and response to radiation therapy in 55 patients with acquired immunodeficiency syndrome. *J Neurosurg* 1990;73:206–11.

69. Galetto G, Levine A. AIDS-associated primary central nervous system lymphoma. Oncology Core Committee. AIDS Clinical Trials Group. *JAMA* 1993;269:92–3.

70. Formenti SC, Gill PS, Lean E, et al. Primary central nervous system lymphoma in AIDS. Results of radiation therapy. *Cancer* 1989;63:1101–7.

71. Nisce LZ, Kaufmann T, Metroka C. Radiation therapy in patients with AIDS-related central nervous system lymphomas (Letter). *JAMA* 1992;267:1921–2.

72. Katzman R: The prevalence and malignancy of Alzheimer's disease: a major killer. *Arch Neurol* 1976;33:217.

73. Keefover RW. The clinical epidemiology of Alzheimer's disease. *Neurol Clin* 1996;14:337–52.

74. McKhann G, Drachman D, Folstein M, et al. Clinical diagnosis of Alzheimer's disease. Report of the NINCDS/ADRDA Work Group under the auspices of Department of Health and Human Services Task Force on Alzheimer's Disease. *Neurology* 1984;34:939.

75. World Health Organization. *The ICD–10 Classification of Mental and Behavioral Disorders: Diagnostic Criteria for Research (DCR–10)*. Geneva, World Health Organization, 1993.

76. American Psychiatric Association, Committee on Nomenclature and Statistics. *Diagnostic and Statistical Manual of Mental Disorders (Fourth revision) (DSM–IV)*. Washington, DC: American Psychiatric Association, 1994.

77. Hijdra A. Vascular dementia. In Bradley WG, Daroff RB, Fenichel GM, Marsden GD (eds.). *Neurology in Clinical Practice*, 2nd Edition. Butterworth-Heinemann, 1996:1602–10.

78. Hachinski VC, Illiff LD, Zilhka H, et al. Cerebral blood flow in dementia. *Arch Neurol* 1975;32:632–7.

79. Román GC, Tatemichi TK, Erkinjuntti T, et al. Vascular dementia: diagnostic criteria for research studies. Report of the NINDS-AIREN International Work Group. *Neurology* 1993;43:250–60.

80. van Dijk PTM, Dippel DWJ, Habbema JDF. Survival of patients with dementia. *JAGS* 1991;39:603–10.

81. McGonigal GM, McQuade CA, Thomas BM, Whalley LJ. Survival in presenile Alzheimer's and multi-infarct dementias. *Neuroepidemiology* 1992;11:121–6.

82. Bracco L, Gallato R, Grigoletto F, et al. Factors affecting course and survival in Alzheimer's disease. Arch Neurol 1994;51:1213–17.

83. Treves T, Korczyn Ad, Zilber N, et al. Presenile dementia in Israel. *Arch Neurol* 1986;43:26–9.

84. Kokmen E, Chandra V, Schoenberg BS. Trends in incidence of dementing illness in

Rochester, Minnesota, in three quinquennial periods, 1960–1974. *Neurology* 1988;38:975–80.

85. Hier DB, Warach JD, Gorelick PB, Thomas J. Predictors of survival in clinically diagnosed Alzheimer's disease and multi-infarct dementia. *Arch Neurol* 1989;46:1213–16.

86. Berg PC, Danzinger WL, Storandt M, et al. Predictive features in mild senile dementia of the Alzheimer type. *Neurology* 1984;34:563–9.

87. Burns A, Jacoby R, Levy R. Progression of cognitive impairment in Alzheimer's disease. *JAGS* 1991;39:39–45.

88. Ries LAG, Miller BA, Hankey BF, et al. (Eds.). *SEER Cancer Statistic Review 1973–1991: Tables and Graphs.* National Institutes of Health, Pub. 94-2789. Bethesda, National Cancer Institute, 1994.

89. Parker SL, Tong T, Bolden S, et al. *Cancer Statistics, 1997. CA: A Cancer Journal for Clinicians* 1997;47:5–27.

90. Preston-Martin S, Staples M, Farrugia H, et al. Primary tumors of the brain, cranial nerves and cranial meninges in Victoria, Australia, 1982–1990: patterns of incidence and survival. *Neuroepidemiology* 1993;12:270–9.

91. Walker MD, Green SB, Byar DP, et al. Randomised comparisons of radiotherapy and nitrosureas for the treatment of malignant glioma after surgery. *N Engl J Med* 1980;303:1323–9.

92. Green SB, Byar DP, Walker MD, et al. Comparisons of carmustine, procarbazine, and high-dose methylprednisolone as additions to surgery and radiotherapy for the treatment of malignant glioma. *Cancer Treat Rep* 1983;67:1121–32.

93. Davies E, Clarke C, Hopkins A. Malignant cerebral glioma I: survival, disability, and morbidity after radiotherapy. *BMJ* 1996;313:1507–12.

94. Commission for the Control of Epilepsy and its Consequences. *Plan for Nationwide Action on Epilepsy.* Bethesda, MD: US Dept of Health, Education, and Welfare, 1978.

95. Hauser W. Status epilepticus. Epidemiologic considerations. *Neurology* 1990;40 (suppl.2):9–13.

96. Cranford RE, Leppik IE, Patrick B, Anderson CB, Kostrick B. Intravenous phenytoin in acute treatment of seizures. *Neurology* 1979;29:1474–9.

97. Cranford RE, Leppik IE, Patrick B, Anderson CB, Kostick B. Intravenous phenytoin: clinical and pharmacokinetic aspects. *Neurology* 1978;28:874–80.

98. Payne TA, Bleck TP. Status epilepticus. *Crit Care Clin* 1997;13:17–38.

99. DeLorenzo RJ, Pellock JM, Towne AR, Boggs JG. Epidemiology of status epilepticus. *J Clin Neurophysiol* 1995;12(4):316–25.

100. Fowler K. *AIDS Survival Progress. STEP Perspect* 1997;9(1):15–16.

101. Taeuber CM, Rosenwaide I. A demographic portrait of America's oldest old. In: Suzman RM, Willis DP, Manton KG (Eds.). *The Oldest Old.* New York: Oxford University Press, 1992:17.

102. Kurtzke JF. Epidemiology of cerebrovascular disease. In: McDowell FH, Caplan LR (Eds.). *Cerebrovascular Survey Report for the National Institute of Neurological and Communicative Disorders and Stroke (Revised).* White Plains, NY: Burke Rehabilitation Center, 1985:1–34.

9

The clinical trial in efficacy research in neurological diseases

J. van Gijn and M. Vermeulen

Introduction

The introduction of the controlled clinical trial heralded the era of rational treatment. An important landmark was the UK Medical Research Council trial of streptomycin in pulmonary tuberculosis, with random assignment to treatment groups (1), but some forerunners had already used parallel control groups. Among these were James Lind in 1753 (lemons and oranges to prevent scurvy in sailors) (2), Louis in 1835 (bleeding as a treatment for pneumonia, erysipelas or throat inflammation) (3), Fibinger in 1898 (serum for diphtheria, with alternate assignment) (4), and Ferguson, Davey and Topley in 1927 (vaccines for the common cold, with blinding of patients) (5).

The main principles for design and execution of clinical trials are no different for neurology than for other disciplines. Excellent textbooks have been written to explain these even to the uninitiated(6,7). In this chapter we shall therefore not attempt to summarize and paraphrase the principles of clinical trials. Rather we wish to concentrate on a few special subjects. Our choice has been determined mostly by what we have learned through our own mistakes. We start with some issues that apply to clinical trials in general: pragmatic versus explanatory trials, role of sponsoring industries, methods of randomization, and double blind versus single blind design. The second and greatest part of the chapter is dedicated to measurement of outcome in neurology. This is a notorious minefield, perhaps especially for neurological disorders. It is not our aim to cover every field, but again we have made a selection: stroke, Parkinson's disease, multiple sclerosis, polyneuropathy, migraine, and epilepsy. The paragraph about the first subject (stroke) in this *tour d'horizon* of neurology is intertwined with a general discussion about levels at which outcome can be assessed. One of the conclusions is that measures of outcome need not always be disease-specific.

Some general issues in the design of clinical trials

Pragmatic versus explanatory trials
Different phases of clinical studies

Several phases can be distinguished in the evaluation of therapy. Phase I trials are studies in which the safety of treatment is investigated in healthy subjects. In these studies toxic effects that were not apparent from laboratory studies may be detected. Phase I studies often investigate what the safe dose range is. These studies are usually carried out in a few volunteers and belong to the field of clinical pharmacology. Phase II studies are carried out in volunteers or in patients. Some regard the assessment of the optimal dosage in large series of volunteers as phase II studies. Others classify all studies in volunteers as phase I and restrict the classification phase II to studies in patients. The aim of phase II studies is to investigate the likely efficacy of the treatment under scrutiny and to determine the optimal dosage and method of administration via pharmacological indices. Phase III studies are clinical studies in which the effectiveness suggested by phase II studies is put to the test. Phase IV studies are planned postmarketing studies that aim to detect side-effects that occur late, or changes of effectiveness over time.

Another classification

Schwartz, Flamant, and Lellouch described another classification (8). They distinguished explanatory from pragmatic studies. Explanatory studies were considered to be direct extensions of laboratory experimentation. Therefore, research methods have to be controlled with similar rigidity as in the laboratory. For explanatory studies patients are selected in whom the diagnosis has been established with the highest level of certainty, for example a biopsy-proven diagnosis. The route of drug administration is dictated by the highest biological effect, such as intravenous administration, to be certain that high and constant serum levels are reached. Assessment of the effects of treatment are as close as possible to the pathological process, which means repeated biopsies or measurements of biochemical indices. These explanatory studies aim at a better understanding of the effects of treatment at the level of pathology or pathophysiology. In other words, these studies investigate whether the treatment works (in a biological sense). Explanatory studies have more in common with phase II than with phase III studies.

Pragmatic studies are different. These aim to investigate whether patients benefit from treatment. For these studies patients may be selected in whom the diagnosis is suspected, rather than certain. If in practice a biopsy is not carried out to confirm the diagnosis in question, then biopsies are not a requisite for inclusion. If intravenous treatment is not practical because treatment is considered in outpatients, then the effects of oral treatment will be investigated – even when it is known that intravenous treatment results in more reliable serum levels. Assessment of the treatment effects in pragmatic studies is as close as possible to what is relevant for patients. If a treatment is supposed to increase the peripheral blood flow in the legs it is not this flow that is measured but the change in distance the patient is able to walk. Pragmatic studies are similar to phase III studies.

For the design of a study it is of paramount importance first to decide whether an explanatory study or a pragmatic study should be carried out. For the reader of a report of a trial it is also important to distinguish the two types of studies because only pragmatic studies should influence the choice of treatment in practice. Explanatory studies are not always easy to recognize. For instance, patients with subarachnoid hemorrhage are threatened by recurrent hemorrhage. If a treatment aims at the prevention of these recurrent hemorrhages and the effects of treatment on the rate of recurrent hemorrhage is counted, the design of the study is more explanatory than pragmatic. After all, for the patient the relevant question is not whether recurrent hemorrhage occurs but whether or not he or she is better off with treatment, in terms of final outcome. One may argue that the final outcome will improve when recurrent hemorrhages are prevented but this is only the case if recurrent hemorrhages have direct influence on the final outcome and if the treatment has no other effects. In the example of subarachnoid hemorrhage it was shown that treatment did significantly reduce the recurrent hemorrhage rate but that another complication after this type of hemorrhage increased in occurrence to such an extent that overall morbidity and mortality were not different between groups (9). In other words, the treatment worked (explanatory point of view) but did not help (pragmatic point of view).

The assessment of treatment effects should start with explanatory studies. In these studies highly selected groups of patients will be compared. Outcome will be assessed with the most sensitive measures available. If these studies are unable to detect any treatment effect there is no need for large-scale studies with a pragmatic design. If there is a biological effect, pragmatic studies should investigate what the effect of treatment is on the functional status of patients. This means that in explanatory studies measurements will be carried out at the level of the disease process or the organ, but in pragmatic studies at the level of the individual. We shall see that this last requirement is unfulfilled in many fields of neurology.

Role of sponsoring industries

Though sponsors derive certain rights from their investments this does not include the right to exclude clinicians from core activities that should guarantee the quality and credibility of the trial. Not only drawing up the protocol but also storage of the data, planning of interim analyses, and prior definition of subgroups are grave responsibilities that should be shared between sponsor and participants. This shared responsibility should be reflected in the creation of a single steering committee as the highest authority of the study, a body in which all parties are represented. The selection of clinicians in the steering committee should be made by the participants, and not by the sponsoring company. In this day and age it is unacceptable for trial participants to be confronted by changes in the protocol or interim analyses which have been initiated almost entirely by the industry in question, without involvement of an independent steering committee in which the participating physicians are represented. It is not sufficient if the industry appoints one or two clinicians only to keep up appearances, while the operation of the trial remains hidden from the participants to such an extent that great damage is done to the reputation of the trial as well as of the physicians in the masthead.

Trial forms should be sent for checking and inclusion in the database not to the sponsoring company, but to an independent office, run under the direction of one of the clinical participants or of an epidemiologist – provided the people involved have a good track record in independent research. It has been rightly argued that the group responsible for data collection and analysis should be financially independent from the results of the trial (10). If the result of a trial is disappointing, investigators and especially sponsoring industries may be tempted to bury the entire project in a drawer and try to forget about it. It hardly needs emphasis that it is mandatory to report the results or to make them available to meta-analysts.

Participation in sponsored trials may be extremely profitable. Ideally the choice of clinicians about which clinical trials they wish to join should not be influenced by pecuniary motives (11). These decisions should have to do with how burning the issue under investigation is, from the perspective of health care, science, or both.

Methods of randomization

Many methods of randomization exist but it is generally accepted that the use of random number tables is the ideal method. In general it is wise to avoid methods related to characteristics of the study subjects, such as surname or place of recruitment. The reason is that imbalances between the groups may occur, for example when through selection by first letter of surnames some families, with certain genetic factors, dominate in one of the groups. The distribution between the arms of the trial should be truly random for each individual, since this is the best guarantee that prognostic factors are similarly distributed between the groups. The argument that it is possible to check in the phase of the analysis whether the distribution is similar is not quite valid, since this implies that we know and can check for all the prognostic factors. For similar reasons it is not recommended to correct for imbalances of known prognostic factors between the groups since unknown factors may also have influenced the results.

It is also important that randomization is concealed. In the past, trial reports have not always been clear about the method of randomization. If allocation of treatment is random but open, clinicians will know what the treatment is in the next patient. If for example a trial compares aspirin with an anticoagulant, a clinician may decide not to include the next eligible patient, who happens to be old, when the next treatment is the anticoagulant. In articles on clinical studies, information on whether or not random allocation was used is always given but not the method of randomization (12,13). In a meta-analysis from the Cochrane Pregnancy and Childbirth Database, trials in which concealment was either inadequate or unclear (did not report or incompletely reported a concealment approach) yielded significantly larger estimates of treatment effects than trials in which authors reported adequately concealed treatment allocation (14). The results of comparisons of treatment without concealed randomization should therefore not be trusted.

Even if allocation is concealed and random number tables are used the method may be suboptimal. This is the case when informed consent is asked after randomization. Some clinicians prefer to inform the patient of the trial when randomization to one of the treatment arms has already been carried out. The patient is informed about the trial and immediately the patient is told to what treatment he has been randomized. Although the treatment allocation was concealed this procedure may cause imbalances between the groups by refusal of the patients. Such refusal may be induced by the clinician, when the side-effects of treatment to which the patient was randomized are overemphasized. If for example an aged patient is randomized to an anticoagulant the clinician may deliberately or perhaps inadvertently stress the side-effects of this treatment when informing the patient.

Double-blind versus single-blind design

The advent of randomized, controlled, double-blind trials constitutes one of the great advances of medicine in the 20th century. So much has this notion been impressed on every physician from his student days onwards, that some regard any departure from this sanctified principle as detestable heresy. Indeed the process of randomization itself should be rigorously adhered to, in that adequate concealment excludes any influence of the participating trialist (14). But the double-blind approach is practicable only when the treatment arms in the trial are of a similar nature. In some cases the use of placebos can be impracticable or even unethical. In fact the archetype of clinical trials, the UK Medical Research Council Trial of streptomycin for the treatment of pulmonary tuberculosis in 1948 was only partially blinded, as the need for four intramuscular injections daily for 4 months precluded the use of a placebo (1). Hill defended the design (blinded evaluation of X-rays) with the comment that "in a controlled trial, as in all experimental work, there is no need in the search for precision to throw common sense out of the window" (15). Similarly, trials of cytotoxic drugs in patients with cancer are seldom double-blind; the complicated dose schedules, the frequency of unpleasant and serious side-effects and subsequent dose modifications make it necessary for the attending physician to know a patient's therapy (6). Another example is a trial of surgery versus no surgery: in the two epoch-making trials of carotid endarterectomy only the outcome assessment was blinded (16,17).

Even when two medical treatments are compared a double-blind design is not necessarily the best. For example, if the efficacy of oral anticoagulants in the prevention of stroke is compared with the standard regimen of aspirin, double-blinding would imply the use of double dummies, all patients would have to visit an anticoagulation clinic, and co-medication would in all patients have to be adapted to concurrent use of anticoagulants. In that situation the study addresses the pharmacological question of whether tablets containing anticoagulants or those with aspirin are better in the prevention of stroke and other important vascular events. Practicing physicians, however, will wish to compare strategies rather than tablets and will not choose to contaminate aspirin prophylaxis with the hassle of anticoagulation (18). In brief, when the measure of outcome is reasonably objective and can be made completely independent from the study subject and the trialist, blinding of either is not crucial (19).

Measurement of outcome in neurological disorders

However well designed and ethically well thought-out, any result obtained in clinical research needs to be considered from the perspective of future patients. Accordingly, the effect of the proposed intervention should be relevant to patients. How then should effect be measured? What outcome is relevant and from which or whose perspective? Below we shall elaborate on different levels of measurement (Table 9.1) and on some specific instruments, in relation to a few important categories of neurological disease. Stroke is our first example, for which category of diseases we shall explain the levels of measurement in more detail.

Levels of measurement: the example of stroke
The disease process

This level of measurement reflects the function of molecules, cells, or organs. For ischemic stroke the severity of disease might be conveniently expressed at this level by the volume of infarcted tissue on computed tomography or magnetic resonance imaging. The limitations of this measure are immediately evident by the

Table 9.1. Levels of assessment of outcome

I. The disease process (occurrence of biological events)
II. Impairments (performance at the level of the organ)
III. Disability (performance at the level of the person)
IV. Handicap (performance at individual and social level)
V. Quality of life (subjective well-being)

contrast between a patient with a small infarct in the midbrain who is comatose and a patient who has a large infarct in a cerebellar hemisphere but little or no disability. Correlation between the size of the lesion and the severity of neurological deficits is better within a cerebral hemisphere (20). For example, outcome after so-called lacunar infarcts is generally better than after large cortical infarcts. Yet there are frequent exceptions on both sides, by the intricate balance between functional differentiation and the capacities for compensation of less localized (cognitive) functions. This makes it often impossible to predict confidently from a scan how the patient is doing.

Impairments

The next step in the spectrum of outcome measures is the effect the condition has on patients. Scales have been designed for measuring tremor, aphasia, muscle power, intellectual performance, and many other specific functions that can be disturbed by disease. Doctors are often attracted to this kind of measurement, because the grades of these scales seem to lend some kind of objectivity to clinical impressions. In an attempt to overcome the limitations of measuring only a single function, many groups of researchers have developed composite scales, in which many different impairments have been incorporated. Such composite scales exist not only for stroke but for many other specific conditions. The neurologists who have designed or used these scales assume that the sum of all the separate elements in the scale will add up to a meaningful picture of the patient as a whole. Regrettably, this assumption is incorrect.

The first problem with disease-specific scales is the choice of the separate elements. Many scales ignore important aspects. For instance, stroke scales mostly reflect the conventional neurological examination and take no account of depression or cognitive defects such as impaired concentration or loss of initiative, whereas these symptoms may be very distressing. On the other hand, disease scales often include elements of the neurologic examination that are quite useful for localizing a lesion in the nervous system but that are completely irrelevant from the patient's point of view, such as Babinski signs, muscle rigidity, or fasciculations.

The most serious deficiency of composite scales for specific diseases is that the scores for separate functions can never add up to something meaningful (21). Weighting of different items is a futile attempt to solve this problem, because overall performance results from a complex interaction between different "functions." Not the least of this is intellectual function, which is grossly neglected in many scales of neurological disease, whereas motor aspects are overrated. Everyday life consists of a multitude of tasks that are integrated and difficult to separate.

Measuring impairment can be useful in the early stages of research, when the question is whether a particular mode of treatment has some biological effect at all (8). For instance, if some imaginary new drug might favorably influence the muscle defect in Duchenne muscular dystrophy, it is reasonable to start by studying the effects on the power of one particular muscle. But when the question is whether the drug should be given to all patients with the disease the measure of outcome should include disability. In short, the patient is more than the sum of his signs (21). A higher, more integrated level of measurement is needed, that is, scales should measure function not at the level of the organ (impairments) but at the level of the person (disability scales).

Many favor outcome measures at the level of impairments, or even at that of the disease process. These are of little relevance to the patient but may impress the unwary because they are "objective," can be quantified, and often lend themselves to statistical massage from which some significant advantage can be made to emerge. In the past, drugs have been licensed merely on the basis of such dubious benefits. Most licensing bodies now firmly and sensibly take the position that new drugs for neurological diseases are allowed only if an effect on at least disability has been demonstrated.

Disability

According to the international classification of the World Health Organization (22), disability represents function at the level of the person; it is "the restriction or lack (resulting from an impairment) of the ability to perform tasks, within the physical and social environment." A great advantage of disability scales is that these integrate not only different impairments but also different diseases; it is often thought that this generalizability is at the cost of sensitivity, but with a sufficient number of patients a simple scale with a few meaningful categories may suffice for picking up effects of interventions.

Most disability scales measure essential tasks in activities of daily living (ADL), such as toilet use, walking, dressing, and managing stairs. The large number of existing ADL scales testifies that this level of measurement has its own difficulties. The Barthel index is the most widely used in stroke patients, and it has proved reliable on repeated testing (23–25). The scale is hierarchical, in the sense that an

Table 9.2. Oxford Handicap Scale (32)

Grade	Description (abridged)
0	No symptoms
1	Only symptoms
2	Some restriction of lifestyle, but independent
3	Partly dependent
4	Dependent, but no constant attention required
5	Fully dependent

ascending order of difficulty can be attributed to the activities listed, from bowel continence to taking a bath (26). Cultural differences may interfere with this fixed order. For instance, bathing is relatively easy in the United States, because this means taking a shower rather than immersing oneself into a tub from the neck down, and in Japan feeding oneself is the easiest activity instead of being moderately difficult, because this involves picking up pieces of meat without the necessity of cutting it (27).

Yet there is more to life than getting into the bath on one's own. Also ADL scales measure only what patients can do, and not what they actually do do when left to care for themselves. The true degree of independence is more accurately reflected by scales that do not specify separate tasks, such as the Rankin scale (28), the Glasgow Outcome Scale (29), and the Karnofsky Index (30). Some have called this type of scale performance scales, as opposed to capacity scales (31). In its original form the Rankin scale contained the term "walking" and was therefore something of a hybrid with ADL scales, but this has been remedied in a recent modification named the Oxford Handicap Scale (Table 9.2) (32).

Although some of the elements of the Oxford Handicap Scale indeed refer to social roles ("lifestyle") or even to quality of life (symptoms without impairment or disability), the emphasis is on (in)dependence and the scale should perhaps more appropriately be classified among the measures of disability (33). Some other performance scales also overlap with the measurement of handicap because they refer to work (Karnofsky Index) or to other social interactions (Frenchay Activities Index (34,35)). The Glasgow Outcome Scale is more exclusively concerned with (in)dependence (29), and is reasonably reliable (36). A great advantage of performance scales in multicentre trials is that these can be applied without the patient being examined or even seen; interviews by telephone proved satisfactory in one study (37), and probably even postal questionnaires can be used.

Handicap and "quality of life"

Whereas impairment and disability can be assessed more or less objectively, measuring handicap addresses the social consequences of impairment and disability, in the domains of, for instance, relationships, occupation and economic independence, and leisure activities (22). On the whole, the measurement of handicap has been less well conceptualized and tested than that of impairments or disabilities.

The most comprehensive and at the same time most subjective measure of outcome is quality of life. It refers to a person's sense of well-being and life satisfaction, and includes all physical, social, and emotional domains of life. At this level of measurement it is the patient and no longer the doctor who determines to what extent the disease interferes with the desired lifestyle. Oncologists have been leading this field of research, because they are continuously confronted by the question of at what cost prolongation of life should be obtained (38). Quality of life depends on many more factors than outcome measured at lower levels of integration. It is therefore possible that people without disability report a worse quality of life than people with disability. In fact correlations with quality of life become increasingly worse as measurement moves from "handicap" (modified Rankin scale) to disability (Barthel scale), and from disability to impairments ("stroke scales") (39). Quality of life can be measured by a variety of instruments, depending on the research question (40). Extensive questionnaires are the Sickness Impact Profile and the Nottingham Health Profile (41,42), yet these are feasible in stroke patients (43). At the other end is something as simple as a visual analogue scale (44). The Health Utility Index and the EuroQol questionnaire are examples of instruments designed to provide a single numerical index of outcome (45,46).

Multiple sclerosis

The number and extent of lesions on MRI scanning has been used as a surrogate measure for the efficacy of medical interventions. Such lesions appear with greater frequency than clinical relapses (47,48). An effect of treatment shown at the level of the disease process informs us that the intervention has a biological effect ("works") but not that patients benefit from this treatment. In cross-sectional studies the correlation between lesion load (T2 weighted) and disability (usually the EDSS scale – see below) was found weak at best (49,50), or even nonexistent (51). Longitudinal studies showed a good correlation between the two when the study group consisted of patients with isolated clinical syndromes suggestive of multiple sclerosis (MS) (52,53), but the relation was much more inconspicuous for patients with definite MS (50,54). The explanation for the disparity is two-fold. One reason is that T2-weighted images cannot reliably identify demyelination and axonal loss within plaques, whereas these two processes are largely responsible for clinical manifestations of disease (55). The other is that spinal cord lesions are not accounted for, despite the large contribution of such lesions to the patient's functional health status (56). Special MRI techniques can perhaps improve the specificity of abnormalities (57); these include measurement of N-acetyl-aspartate levels on proton MR spectroscopy, enhancement with gadolinium (58), and determination of magnetization transfer ratio (59).

The most well-known and widely used *clinical measure* for measuring outcome in clinical trials of patients with MS is the Kurtzke Extended Disability Scale (EDSS) (60). Unfortunately, this instrument has severe imperfections (61–63). Firstly its design reflects impairment rather than disability, with heavy weighting towards ambulation. Therefore the scale is insensitive to symptoms such as fatigue (64,65), and also to changes in mood and in interaction with relatives or other persons (65). Secondly in its practical application the interrater variability is often as high as 1.0 to 1.5 steps out of the 0–10 steps available (66,67). Therefore many neurologists question the wisdom of the speed with which health authorities in some countries have ratified the introduction of interferon-β–1a for the treatment of relapsing MS (68,69), a decision based on only a single clinical trial that used the EDSS and demonstrated a marginal slowing of progression (70). Finally, the progression of disability across the scale is nonlinear. Especially in the middle range the separation between grades is narrow. It is disturbing that major journals continue to publish trial reports where the EDSS is statistically treated as an interval scale, as for inches or miles (71). Special (nonparametric) statistical methods can be used for comparison between groups, but in studies where the outcome event is defined as progression of one step on the EDSS (70), the problem remains that one step is different from another.

A recently developed alternative for the EDSS is the Cambridge Multiple Sclerosis Basic Score (CAMBS) (72). It considers four aspects of the illness as it affects the patient. The first part consists of an overall appraisal of clinical symptoms and disability, the second measures current remission/relapse status, the third describes progression over the year before assessment, and the fourth component addresses handicap. The parts for disability, relapse, and handicap consist of a simple score between 1 and 5, and they can be completed by patient or carer without the need for physical examination or even attending a clinic. The scale is promising but so far it has undergone limited validation. The same applies to a recently published measure for the quality of life in patients with MS (73).

Parkinson's disease

Parkinson's disease is a slowly progressive degenerative disorder resulting in slowness of movement, rigidity, tremor, and abnormalities of posture. In addition, cognitive disorders may develop such as poor memory, impaired visuospatial function and slow mentation. Initially there is a good response to treatment with levodopa but after approximately 5 years of treatment response fluctuations may occur. These fluctuations make the assessment of the functional status even more difficult. The assessment scales most often used in clinical studies will be discussed in historical order.

The Schwab and England scale

This scale, first used in the 1950s but not formally described until 1969, scores the patient's ability over the preceding week on the basis of information obtained from the patient and relatives (74). It has 11 steps and ranges from completely independent (100%) to bedridden, while swallowing, bladder, and bowels are not functioning (0%). Each step of increasing dependency is 10% lower, suggesting that the differences between the steps are equal but this is very unlikely. The problem with this scale is that the choice between the description of the different grades is often difficult. An advantage is that this scale does not mix different entities like impairment and disability, which is common in scales that have been recommended later.

North Western University Disability Scales

In 1961 Canter and colleagues described a method for the evaluation of disability in Parkinson's disease (75). The authors had recognized already the problem of many other scales, which is apparent from their conclusion that the major disadvantage of the scale developed by Fairman and Schwab was its pooling of performance items (e.g., locomotion) and primary manifestations (e.g., rigidity) into a single percentage score. This criticism has been forgotten, since in 1992 a group of experts recommended to use the Unified Parkinson's disease rating scale which is a typical example of a similarly mixed scale (76). The North Western Disability Scales have been criticized for not being specific for Parkinson's disease. Moreover, although the scale had good reliability in the original study it was felt this could not be sustained (77).

Hoehn and Yahr grades

This scale gives information on the severity of the disease and distinguishes only a few broad categories (78). This kind of scale can probably not be used in studies aiming to investigate the effectiveness of treatment. The scale has often been used for detecting differences between groups of patients at the beginning of a study in which treatments are compared.

Webster Rating Scale

This is a typical example of a scale in which different issues as impairment and disability have been mixed (79). This scale includes for instance rigidity but also self-care.

Unified Parkinson's Disease Rating Scale (UPDRS)

This scale is widely recommended (76). It is hardly possible to publish the results of a study on the effectiveness of treatment in patients with Parkinson's disease and not having used the UPDRS. Despite having been rather recently developed, this scale has many disadvantages in comparison with earlier developed scales. First of all the scale is extremely complex. In addition to the Hoehn and Yahr staging and the Schwab and England scale which are both included, 42 other items have to be tested. These include vivid dreaming, salivation, freezing when walking, numbness, facial expression, and gait. The experts should be persuaded that the UPDRS must be replaced by a true, integrated disability scale which is also reliable and valid.

Which scale in Parkinson's disease?

The review of the scales used in Parkinson's disease shows that in the field of movement disorders there is little awareness that scales should measure either impairment or disability and that the choice of these scales depends on the type of question that has to be answered. Outcome measures in an explanatory study will be different from those in pragmatic studies. There is a need for a reliable disability scale applicable in Parkinson's disease. These scales are not only necessary for clinical trials but also for the evaluation of treatment in practice. Apart from the measurement of impairment, disability, or handicap, quality of life measures may be informative about the impact the disease has on the patient. A generic health status measure showed that the disease has considerable impact on general levels of functioning and well-being, but areas not contained in the generic measures were also found to be relevant in this group of patients (80). Therefore more disease-specific measures give better information on the impact of Parkinson's disease (81).

Polyneuropathy

Disorders of peripheral nerves cause weakness, sensory disturbances, or both. Symptoms in these patients may range from purely motor to purely sensory and from slight numbness and weakness in the feet to complete loss of muscle strength including respiratory muscles, as for instance in Guillain–Barré syndrome. Molenaar and colleagues stressed that the choice of outcome measures should not depend on whether the neuropathy is predominantly sensory or motor but should be dictated by the aim of the study (82). Outcome measures in explanatory studies should measure organ dysfunctions, for instance by electrophysiological techniques, by measures that detect changes in muscle strength, or in the perception of vibration or thermal stimuli. These are measurements at the level of impairment. In pragmatic studies the patient's functional performance should be measured, usually at the level of disability. From a review of the medical literature between 1978 and 1993 it was evident that the choice of outcome measures in patients with peripheral neuropathy often was not appropriate (82). In several studies impairment measures were used but the conclusion was not limited in that the results only showed that treatment had a beneficial effect on peripheral nerve function. The authors usually concluded that the treatment had a beneficial effect on the patient and therefore this treatment was recommended without evidence from a pragmatic study.

In the published recommendations of an authoritative consensus meeting on standards in diabetic neuropathy the differences between impairment and disability remained unnoticed (83). Instead, emphasis was put on sensitivity and objectivity of measurements. The authors stressed that because of the relative subjectivity and imprecision of the clinical measures confirmation by so-called objective measures was required, such as electrodiagnostic tests, quantitative tests of sensory and autonomic function, or morphometric tests. Objectivity is undoubtedly important but for clinical studies on which treatment recommendations have to be based scales reflecting the functional status of patients are far more important, provided the reliability and validity of these scales have been tested and found acceptable. The notion of functional measures was not considered in the recommendations of the consensus meeting (83). At first sight it may appear as if a measure of functional health was considered since a neurologic disability scale was recommended but this scale is in fact not a disability scale but a composite of cranial nerve function, reflexes, muscle strength, and sensory disturbances.

The review of outcome measures in clinical trials in patients with peripheral neuropathies showed that disability or handicap measures were used in only two of 54 studies in patients with diabetic neuropathy, in two of six studies in patients with chronic inflammatory demyelinating polyneuropathy, and in none of five studies in a mixed group of patients. In contrast, in all eight studies in patients with Guillain–Barré syndrome, disability scales were used (82). This is difficult to understand since there are no valid reasons why measurements in the chronic phase of Guillain–Barré syndrome should be different. We conclude that in the field of peripheral neuropathy much more attention should be paid to a proper choice of outcome measures.

Epilepsy

Traditionally, outcome in patients with epilepsy has been measured in terms of the frequency of seizures. This custom applies to individual patient care as well as to studies about medical treatment (84), surgical treatment (85), and epidemiological surveys (86). The severity of seizures and adverse effects of antiepileptic drugs are often also recorded, but such yardsticks are difficult to integrate. Attempts have been made to create a composite index of impairments (87), but weighting the different problems remains difficult. Another disadvantage is that such scales typically reflect the physicians' point of view, which is not necessarily the same as the patients'. Severely handicapped people may adapt to their situation and do not pity themselves as much as others do (88); conversely many neurologists view a monthly frequency of complex partial seizures and mild side-effects of drugs as "acceptable," whereas for themselves or their colleagues they would regard such symptoms as "unacceptable," given the risk of a seizure during a procedure or medical staff meeting, the inability to drive, and the impaired concentration by the drugs (89). Epilepsy may negatively affect the fulfilment of a patient's chosen way of life in many different ways: anticipation and fear of seizures, their perception of the reaction of other people, the need to take drugs regularly, often in the presence of others, behavioral and cognitive problems caused by the disorder itself or by antiepileptic drugs, and sometimes co-existent impairments associated with an underlying brain disorder.

The ultimate goal in the management of epilepsy is to improve functioning and well-being, through a reduction of seizure frequency, seizure severity, and side-effects from antiepileptic drugs. Therefore integrated measures of health-related quality of life are most suited for assessing the success of any type of intervention (90). Several such measures have been developed and proved reliable and valid in patients with epilepsy (91–94). For children a similar instrument has been devised, which takes account of the special aspirations in childhood and the relatively great impact on the family (95). A comparative study of different outcome measures was carried out for patients who underwent surgery to control their epilepsy (90). Previously published, seizure-specific measures markedly varied in relation to the external standard of health-related quality of life. For example, the quality of life of seizure-free patients was considerably better than that of patients having only auras, whereas the latter category of patients is often classified as "seizure-free." Similarly, simple partial seizures may be more distressing than complex partial seizures as patients are conscious of the unpleasant effects (89).

We do not plead that counting seizures should be abandoned, but the impact of epilepsy and its treatment on patients' lives differs so widely, depending on the professional background and the social structure in general, that research on any type of intervention in epilepsy should include measurement of the quality of life.

Migraine

Migraine, or attacks of headache in general, is another example of a paroxysmal disorder that has a far wider impact on patients' lives than can be expressed by the number of attacks. Often studies about the management of migraine attacks are even more narrowly focused than those in epilepsy research, in that the objective is limited to the treatment of single episodes (96–99), or of the one that follows the next day (100). Only when prophylactic drugs are the subject of study does the time frame become a bit wider, but such "migraine diaries" seldom exceed a few weeks (101,102). The most blatant defect in both types of studies is the total disregard for the disruptive effect of migraine attacks on the patient's life in the long term.

REFERENCES

1. Medical Research Council. Streptomycin treatment of pulmonary tuberculosis. *BMJ* 1948;ii:769–82.
2. Lind J. *A Treatise of the Scurvy.* Edinburgh: Sands, Murray & Cochran, 1753.
3. Louis PCA. *Recherches sur les Effets de la Saignée.* Paris: de Mignaret,1835.
4. Fibinger J. Om serumbehandlung af difteri. *Hospitalstidende* 1898;6:309–25, 338–50.
5. Ferguson FR, Davey AFC, Topley WWC. The value of mixed vaccines in the prevention of the common cold. *J Hyg* 1927;26:98–109.
6. Pocock SJ. *Clinical Trials – A Practical Approach.* Chichester: John Wiley, 1983.
7. Sackett DL, Haynes RB, Guyatt GH, et al. *Clinical Epidemiology – A Basic Science for Clinical Medicine.* 2nd edition. Boston: Little, Brown and Company, 1991.
8. Schwartz D, Lellouch J. Explanatory and pragmatic attitudes in therapeutic trials. *J Chronic Dis* 1967;20:637–48.
9. Vermeulen M, Lindsay KW, Murray GD, et al. Antifibrinolytic treatment in subarachnoid hemorrhage. *N Engl J Med* 1984;311:432–7.
10. Bogousslavsky J. Acute stroke trials: from Morass to Nirvana? *Cerebrovasc Dis* 1995;5:3–6.
11. Fergus M, Stephens R. Marketing clinical trials. *Lancet* 1996;348:111–12.
12. Altman DG, Dore CJ. Randomisation and baseline comparisons in clinical trials. *Lancet* 1990;335:149–53.
13. Schulz KF, Chalmers I, Grimes DA, Altman DG. Assessing the quality of randomization from reports of controlled trials published in obstetrics and gynecology journals. *JAMA* 1994;272:125–8.
14. Schulz KF, Chalmers I, Hayes RJ, Altman DG. Empirical evidence of bias. Dimensions of methodological quality associated with estimates of treatment effects in controlled trials. *JAMA* 1995;273:408–12.
15. Hill AB. Medical ethics and controlled trials. *BMJ* 1963;i:1043–9.
16. European Carotid Surgery Trialists' Collaborative Group. MRC European Carotid Surgery Trial: interim results for symptomatic patients with severe (70–99%) or with mild (0–29%) carotid stenosis. *Lancet* 1991;337:1235–43.

17. North American Symptomatic Carotid Endarterectomy Trial Collaborators. Beneficial effect of carotid endarterectomy in symptomatic patients with high-grade carotid stenosis. *N Engl J Med* 1991;325:445–53.

18. Algra A, van Gijn J. Science unblinded [letter]. *Lancet* 1994;343:1040.

19. Anonymous. Blinded by science. Lancet 1994;343:553–4.

20. Miller LS, Miyamoto AT. Computed tomography: its potential as a predictor of functional recovery following stroke. *Arch Phys Med Rehabil* 1979;60:108–9.

21. van Gijn J, Warlow CP. Down with stroke scales! Cerebrovasc Dis 1992;2:244–6.

22. World Health Organization. *International Classification of Impairments, Disabilities, and Handicaps.* Geneva: WHO, 1980.

23. Granger CV, Dewis LS, Peters NC, Sherwood CC, Barrett JE. Stroke rehabilitation: analysis of repeated Barthel index measures. *Arch Phys Med Rehabil* 1979;60:14–17.

24. Collin C, Wade DT, Davies S, Horne V. The Barthel ADL Index: a reliability study. *Int Disabil Stud* 1988;10:61–3.

25. de Haan R, Limburg M, Schuling J, Broeshart J, Jonkers L, van Zuylen P. [Clinimetric evaluation of the Barthel Index, a measure of limitations in daily activities] Klinimetrische evaluatie van de Barthel-index, een maat voor beperkingen in het dagelijks functioneren. *Ned Tijdschr Geneeskd* 1993;137:917–21.

26. Wade DT, Hewer RL. Functional abilities after stroke: measurement, natural history and prognosis. *J Neurol Neurosurg Psychiatry* 1987;50:177–82.

27. Chino N. Efficacy of Barthel index in evaluating activities of daily living in Japan, the United States, and United Kingdom. *Stroke* 1990;21:II64–5.

28. van Swieten JC, Koudstaal PJ, Visser MC, Schouten HJ, van Gijn J. Interobserver agreement for the assessment of handicap in stroke patients. *Stroke* 1988;19:604–7.

29. Jennett B, Bond M. Assessment of outcome after severe brain damage: a practical scale. *Lancet* 1975;i:480–4.

30. Karnofsky DA, Burchenal JH. The clinical evaluation of chemotherapeutic agents in cancer. In: Macleod CM, (ed.) *Evaluation of Chemotherapeutic Agents.* New York: Columbia University Press, 1949:191–205.

31. Task force on stroke impairment, and task force on stroke handicap. Symposium recommendations for methodology in stroke outcome research. *Stroke* 1990;21(suppl.2):68–73.

32. Bamford JM, Sandercock PA, Warlow CP, Slattery J. Interobserver agreement for the assessment of handicap in stroke patients [letter]. *Stroke* 1989;20:828.

33. de Haan R, Limburg M, Bossuyt P, Van der Meulen J, Aaronson N. The clinical meaning of Rankin 'handicap' grades after stroke. *Stroke* 1995;26:2027–30.

34. Holbrook M, Skilbeck CE. An activities index for use with stroke patients. *Age Ageing* 1983;12:166–70.

35. Schuling J, de Haan R, Limburg M, Groenier KH. The Frenchay Activities Index. Assessment of functional status in stroke patients. *Stroke* 1993;24:1173–7.

36. Maas AI, Braakman R, Schouten HJ, Minderhoud JM, van Zomeren AH. Agreement between physicians on assessment of outcome following severe head injury. *J Neurosurg* 1983;58:321–5.

37. Italian Acute Stroke Study Group. Haemodilution in acute stroke: results of the Italian haemodilution trial. *Lancet* 1988;i:318–21.

38. Spitzer WO. State of science 1986: quality of life and functional status as target variables for research. *J Chronic Dis* 1987;40:465–71.

39. de Haan R, Horn J, Limburg M, Van der Meulen JHP, Bossuyt P. A comparison of five stroke scales with measures of disability, handicap, and quality of life. *Stroke* 1993;24:1178–81.

40. de Haan R, Aaronson N, Limburg M, Hewer RL, van Crevel H. Measuring quality of life in stroke. *Stroke* 1993;24:320–7.

41. Bergner M, Bobbitt RA, Carter WB, Gilson BS. The Sickness Impact Profile: development and final revision of a health status measure. *Med Care* 1981;19:787–805.

42. Hunt SM, McKenna SP, McEwen J, Backett EM, Williams J, Papp E. A quantitative approach to perceived health status: a validation study. *J Epidemiol Community Health* 1980;34:281–6.

43. Visser MC, Koudstaal PJ, Erdman RA, Deckers JW, Passchier J, van Gijn J, et al. Measuring quality of life in patients with myocardial infarction or stroke: a feasibility study of four questionnaires in The Netherlands. *J Epidemiol Community Health* 1995;49:513–7.

44. Ahlsio B, Britton M, Murray V, Theorell T. Disablement and quality of life after stroke. *Stroke* 1984;15:886–90.

45. Torrance GW. The measurement of health state utilities for economic appraisal. *J Health Econ* 1986;5:1–30.

46. EuroQuol Group. Euroquol – a new facility for the measurement of health-related quality of life. *Health Policy* 1990;16:199–208.

47. Paty DW, Li DK, Oger JJ, et al. Magnetic resonance imaging in the evaluation of clinical trials in multiple sclerosis. *Ann Neurol* 1994;36 suppl:S95–96.

48. Paty DW, Li DK, the UBC MS/MRI Study Group, and the IFNB Multiple Sclerosis Study Group. Interferon beta–1b is effective in relapsing-remitting multiple sclerosis. ii. MRI analysis results of a multicenter, randomized, double-blind, placebo-controlled trial. *Neurology* 1993;43:662–7.

49. van Walderveen MA, Barkhof F, Hommes OR, Polman CH, Tobi H, Frequin ST, et al. Correlating MRI and clinical disease activity in multiple sclerosis: relevance of hypo-intense lesions on short-TR/short-TE (T1-weighted) spin-echo images. *Neurology* 1995;45:1684–90.

50. The INFB Multiple Sclerosis Study Group, and the University of British Columbia MS/MRI Analysis Group. Interferon-β-1b in the treatment of multiple sclerosis: final outcome of the randomized controlled trial. *Neurology* 1995;45:1277–85.

51. Thompson AJ, Kermode AG, MacManus DG, et al. Patterns of disease activity in multiple sclerosis: clinical and magnetic resonance imaging study. *BMJ* 1990;300:631–4.

52. Filippi M, Horsfield MA, Morrissey SP, et al. Quantitative brain MRI lesion load predicts the course of clinically isolated syndromes suggestive of multiple sclerosis. *Neurology* 1994;44:635–41.

53. Morrissey SP, Miller DH, Kendall BE, et al. The significance of brain magnetic resonance imaging abnormalities at presentation with clinically isolated syndromes suggestive of multiple sclerosis. a 5-year follow-up study. *Brain* 1993;116:135–46.

54. Filippi M, Paty DW, Kappos L, et al. Correlations between changes in disability and T2-weighted brain MRI activity in multiple sclerosis: a follow-up study. *Neurology* 1995;45:255–60.

55. McDonald WI, Miller DH, Thompson AJ. Are magnetic resonance findings predictive of clinical outcome in therapeutic trials in multiple sclerosis? The dilemma of interferon-beta. *Ann Neurol* 1994;36:14–18.

56. Kidd D, Thorpe JW, Thompson AJ, et al. Spinal cord MRI using multi-array coils and fast spin echo. II. Findings in multiple sclerosis. *Neurology* 1993;43:2632–7.

57. Miller DH, Albert PS, Barkhof F, et al. Guidelines for the use of magnetic resonance techniques in monitoring the treatment of multiple sclerosis. US national MS Society Task Force. *Ann Neurol* 1996;39:6–16.

58. Stone LA, Smith ME, Albert PS, et al. Blood–brain barrier disruption on contrast-enhanced MRI in patients with mild relapsing–remitting multiple sclerosis: relationship to course, gender, and age. *Neurology* 1995;45:1122–6.

59. Gass A, Barker GJ, Kidd D, et al. Correlation of magnetization transfer ratio with clinical disability in multiple sclerosis. *Ann Neurol* 1994;36:62–7.

60. Kurtzke JF. Rating neurologic impairment in multiple sclerosis: an expanded disability status scale (EDSS). *Neurology* 1983;33:1444–52.

61. Willoughby EW, Paty DW. Scales for rating impairment in multiple sclerosis: a critique. *Neurology* 1988;38:1793–8.

62. Hughes RAC, Sharrack B. More immunotherapy for multiple sclerosis. *J Neurol Neurosurg Psychiatry* 1996;61:239–41.

63. Whitaker J, McFarland H, Rudge P, Reingold S. Outcomes assessment in multiple sclerosis clinical trials: a critical analysis. *Multiple Sclerosis* 1995;1:37–47.

64. Vercoulen JHMM, Hommes OR, Swanink MA, et al. The measurement of fatigue in patients with multiple sclerosis – a multidimensional comparison with patients with chronic fatigue syndrome and healthy subjects. *Arch Neurol* 1996;53:642–9.

65. Cella DF, Dineen K, Arnason B, et al. Validation of the functional assessment of multiple sclerosis quality of life instrument. *Neurology* 1996;47:129–39.

66. Goodkin DE, Cookfair D, Wende K, et al. Inter- and intrarater scoring agreement using grades 1.0 to 3.5 of the Kurtzke expanded disability status scale (EDSS). *Neurology* 1992;42:859–63.

67. Francis DA, Bain P, Swan AV, Hughes RAC. An assessment of disability rating scales used in multiple sclerosis. *Arch Neurol* 1991;48:299–301.

68. Mumford CJ. *β*-Interferon and multiple sclerosis: why the fuss? Q J Med 1996;89:1–3.

69. de Haan RJ, Polman CH. Het behandelingseffect van interferon-beta1a en-1b bij multipele sclerose clinimetrisch getoetst. *Ned Tijdschr Geneeskd* 1996;140:2168–71.

70. Jacobs LD, Cookfair DL, Rudick RA, et al. Intramuscular interferon beta-1a for disease progression in relapsing multiple sclerosis. *Ann Neurol* 1996;39:285–94.

71. Fazekas F, Deisenhammer F, Strasser-Fuchs S, Nahler G, Mamoli B. Randomised placebo-controlled trial of monthly intravenous immunoglobulin therapy in relapsing-remitting multiple sclerosis. *Lancet* 1997;349:589–93.

72. Mumford CJ, Compston A. Problems with rating scales for multiple sclerosis: a novel approach – the CAMBS score. *J Neurol* 1993;240:209–15.

73. Lankhorst GJ, Jelles F, Smits RCF, et al. Quality of life in multiple sclerosis: the disability and impact profile (DIP). *J Neurol* 1996;243:469–74.

74. Schwab RS, England AC. Projection technique for evaluating surgery in Parkinson's disease. In Gillingham FJ, Donaldson MC (Eds.). *Third Symposium on Parkinson's Disease.* Edinburgh: Churchill Livingstone, 1969:152–7.

75. Canter CJ, de la Torre R, Mier M. A method of evaluating disability in patients with Parkinson's disease. *J Nerv Ment Dis* 1961;133:143–7.

76. Langston JW, Widner H, Goetz CG, et al. Core assessment program for intracerebral transplantations (capit). *Mov Disord* 1992;7:2–13.

77. Wade DT. Measurement in neurologic rehabilitation. *Curr Opin Neurol* 1993;6:778–84.

78. Hoehn MM, Yahr MD. Parkinsonism: onset, progression and mortality. *Neurology* 1967;17:427–42.

79. Webster DD. Critical analysis of the disability in Parkinson's disease. *Modern Treatment* 1968;5:257–82.

80. Jenkinson C, Peto V, Fitzpatrick R, Greenhall R, Hyman N. Self-reported functioning and well-being in patients with Parkinson's disease: comparison of the short-form health survey (SF-36) and the Parkinson's disease questionnaire (PDQ–39). *Age Ageing* 1995;24:505–9.

81. de Boer AG, Wijker W, Speelman JD, de Haes JC. Quality of life in patients with Parkinson's disease: development of a questionnaire. *J Neurol Neurosurg Psychiatry* 1996;61:70–4.

82. Molenaar DSM, de Haan R, Vermeulen M. Impairment, disability, or handicap in peripheral neuropathy: analysis of the use of outcome measures in clinical trials in patients with peripheral neuropathies. *J Neurol Neurosurg Psychiatry* 1995;59:165–9.

83. Albers JW, Andersen H, Arezzo JC, et al. Diabetic polyneuropathy in controlled clinical trials: consensus report of the Peripheral Nerve Society. *Ann Neurol* 1995;38:478–82.

84. Lhoir A. Vigabatrin in uncontrolled seizures: Belgian clinical experience. The Belgian vigabatrin evaluation group. *Clin Neurol Neurosurg* 1994;96:42–6.

85. Walczak TS, Radtke RA, McNamara JO, et al. Anterior temporal lobectomy for complex partial seizures: evaluation, results, and long-term follow-up in 100 cases. *Neurology* 1990;40:413–8.

86. Hart YM, Shorvon SD. The nature of epilepsy in the general population. I. Characteristics of patients receiving medication for epilepsy. *Epilepsy Res* 1995;21:43–9.

87. Lammers MW, Hekster YA, Keyser A, et al. Clinimetric analysis of treatment objectives and clinical status: individualized treatment in epileptic patients. *Epilepsia* 1994;35:1271–8.

88. Stensman R. Severely mobility-disabled people assess the quality of their lives. *Scand J Rehabil Med* 1985;17:87–99.

89. Devinsky O. Outcome research in neurology: incorporating health-related quality of life [editorial comment]. *Ann Neurol* 1995;37:141–2.

90. Vickrey BG, Hays RD, Engel J, Jr., et al. Outcome assessment for epilepsy surgery: the impact of measuring health-related quality of life. *Ann Neurol* 1995;37:158–66.

91. Chaplin JE, Yepez R, Shorvon S, Floyd M. A quantitative approach to measuring the social effects of epilepsy. *Neuroepidemiology* 1990;9:151–8.

92. Collings JA. Psychosocial well-being and epilepsy: an empirical study. *Epilepsia* 1990;31:418–26.

93. Vickrey BG. A procedure for developing a quality-of-life measure for epilepsy surgery patients. *Epilepsia* 1993;34 Suppl.4:S22–7.

94. Baker GA, Smith DF, Dewey M, Jacoby A, Chadwick DW. The initial development of a health-related quality of life model as an outcome measure in epilepsy. *Epilepsy Res* 1993;16:65–81.

95. Hoare P, Russell M. The quality of life of children with chronic epilepsy and their families: preliminary findings with a new assessment measure. *Dev Med Child Neurol* 1995;37:689–96.

96. Anonymous. Treatment of migraine attacks with sumatriptan. The subcutaneous sumatriptan international study group. *N Engl J Med* 1991;325:316–21.

97. Kudrow L, Kudrow DB, Sandweiss JH. Rapid and sustained relief of migraine attacks with intranasal lidocaine: preliminary findings. *Headache* 1995;35:79–82.

98. Cameron JD, Lane PL, Speechley M. Intravenous chlorpromazine vs intravenous metoclopramide in acute migraine headache. *Acad Emerg Med* 1995;2:597–602.

99. Tfelt-Hansen P, Henry P, Mulder LJ, Scheldewaert RG, Schoenen E, Chazot G. The effectiveness of combined oral lysine acetylsalicylate and metoclopramide compared with oral sumatriptan for migraine. *Lancet* 1995;346:923–6.

100. Rapoport AM, Visser WH, Cutler NR, et al. Oral sumatriptan in preventing headache recurrence after treatment of migraine attacks with subcutaneous sumatriptan. *Neurology* 1995;45:1505–9.

101. Jensen R, Brinck T, Olesen J. Sodium valproate has a prophylactic effect in migraine without aura: a triple-blind, placebo-controlled crossover study. *Neurology* 1994;44:647–51.

102. Baischer W. Acupuncture in migraine: long-term outcome and predicting factors. *Headache* 1995;35:472–4.

Part II

Neurological diseases

10

Cerebrovascular ischemic disease

Philip A. Wolf

Etiology

Magnitude of the problem

Stroke is a major clinical manifestation of atherosclerotic cardiovascular disease along with coronary artery disease (CHD) and peripheral arterial disease. Ischemic cerebrovascular disease accounts for more than 85% of all clinical stroke events with the remainder divided approximately equally between intracerebral hemorrhage (ICH) and subarachnoid hemorrhage (SH). Stroke is the third leading cause of death in most developed countries, accounting for approximately one in 15 deaths. In the United States, nearly 150 000 persons died of stroke in 1995, amounting to one death every 3.4 minutes. Stroke mortality is heterogeneous, is greater among the elderly, in men, and in African–Americans (1). Even within discrete age and sex groups sizable regional variations in mortality exist between and within nations. In the southeastern United States, stroke death rates are approximately 1.4 times greater than the US average (2).

Secular trends in mortality

In the United States, death rates from stroke fell steadily at approximately 1% per year from 1915 (when such data became available) until 1968. The pace of decline then accelerated, averaging 5–7% annually; between 1972 and 1990 US death rates from stroke fell a remarkable 65%. This rapid decline more than counter-balanced the aging of the population; as a result, the *number* of persons dying from stroke also declined steadily. However, the decline in both the numbers and in the age-adjusted death rates for stroke reached a nadir in 1992–1993 and seem to be rising since then for the first time since 1915 (Figure 10.1) (3). This declining mortality results from reduced severity of stroke and, perhaps, from a falling stroke incidence. In several defined populations, notably Olmsted County (Rochester, MN), there has been a documented decline in stroke incidence which decreased from 205 per 100 000 in the 1955–1959 quinquennium to 128 per 100 000 in the period 1975–1979. However, incidence rose to 153 per 100 000 in

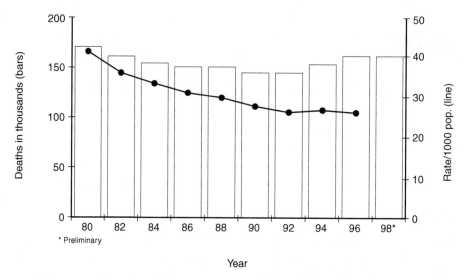

Figure 10.1 Mortality from stroke, United States 1980–1998. From *Vital Statistics of U.S.*, National Centers of Health.

1980–1984 and has remained constant since then while national mortality rates continued to fall through 1991. The continued decline in death rates coincident with stable incidence is consistent with a decline in stroke case fatality rates, presumed to result from reduced stroke severity. In five rural North Carolina counties studied in the periods 1970–1973 and 1979–1980, one-year survival following stroke increased from 49% to 62% (4). Improved detection of milder cases, largely through improved brain imaging, may also have contributed to the apparent reduction in stroke severity.

Disability

It is apparent that stroke is more disabling than lethal and is the leading cause of neurologic disability in the elderly. Of the 500 000 estimated initial strokes in 1996, there were approximately 3 900 000 stroke survivors in the United States, many of whom required chronic care (3). Among long-term (6 months +) stroke survivors, 48% were hemiparetic, 22% were unable to walk, 24% to 53% reported complete or partial dependence on activity of daily living (ADL) scales, 12% to 18% were aphasic, and 32% were clinically depressed (5,6). The average health care costs (inpatient and outpatient) for cerebral infarction have been estimated at $8000 to $16 500, for subarachnoid hemorrhage between $27 000 and $32 911, and for intracerebral hemorrhage to be between $11 100 and $12 881. While impressive, they do not include the additional costs associated with residual morbidity following stroke (lost work, additional nursing care, etc.). If these are included, total cost of stroke to the US is crudely estimated to have been $37.8 billion in 1990 (3).

Diagnosis

The diagnosis of stroke requires differentiation from other diseases of the brain of acute onset based on clinical history, neurologic exam, and brain imaging. Differentiating infarction from hemorrhage is now rather easily accomplished by computerized tomography (CT) scan; determining the specific infarction subtype, however, is more difficult. Despite intensive workup, in approximately one-third of infarcts the precise underlying mechanism cannot be determined – a group labeled *infarction of undetermined cause (IUC)*.

Ischemic stroke mechanism

At least two-thirds of ischemic strokes result from atherothrombotic occlusive disease while embolism from a documented cardiac source and infarction of undetermined cause constitute the balance (7). Atherothrombosis results from: atherosclerosis affecting the large and medium size arteries to the brain, extracranial and intracerebral; and lipohyalinosis affecting small penetrating arteries within the brain. A substantial portion of ischemic strokes, estimated at between 15 and 30%, result from embolism from a cardiac source. Since the cardiac diseases predisposing to embolism chiefly result from atherosclerosis affecting the coronary arteries and ascending aorta, precursors of atherosclerosis underlie both atherothrombotic and embolic stroke.

Prognosis

Outcome following stroke varies widely according to mechanism or subtype of the stroke. Outcome is also adversely affected by the development of a second (or more) stroke with attendant increase in physical disability and decrease in cognitive function. Such recurrences are quite frequent, occurring in approximately 25% during the first 2 years following the initial stroke. Strokes resulting from hemorrhage, intraparenchymatous and subarachnoid, are fatal in about half the cases and hemorrhage survivors often have severe permanent disability. Cerebral infarction accounts for approximately 85% of all strokes. Case-fatality rates vary widely among ischemic stroke subtypes ranging from less than 5% for lacunar infarcts to 25% in large artery and cardioembolic ischemic strokes. Overall, stroke is more disabling than lethal and is the leading cause of adult neurologic disability and a key diagnosis leading to institutionalization. Physical disability and dementia frequently follow stroke, leading to loss of independence and, as far as the stroke survivor and the family is concerned, the end of useful life.

Intervention

While treatment of acute stroke is being actively pursued it is likely the major impact on reducing death and disability from cerebrovascular disease will come from prevention. Modification of factors predisposing to initial or recurrent stroke holds the key to stroke prevention. Many stroke precursors remain incompletely understood: genetic influences, clotting factors, blood lipids, inflammatory markers, infectious agents, homocyst(e)ine level, nutritional factors, and others. However, a number of key risk factors for stroke have been identified and their impact estimated (1). Although a full discussion of stroke precursors and their interaction is beyond the scope of this chapter, it is important to highlight those modifiable risk factors known to predispose to stroke where intervention has been shown to reduce stroke occurrence. *Hypertension* is the principal risk factor for ischemic stroke with risk rising in proportion to level of blood pressure, systolic as well as diastolic. Reducing elevated pressures, even mild elevations of systolic pressure, has been shown to reduce stroke incidence in direct proportion to the degree of blood pressure reduction (8–10). Although incidence is highest at the extreme upper levels of the blood pressure range, most stroke occurs at moderately elevated blood pressure which is the most prevalent in middle aged and older individuals. In a recent survey of a stratified sample of the United States population, approximately 50 million Americans were estimated to have hypertension, according to the JNCVI criteria (11). Of these 50 million persons, only 10.5 million were known to be hypertensive, were actively treated and their hypertension was controlled. Thus, in the 1990s in the United States, four out of five hypertensives were either unaware, untreated, or uncontrolled. Reduction of elevated systolic and diastolic blood pressures, in men and women of all ages up to age 85 years, has been repeatedly shown to reduce stroke incidence by approximately 42% (8). Clearly detection and treatment of hypertension is the key preventive measure to reduce stroke.

Cigarette smoking

Risk of stroke is increased about 1.5-fold in cigarette smokers with risk rising with the number of cigarettes smoked. Following smoking cessation, observational studies show risk of stroke falls within 5 years to a level of a person who never smoked (12). In fact, risk is halved within 2 years of smoking cessation regardless of number of cigarettes smoked and the age of the smoker – hence the adage "It's never too late to quit!" (13).

Physical activity

Moderate or heavy physical activity is associated with lower rates of stroke in men and women (14). Exercise promotes weight reduction and fitness with attendant reduction in other risk factors including a greater receptiveness to smoking cessation advice.

Atrial fibrillation

Dramatic reduction in stroke, in excess of two-thirds risk reduction, has been achieved with warfarin anticoagulation in a half-dozen primary and secondary trials of patients with nonrheumatic atrial fibrillation (15). In clinical trials, it was apparent risk of stroke could be achieved safely with careful monitoring of the International Normalized Ratio (INR maintained above 2 and below 3) and patient selection. Other possible risk factors: elevated plasma homocysteine may be reduced with folic acid and pyridoxine (vitamin B6) supplementation (16); treatment with pravastatin or simvistatin in coronary patients with elevated total and LDL-cholesterol levels substantially reduces stroke rates by 20–30% (17,18); and weight loss in obese persons may be expected to reduce glucose intolerance and blood pressure and thereby prevent stroke.

Implications for clinical practice

It is not difficult to identify the stroke-prone individual. The presence of certain nonmodifiable personal characteristics: African–American race; parental history of stroke; advanced age; residence in a high stroke incidence geographic region; evidence of subclinical cardiovascular disease; echocardiographic markers of increased stroke risk (1); and prior diabetes and cardiovascular disease, helps to identify those at increased stroke risk. Persons with a prior stroke or recent episode of transient cerebral ischemia (TIA) are at particularly high risk. These TIA or stroke survivors with symptomatic significant extracranial carotid stenosis have been shown to benefit from carotid endarterectomy performed by expert surgeons with documented low complication rates (19–22). In addition, there may be modifiable risk factors: elevated systolic and/or diastolic blood pressure levels; cigarette smoking; physical inactivity; nonrheumatic atrial fibrillation; for which risk factor modification should be strongly urged. A quantitative assessment of stroke risk may be obtained using a stroke risk profile, such as that based on Framingham Study data, where increased probability of stroke is apparent even in persons with borderline levels of multiple risk factors (23). Using the risk profile, both the physician and patient may tabulate the stroke risk score and view the level of increased risk and potential benefit of elevated blood pressure reduction, smoking cessation, and warfarin use in atrial fibrillation. Aspirin has been shown to reduce ischemic stroke recurrence by approximately 20%, and other antiplatelet agents such as ticlopidine and more recently clopidogrel have even greater efficacy for stroke prevention (24–26). Less certain is the use of vitamins, notably folic acid and pyridoxine, to reduce plasma homocysteine. Pravastatin or simvistatin have been shown to reduce stroke rates in high stroke-risk patients with evidence of coronary artery disease who have elevated total and LDL-cholesterol (17,18).

There is much to be learned about factors which predispose to stroke and therapeutic measures which will reduce the incidence of stroke and the attendant death and disability. However, at present what is already known is not being utilized by physicians and patients with sufficient diligence. It is likely far greater reductions in stroke incidence can be achieved by application of proved therapies or risk factor reduction measures than is currently being done. It is estimated that more than half the initial strokes in the United States could be prevented by treating hypertension, achieving cigarette smoking cessation, and assiduously treating atrial fibrillation with warfarin (27). Newer measures promise to provide additional benefits, but only if they are applied with vigor and resolve by physicians.

REFERENCES

1. Sacco RL, Benjamin EJ, Broderick JP, et al. Risk factors, Panel. Stroke 1997;28(7):1507–17.
2. Howard G, Evans GW, Pearce K, et al. Is the stroke belt disappearing? An analysis of racial, temporal, and age effects. *Stroke* 1995;26:1153–8.
3. American Heart Association. *Heart and Stroke Facts Statistics: 1997 Statistical Supplement.* Dallas: American Heart Association, 1997.
4. Howard G, Toole JF, Becker C, et al. Changes in survival following stroke in five North Carolina counties observed during two different periods. *Stroke* 1989;20:345–50.
5. Gresham GE, Fitzpatrick TE, Wolf PA, McNamara PM, Kannel WB, Dawber TR. Residual disability in survivors of stroke: The Framingham Study. *N Engl J Med* 1975;293:954–6.
6. Gresham GE, Kelly-Hayes M, Wolf PA, Beiser AS, Kase CS, D'Agostino RB. Survival and functional status 20 or more years following first stroke: The Framingham Study. *Stroke* 1998;29:793–7.
7. Sacco RL, Ellenberg JH, Mohr JP, et al. Infarcts of undetermined cause: The NINCDS Stroke Data Bank. *Ann Neurol* 1989;25:382–90.
8. Collins R, Peto R, MacMahon S, et al. Blood pressure, stroke, and coronary heart disease. Part 2, Short-term reductions in blood pressure: overview of randomised drug trials in their epidemiological context. *Lancet* 1990;335:827–38.

9. SHEP Cooperative Research Group. Prevention of stroke by antihypertensive drug treatment in older persons with isolated systolic hypertension. Final results of the Systolic Hypertension in the Elderly Program (SHEP). *JAMA* 1991;265:3255–64.

10. Staessen J, Amery A, Birkenhager W, et al. Syst-Eur – a multicenter trial on the treatment of isolated systolic hypertension in the elderly: first interim report. *J Cardiovasc Pharmacol* 1992;19:120–5.

11. The Sixth Report of the Joint National Committee on Prevention, Detection, Evaluation, and Treatment of High Blood Pressure (JNC VI). *Arch Intern Med* 1997;157:2413–46.

12. Shinton R, Beevers G. Meta-analysis of relation between cigarette smoking and stroke. *BMJ* 1989;298:789–94.

13. Wolf PA, D'Agostino RB, Kannel WB, Bonita R, Belanger AJ. Cigarette smoking as a risk factor for stroke. The Framingham Study. *JAMA* 1988;259:1025–9.

14. Gillum RF, Mussolino ME, Ingram DD. Physical activity and stroke incidence in women and men. The NHANES. I: Epidemiologic Follow-Up Study. *Am J Epidemiol* 1996;143:860–9.

15. Atrial Fibrillation Investigators. Risk factors for stroke and efficacy of antithrombotic therapy in atrial fibrillation. *Arch Intern Med* 1994;154:1449–57.

16. Boushey CJ, Beresford SAA, Omenn GS, Motulsky AG. A quantitative assessment of plasma homocysteine as a risk factor for vascular disease. Probable benefits of increasing folic acid intakes. *JAMA* 1995;274:1049–57.

17. Sacks FM, Pfeffer MA, Moye LA, et al. The effect of pravastatin on coronary events after myocardial infarction in patients with average cholesterol levels. Cholesterol and Recurrent Events Trial investigators. *N Engl J Med* 1996;335:1001–9.

18. Scandinavian Simvastatin Survival Study Group. Randomised trial of cholesterol lowering in 4444 patients with coronary heart disease: the Scandinavian Simvastatin Survival Study (4S). *Lancet* 1994;344:1383–9.

19. North American Symptomatic Carotid Endarterectomy Trial Collaborators. Beneficial effect of carotid endarterectomy in symptomatic patients with high-grade carotid stenosis. *N Engl J Med* 1991;325:445–53.

20. European Carotid Surgery Trialists' Collaborative Group. Randomised trial of endarterectomy for recently symptomatic carotid stenosis: final results of the MRC European Carotid Surgery Trial (ECST). *Lancet* 1998;351:1379–87.

21. Asymptomatic Carotid Atherosclerosis Study Executive Committee. Endarterectomy for asymptomatic carotid artery stenosis. *JAMA* 1995;273:1421–8.

22. Barnett HJM, Eliasziw M, Meldrum HE, Taylor DW. Do the facts and figures warrant a 10-fold increase in the performance of carotid endarterectomy on asymptomatic patients? *Neurology* 1996;46:603–8.

23. Wolf PA, D'Agostino RB, Belanger AJ, Kannel WB. Probability of stroke: a risk profile from the Framingham Study. *Stroke* 1991;22:312–18.

24. Antiplatelet Trialists' Collaboration. Collaborative overview of randomized trials of antiplatelet therapy. I: Prevention of death, myocardial infarction, and stroke by prolonged antiplatelet therapy in various categories of patients. *BMJ* 1994;308:81–106.

25. Hass WK, Easton JD, Adams HP, Jr., et al. A randomized trial comparing ticlopidine hydrochloride with aspirin for the prevention of stroke in high-risk patients. Ticlopidine Aspirin Stroke Study Group. *N Engl J Med* 1989;321:501–7.

26. CAPRIE Steering Committee. A Randomised, Blinded, Trial of Clopidogrel Versus Aspirin in Patients at Risk of Ischaemic Events (CAPRIE). *Lancet* 1996;348:1329–39.

27. Gorelick PB. Stroke prevention, an opportunity for efficient utilization of health care resources during the coming decade. *Stroke* 1994;25:220–4.

11

Vascular dementia

Richard K. Chan and Vladimir C. Hachinski

Introduction

Improvement in overall standard of living and advances in medical sciences have led to significant improvements in life expectancy in the last century. With the aging of the population, dementing illness becomes an important cause of concern in developed countries. After Alzheimer's disease, vascular dementia is the second most common cause of dementia (1).

The incidence and prevalence of vascular dementia in young individuals are unknown. They are expected to be low since cerebrovascular diseases are uncommon in individuals less than 50 years old. Depending on the instrument used in the diagnosis and the age of the study population the prevalence of vascular dementia in the geriatric population ranges from 1–5% (1–8). The incidence of dementia in the elderly population is about 0.5–1.5 per 100 person-years (7).

Etiology

The name "vascular dementia" implies that the dementia is secondary with interference to the vascular supply of the brain. This may take the form of cerebral infarct or intracerebral hemorrhage. Although vascular events such as subdural hematoma or subarachnoid hemorrhage (without concomitant intracerebral hemorrhage or infarct) can cause significant decline of cognitive state, they are not, by convention, considered to be causes of vascular dementia. The causes of vascular dementia are listed in Table 11.1.

Single, strategic infarct can cause significant cognitive deficit in patients (Table 11.2). Recurrent cerebral infarctions are by far the more common cause of vascular dementia. The infarcts may involve the cerebral cortex, the cerebral white matter, or the deep gray nuclei. Infarcts affecting the brainstem and/or cerebellum, by themselves, do not cause cognitive impairment. As indicated in Table 11.1, cerebral infarcts are results of thromboembolic occlusion of cerebral arteries or hypoperfusion from many causes.

Table 11.1. Causes of vascular dementia

	Predisposing causes/diseases
Cerebral infarctions	
Large vessel disease	Carotid artery atherosclerosis
	Vasculitis
Small vessel disease	Familial/genetic (e.g., CADASIL)
	Hypertension
	Diabetes mellitus
Cardioembolism	Myocardial ischemia/infarct
	Myocardiopathy
	Arhythmia (atrial fibrillation, paroxysmal atrial tachycardia)
	Valvular heart disease (mitral stenosis)
Hemodynamic	Watershed infarct
	Global ischemia (e.g., during cardiac arrest, open heart surgery)
Cerebral hemorrhage	
Lobar hemorrhage	Amyloid angiopathy
	Hypertension
Subcortical/deep gray matter hemorrhage	Hypertension

Table 11.2. Strategic single infarct dementia

1. Middle cerebral artery territory
   a. Angular gyrus infarct
   b. Frontal or parietal lobe infarct with aphasia

2. Anterior cerebral artery territory
   a. Mesial frontal infarct (usually bilateral, with abulia, dyspraxia, memory impairment, and/or transcortical motor aphasia)
   b. Basal forebrain infarct

3. Posterior cerebral artery territory
   a. Bilateral mesial temporal lobe involvement
   b. Thalamus

Intracerebral hemorrhage leads to focal neuronal fallout. As with the case of cerebral infarction, when the neuronal loss involves a strategic location, or when multiple domains are involved, dementia ensues. Amyloid angiopathy deserves special attention. In this disease, recurrent cortical hemorrhages are associated with amyloid deposits in the vessel walls of the intracerebral arterioles. The affected patients often have premorbid decline in cognitive state. This is one condition where the distinction between vascular and degenerative dementia cannot be clearly delineated.

Diagnosis

The diagnosis of vascular dementia starts with a detailed history and careful clinical examination. It is important to interview the family members, and occasionally fellow workers, to assess the extent of disability due to the cognitive problem. A general examination is helpful in detecting systemic illness that might cause cognitive problems. The neurological examination is focused, paying particular attention to the presence of focal upper motor neuron signs (hypertonia, hyper-reflexia, hemiparesis, etc.) and primitive reflexes (palmomental reflex, grasp reflex, rooting reflex, etc.). Assessment of the mental processes can be performed using one of several bedside mental status assessment scales. Folstein's mini-mental status examination (9) is easy to administer; a score of less than 24 usually signifies significant cognitive deficit. The Mattis dementia scale (10) is another tool to assess cognitive function.

Any patient with cognitive deficit should be investigated to detect a treatable (and potentially reversible) dementia (11). Basic investigations should include a thyroid function assessment, serum vitamin B12 level, syphilis serology, and computed tomographic scan or magnetic resonance imaging study of the brain. Examination of the cerebrospinal fluid and electroencephalogram may also be needed in selected patients. Neuropsychological assessment is useful in defining the extent and type of cognitive deficit.

The diagnosis of vascular dementia requires the demonstration of socio-professional handicap and demonstrable causal link to vascular disease of the brain. Diagnosis sometimes appears much simpler than it really is. In practice, it can be difficult for the clinicians to assess socio-professional handicap from ignorant family members. It is even more difficult to prove a causal link between cerebrovascular disease and dementia, since the presence of vascular lesions in the brain does not always cause vascular dementia (11). Well-established dementia may be due to underlying degenerative brain disease that is not apparent on routine investigation. The distinction between vascular dementia and degenerative dementia is difficult and erroneous in cases of mixed dementia. The diagnosis of vascular dementia is thus, by necessity, a clinical one.

The Hachinski Ischemic Scale is the first attempt at differentiating vascular dementia from Alzheimer's disease (12). This is a 13-item scale, and a score of more than 6 is usually indicative of a multi-infarct state. This scale has acceptable sensitivity and specificity in defining degenerative or vascular dementia, but is unable to define mixed type dementia or subtypes of vascular dementia (13). Subsequent instruments in diagnosis of vascular dementia were variants from the Hachinski's scale, but incorporating the criteria of dementia at the same time. The two most commonly used instruments are the DSM–III classification (14) and the NINDS–AIREN criteria (15) for vascular dementia. The three instruments are shown in Table 11.3.

Prognosis

Vascular dementia, not unlike Alzheimer's disease, is progressive. In part, patients with vascular dementia are prone to recurrent stroke with further worsening of the cognitive state. In addition, there may be changes in the cellular level that appears to contribute to ongoing neuronal loss and loss of cerebral function. This includes inflammatory changes and elaboration of cytokines (16).

The rate of progression varies widely among the afflicted. In some individuals the cognitive deficit appears to be static over years; in others, the cognitive deficit worsens rapidly over months. The factors that determine the rate of progression are poorly understood. It is known, however, that a new stroke can cause an acute decline in cognitive state. The clinical presentation is thus that of stepwise progression, considered to be characteristic of vascular dementia (12,14,15).

Intervention

Vascular dementia is irreversible once established. There is no proven therapy or procedure that halts the progressive nature of the disease. Nootropics (e.g., "Hydergine," dihydroergotoxine, etc.) have not been shown to significantly bene-fit patients with vascular dementia. There is ongoing research for agents that can slow down the rate of cognitive decline. The cognitive state often worsens con-siderably with every vascular event, and there are theoretical grounds for preven-ting recurrence of cerebrovascular events in the hopes of slowing down the rate of cognitive decline.

In patients with known symptomatic cerebral infarctions, acetylsalicylic acid, ticlopidine and warfarin have been shown to reduce the risk of recurrent stroke (17). In patients with cerebral infarcts that were asymptomatic, the same is probably true. Antithrombotics should be prescribed in patients with vascular dementia due to cerebral infarcts although no trials had been or will be conducted to show that antithrombotics retard the rate of cognitive decline. In patients with proven cardioembolic stroke, warfarin is superior to acetylsalicylic acid and ticlopidine (18). In patients with severe internal carotid artery stenosis that is symptomatic, carotid endarterectomy reduces the risk of ipsilateral stroke (19). When the underlying cerebral pathology is due to small vessel disease, it is not known if antithrombotics or carotid endarterectomy could prevent recurrent ischemic event. Treatment of concomitant diabetes mellitus and hypertension are important and may reduce the risk of recurrent ischemic insults to the brain.

The patients with vascular dementia secondary to primary intracerebral hemorrhage are often clinically challenging. Antithrombotics should be avoided although they are not absolutely contraindicated. Prevention of subsequent hemorrhage depends on control of hypertension. There is no known effective intervention for amyloid angiopathy.

Depression is common in patients with vascular dementia, and often causes further worsening of the cognitive state. Antidepressants should be prescribed for patients with symptomatic or subclinical depression. Patients with severe cognitive deficit may develop behavioral or sleep disorders. Treatment with psychoactive agents and sedatives may be required. The clinicians should, however, be aware that these drugs may worsen the cognitive deficits.

Implication for clinical practice

The population is aging worldwide. Over the next few decades, the proportion of elderly people in the population will increase gradually. With this gradual shift in the age structure of the population, the clinicians will see more cases of dementia. As an example, in Canada the number of individuals with dementia will rise to 592 000 in the year 2021, compared to the estimated 252 600 in 1991 (4). About one-third of the demented individuals will have vascular dementia.

Cognitive decline from vascular dementia is not reversible, and tends to be progressive despite currently available treatment. It is far more important to prevent vascular dementia than to savage cerebral function once dementia has occurred. Almost one-third of elderly patients with recent cerebral hemispheric infarcts developed vascular dementia (20). Prevention of the first stroke is thus a clinically desirable goal. Individuals at high risk of stroke, especially those with transient ischemic attacks, should be managed aggressively. This may include prescription of an antithrombotic, carotid endarterectomy, treatment of concomitant cardiovascular disease and/or modification of vascular risk factors.

Patients who have already suffered one or more strokes may have cognitive deficit, and yet not severe enough to seriously affect their lives. Using the currently available diagnostic criteria, none of these patients would qualify for the diagnosis of vascular dementia. We have elected to use the term "vascular cognitive impairment" to describe these patients (21). Given time, patients with vascular cognitive impairment may worsen into the state of vascular dementia. Active interventions are therefore indicated in patients with either vascular cognitive impairment or vascular dementia to retard the rate of cognitive decline.

Table 11.3. Diagnostic criteria of vascular dementia

HIS	DSM–III–R	NINDS–AIREN
Established diagnosis of dementia	A. Dementia according to criteria (i)–(v): (i) Demonstrable evidence of impairment in short and long term memory; (ii) One of the following: *impairment in abstract thinking, impaired judgment; other disturbance of higher cortical function (aphasia, apraxia, agnosia or constructional difficulty)*; (iii) Disturbance in A and B significantly interferes with work or usual social activities or relationships with other; (iv) Not occurring during the course of delirium; (v) Either (1) evidence from the history, physical examination, or laboratory tests of a specific organic factor (or factors) judged to be etiologically related to the disturbance; OR (2) in the absence of such evidence, an etiological organic factor can be presumed if the disturbance cannot be accounted for by any nonorganic mental disorder.	1. Dementia fulfilling criteria a–d: a. Impairment of memory. b. Deficit in at least two of the following cognitive domains: *orientation, attention, language, visuospatial function, executive functions, motor control, and praxis.* c. Deficit severe enough to interfere with activities of daily living (and not due to physical effect of stroke alone). d. Exclusion criteria: *Cases with disturbance of consciousness, delirium, psychosis, severe aphasia, or major sensorimotor impairment precluding neuropsychology testing. Also excluded are systemic disorders or other brain diseases (such as Alzheimer's disease) that in and of themselves could account for deficits in memory and cognition.*
Focal neurological symptoms (2) Focal neurological signs (2)	C. Focal neurological signs and symptoms.	2. Presence of CVD, defined by one or both of the following: a. Focal signs on neurological examination. b. Evidence of relevant CVD by brain imaging.
History of strokes (2)	D. Evidence of significant CVD that is judged to be etiologically related to the disturbance (based on history and physical examination).	3. One or more of the following to infer relationship between dementia and CVD: a. Onset of dementia within three months following a recognized stroke.

Abrupt onset (2)

Stepwise deterioration (1)

Fluctuating course (2)

Somatic complaints (1)

Relative preservation of personality (1)

Emotional incontinence (1)

Nocturnal confusion (1)

Depression (1)

History of hypertension (1)

Evidence of associated atherosclerosis (1)

A score of >6 indicates a high likelihood of VaD.

B. Stepwise deterioration course with "patchy" distribution of deficits early in the course

b. Abrupt onset of cognitive deficits.

c. Fluctuating, stepwise progression of cognitive deficits.

4. Histopathological features, including:

a. histopathologic evidence of CVD obtained from biopsy or autopsy: AND

b. absence of neurofibrillary tangles and neuritic plaques exceeding those expected for age.

VaD: Criteria A–D

Definite VaD: 1 + 2a + 2b + 3 + 4 + absence of other clinical or pathological disorder capable of producing dementia.

Probable VaD: 1 + 2a + 2b + 3

Possible VaD: 1 + 2a + 3,

OR 1 + 2a + 2b,

OR 1 + 2a + 2b + subtle onset and variable course (plateau or improvement)

NINDS–AIREN (15); CVD = Cerebrovascular disease; DSM–III–R = Diagnostic and Statistical Manual of Mental Disorders, Third Edition – Revised (14); HIS = Hachinski's Ischemic Scale (12); MMSE = Mini-mental Status Examination (9); VaD = Vascular dementia.

It is important for clinicians to differentiate vascular dementia from dementia due to degenerative brain disease. Prevention of recurrent strokes may lead to a slower rate of cognitive decline, thereby carrying a better prognosis compared to Alzheimer's disease or the other degenerative type dementias. Patients with severe dementia often require institutional care. Patients with mild to moderate cognitive impairment can continue living at home, with varied level of support from their families and community agencies. In all cases, antithrombotics should be prescribed to prevent further cerebral vascular events. Modification of vascular risk factors should also be incorporated in the standard care. Patients with severe symptomatic carotid artery stenosis and reasonable cognitive status should be offered carotid endarterectomy. Surgery should be withheld in patients with severe cognitive deficit or who are dependent on others for activities of daily living.

There is active interest in looking for agents that might retard the rate of deterioration in vascular dementia. Several agents have shown promise in preclinical studies, and a few have been tested in humans. These drugs are still under investigation at this time. Not having a proven treatment, patients should be encouraged to participate in well-designed clinical trials to help find a treatment for vascular dementia.

REFERENCES

1. Hebert R, Brayne C. Epidemiology of vascular dementia. *Neuroepidemiology* 1995;14:240–57.
2. Roelands M, Wostyn P, Dom H, Baro F. The prevalence of dementia in Belgium: a population-based door-to-door survey in a rural community. *Neuroepidemiology* 1994;13:155–61.
3. Ebly EM, Parhad IM, Hogan DB, Fung TS. Prevalence and types of dementia in the very old: results from the Canadian Study of Health and Aging. *Neurology* 1994;44:1593–600.
4. Canadian Study of Health and Aging: study methods and prevalence of dementia. *Can Med Assoc J* 1994;150:899–913.
5. Ott A, Breteler MM, van Harskamp F, Claus JJ, et al. Prevalence of Alzheimer's disease and vascular dementia: association with education. The Rotterdam study. *BMJ* 1995;310:970–3.
6. Liu HC, Lin KN, Teng EL, et al. Prevalence and subtypes of dementia in Taiwan: A community survey of 5297 individuals. *J Am Geriatr* 1995;43:144–9.
7. Brayne C, Gill C, Huppert FA, et al. Incidence of clinically diagnosed subtypes of dementia in an elderly population. Cambridge Project for Later Life. *Br J Psychiatry* 1995;167:255–62.
8. White L, Petrovitch H, Ross GW, et al. Prevalence of dementia in older Japanese–American men in Hawaii: The Honolulu–Asia Aging Study. *JAMA* 1996;276:955–60.
9. Folstein MF, Folstein SE, McHugh PR. Mini-mental state: a practical method for grading the cognitive state of patients for the clinician. *J Psychiatr Res* 1975;12:189–98.

10. Mattis S. *Dementia Rating Scale: Professional Manual*, Odessa, Florida: Psychological Assessment Resources Inc., 1988.

11. Chan RKT, Hachinski VC. The other dementias. In Johnson RT, Griffin JW (eds.). *Current Therapy in Neurologic Disease*, 5th edition. St. Louis: Mosby, 1997.

12. Hachinski V, Lassen NA, Marshall J. Multi-infarct dementia. *Lancet* 1974;2:207–9.

13. Pantoni L, Inzitari D. Hachinski's Ischemic score and the diagnosis of vascular dementia: a review. *Ital J Neurol Sci* 1993;14:539–46.

14. American Psychiatric Association. *Diagnostic and Statistical Manual of Mental Disorders*, 3rd edition, Revised (DSM–III–R). Washington, DC: American Psychiatric Association, 1987.

15. Roman GC, Tatemichi TK, Erkinjuntti T, et al. Vascular dementia: diagnostic criteria for research studies. Report of the NINDS–AIREN International Workshop. *Neurology* 1993;43:250–60.

16. Djuricic BM, Kostic VS, Mrusulja BB. Prostanoids and ischemic brain edema: human and animal study. *Neurology* 1992;42:437–47.

17. Gorelick PB. Stroke prevention. Arch Neurol 1995;52:347–55.

18. Yanagihara T, Whisnant. Prevention of cardioembolic stroke with anticoagulant therapy. *Ann Neurol* 1996;39:281–2.

19. Goldstein LB, Matchar DB, Hasselblad V, McCrory DC. Comparison and meta-analysis of randomized trials of endarterectomy for symptomatic carotid artery stenosis. *Neurology* 1995;45:1965–70.

20. Censori B, Manara O, Agostinis C, et al. Dementia after first stroke. *Stroke* 1996;27:1205–10.

21. Hachinski V. Vascular cognitive impairment: a new approach to vascular dementia. *Baillières Clin Neurol* 1995;4:357–76.

12

Alzheimer's disease

Ingmar Skoog and Kaj Blennow

Introduction

Alzheimer's disease (AD), alone or in combination with other disorders, is probably the most common form of dementia. It is characterized by an insidious onset with slowly progressive impairments in intellectual functions and changes in personality and emotions (1). The neuropathology shows extensive neuronal loss and deposition of extracellular senile plaques (SP) and intracellular neurofibrillary tangles (NFT) in the hippocampus and the frontal and temporal cortex, while the motor cortex is spared (2). In this chapter, we will describe the frequency of this disorder, the current hypotheses regarding its etiology, the diagnostic challenges, its prognosis, and current and future possibilities for treatment.

Frequency

The prevalence rates of AD differ as may be seen in Table 12.1 (3–15), mostly as a function of methodological differences between studies. All published studies report, however, that the prevalence of dementia and AD increases steeply with increasing age. In most studies, the prevalence is higher in men than in women among younger old people, and higher among women than among men in the very old. Regarding geographical distribution, the prevalence of dementia is similar in most parts of the world, but there are differences concerning the type of dementia. The prevalence of AD is generally higher in Western European countries and lower in Asia and Eastern Europe, while the opposite pattern is found for multi-infarct dementia (3). One explanation for the variation may be different rates of cerebrovascular disorders in different countries. Recently, the Honolulu-Asia Aging study reported that the prevalence of AD in Japanese–American men was similar to that in Americans of European ancestry while the prevalence of vascular dementia approached that observed in Japanese studies (16). This may indicate that environmental or cultural exposure influences the development of AD. This suggestion is supported by the finding that the prevalence of AD is much

Table 12.1. Prevalence of dementia and Alzheimer's disease

| | Country | Sex | Percentage of individuals with dementia, by age group | | | | | Proportion (%) with Alzheimer's disease among the demented |
			70–74	75–79	80–84	85–89	90 +	
Jorm et al. (3)	all	all	3	6	11	21	39	
Fratiglioni et al. (4)	Sweden	men		5	10	14	22	46
		women		6	10	22	34	55
Ott et al. (5)	Holland	men	2	6	14	28	41	58
		women	2	6	19	33	41	79
Rocca et al. (6)	Italy	men	4	9	26	43		20
		women	3	8	11	33		54
O'Connor et al. (7)	Britain	all		4	11	19	33	75
Aevarsson and	Sweden	men				27[‡]/25[§]		44[‡]/44[§]
Skoog (8)		women				31[‡]/46[§]		44[‡]/45[§]
Evans et al. (9)	USA	all	3*	19[†]		47[¶]		91
Bachman et al. (10)	USA	men	4	3	10	12[¶]		38
		women	1	4	11	28[¶]		63
Ebly et al. (11)	Canada	men				19	37	71
	Canada	women				25	47	76
Hendrie et al. (12)	USA	all	3*	11[†]		32[¶]		74
	Nigeria	all	1*	3[†]		10[¶]		64
Zhang et al. (13)	China	men		4[†]		17[¶]		
		women		14[†]		28[¶]		
Ueda et al. (14)	Japan	men	4	1	15	42[¶]		26
		women	1	7	15	38[¶]		26
Shaji et al. (15)	India	men	0.5	4	11	18	29	26
		women	2	3	15	15	36	51

Age groups studied: *, 65–74; [†], 75–84; [‡], 85; [§], 88; [¶], 85 +.

lower among Africans living in Nigeria than among those living in the USA (12).

The incidence of AD was recently reviewed in two meta-analyses. Gao et al. (17) used mixed-effect models in their meta-analysis to accommodate the heterogeneity of the studies. Incident AD was associated with a significant quadratic age effect indicating that the increase in incidence rates slows down with the increase in age, although there is no sign of a decline in the incidence rates themselves. Jorm et al. (18) used a loess-curve fitting to analyze data from 23 published studies reporting age-specific incidence data and found that the incidence of AD rose exponentially

Table 12.2. Incidence of dementia

| | Country | Sex | Rate per 1000 years, by age group | | | | | Proportion (%) with Alzheimer's disease among the demented |
			70–74	75–79	80–84	85–89	90+	
Gao et al. (17)	all	all	8	18	34	53	73	
Jorm and Jolley (18)	Europe mild+	all	18	33	60	104	180	
	East Asia mild+	all	7	15	33	72		
	Europe moderate	all	6	12	22	38	66	
	USA moderate	all	5	11	18	28		
Fratiglioni et al. (19)	Sweden	men		12	33	25	15	48
		women		20	43	72	87	79
Ott et al. (20)	Holland	men	5	15	25	29	26	58
		women	4	18	25	50	77	79
Aevarsson and Skoog (21)	Sweden	men				90		38
		women				103	44	
Paykel et al. (22, 23)	Britain	men		15	71	29	0	64 (both sexes)
		women		27	36	112	89	
Hebert et al. (24)	USA		10	20	33	84*		
Bachman et al. (25)	USA	men	28	57	58	175*		63 (both sexes)
		women	26	49	93	100*		
Aronson et al. (26)	USA	men		7	24	72*		73 (both sexes)
		women		17	41	53*		
Yoshitake et al. (27)	Japan	all	4	20	22	87		Men: 24 Women: 51

Age group studied: *, 85 +.

up to the age of 90 years, with no sign of leveling off. Both these meta-analyses, and several individual studies (Table 12.2) (17–27), report that the incidence of AD is higher among women after the age of 85. East Asian countries tend to report a lower incidence of AD than studies from Western Europe and North America.

Using the 1991 Canadian life table and estimates of the prevalence of dementia from the Canadian Study of Health and Aging, Hill et al. (28) reported that women's expectations of life with dementia and of life in institutions were more than twice the corresponding expectations for men. The difference between the sexes was greater for AD than for any other type of dementia. The Framingham study (29) used a modified survival analysis to estimate both cumulative incidence and the sex-specific remaining lifetime risk estimates for quinquennial age groups above age 65 years. The lifetime risk of AD or other dementias was higher in women than in men. In 65-year-olds, the remaining lifetime risk of AD was 6% in men and 12% for women.

Etiology

The etiology of AD is largely unknown and is probably multifactorial. Therefore, several theories exist, some of which are reviewed here.

The β-amyloid protein is one of the characteristic components of the extracellular senile plaques SP (30) and is also deposited in the brain of AD patients. It is a breakdown product from membrane-associated precursors, the amyloid precursor protein (APP) (31). Most investigators consider amyloid deposition to be a "central event" in the pathogenesis of AD (32,33), starting a cascade which results in neuronal destruction. Individuals with Down's syndrome exhibit severe AD neuropathology by age 40 (34). The dominant chromosomal aberration in Down's syndrome is a trisomy of the long arm of chromosome 21, the site of the APP gene. Alzheimer pathology in Down's syndrome is probably caused by an overexpression of this gene. Cerebral trauma, a risk factor for AD (35–39), results in an increased deposition of β-amyloid (40,41). The amyloid hypothesis has been challenged (42–44) as deposition of β-amyloid in the brain is found in normal aging, in patients with Down's syndrome, and in several other brain disorders without evidence of neuronal damage or dementia during life (45,46).

Intracellular neurofibrillary tangles (NFTs) are mainly composed of paired helical filaments (PHFs), containing an abnormally hyperphosphorylated form of tau protein (PHFtau) (47,48). The normal tau protein binds to tubulin promoting the assembly and stability of the microtubules (49). Hyperphosphorylated PHFtau dissociates from the microtubules, is distributed within the neuron and is cleaved to smaller fragments which become ubiquitinated and polymerize into insoluble PHFs. The role of NFTs in the etiology of AD has also been challenged as they are found in several other disorders (50) and in nondemented elderly persons (51), and as normal tau often exists in a highly phosphorylated state (52).

A marked synaptic loss in the hippocampus and in several cortical regions is found in AD (53–55) and correlates better with clinical measures of dementia than SP and NFT (56–58). A high level of education, a protective factor for AD (5,13,59), has been suggested to increase the density of neocortical synapses (60).

Lesions in the cerebral microvessels, e.g., amyloid angiopathy (61,62) and degeneration of the endothelium (63,64), and increased vascular permeability with protein extravasation in brain parenchyma (65,66) are found in AD. Endothelial degeneration has been related to the location and number of SP (63). A blood–brain barrier dysfunction may be involved in the pathogenesis of AD (61,67–69) by increasing the possibility that substances from serum reach the brain (61,65,67).

Disturbances in the cholinergic, serotonergic, noradrenergic, dopaminergic, glutaminergic, and neuropeptic neurotransmitter systems are described in AD (70). The cholinergic system shows the most consistent and pronounced deficits, and correlates with the cognitive function (70,71). Smoking increases the density of cholinergic nicotine receptors in the brain, which may be the explanation for the inverse relationship reported between smoking and AD (72), although this finding may also be due to diagnostic criteria of AD (73). However, Ott et al. (74) recently reported that current smoking doubled the incidence of dementia and AD. Smoking was a strong risk factor for AD only in individuals without the apolipoprotein E (apoE) $\varepsilon 4$ allele, but had no effect in participants with this allele.

Alzheimer's disease is consistently associated with a family history of dementia (59, 75–79). Genetic studies in families with autosomal dominant inheritance for AD, accounting for less than 1% of all AD cases, have shown that mutations on the genes encoding APP on chromosome 21, presenilin-1 on chromosome 14, and presenilin-2 on chromosome 1 segregate with AD (80). In all of these families, the symptoms have an early onset (around 40–60 years of age). These mutations may increase the production of APP and elevate the levels of β-amyloid aggregates. There are six different APP mutations responsible for AD. All of these are missense mutations giving rise to amino acid substitutions on codons 692, 670/671, 716, and 717 of APP (80). In vitro studies suggest that these mutations may result in an increased production of total β-amyloid (codon 670/671) or a selective increase in the longer form β-amyloid$_{(42-43)}$ (codon 716 and 717) (81). The increased production of β-amyloid$_{(42-43)}$ is believed to lead to an increased deposition of β-amyloid, with development of SP. This hypothesis is supported by the finding that transgenic animals overexpressing mutant APP show an increase in β-amyloid$_{(42-43)}$ with concomitant deposits of β-amyloid in the brain (80). Presenilin-1 and presenilin-2 are both serpentine proteins, spanning the membrane 6–9 times, with a high degree of homology (82). Both proteins are located in the endoplasmic reticulum, Golgi apparatus and nuclear membrane in the cell, and are, within the brain, mainly expressed in neurons (83). The precise function of the proteins is unknown, but they have been suggested to have a role in intracellular trafficking of proteins (84) and in neuronal apoptosis (85). Similar to the APP mutations, the presenilin mutations may result in an increased production of β-amyloid$_{(42-43)}$, which may lead to an increased deposition of β-amyloid (86).

Apolipoprotein E (apoE) is a constituent of plasma lipoproteins, and is essential in the redistribution of lipids between cells by mediating the uptake of lipo-proteins by interaction with specific receptors. During 1993, several papers reported an increased frequency of the apoE ε4 allele in both familial and sporadic AD (87–89), a finding which has now been confirmed in numerous papers (90). The association is also confirmed in population-based studies (91–94), although it is weaker than in more selected samples and is reduced in the oldest-old (95–98). The apoE ε4 acts as an independent and specific susceptibility gene for AD and several hypotheses exist for its pathogenic role in AD. ApoE4 purified from plasma was found to bind with higher affinity than apoE3 to Aβ (99), suggesting that ApoE may act as a "pathological chaperone" (100), binding to soluble Aβ, making it insoluble and thus sequestered in the SP. Based on the finding that ApoE4 binds less avidly than ApoE3 to tau protein, it has also been hypothesized that ApoE3 (in contrast to ApoE4) protects against hyperphosphorylation of tau protein and thus the development of paired helical filaments and NFT (101). Last, apoE has a generalized repair function in the brain, involving membrane lipid re-utilization, and apoE4 may have a decreased function in reactive synaptogenesis (102).

A polymorphism consisting of a deletion at the 5' splice site of exon 18 on α2-macroglobulin (α2m) gene was recently found to be genetically linked to AD (103). The allele frequency for the deletion was higher in AD than in unaffected individuals, and seems to predict whether a susceptible individual will develop AD (103). α2m is a serum pan-protease inhibitor localized in SP (104), binds β-amyloid (105), and mediates clearance and degradation of β-amyloid (106,107), suggesting a link to β-amyloid deposition also for this gene.

Inflammatory proteins are found in AD lesions, suggesting that inflammation plays a role in the etiology (108). Several epidemiological studies also report that the use of anti-inflammatory drugs may protect against the development of AD (109–112).

Oxidative stress with the formation of free radicals has been suggested to be involved in the etiology of AD (113,114). β-amyloid induces oxidative stress in neurons (115,116) and endothelial cells (117), possibly by activating the receptor for advanced glycation end products (116). One common explanation for the risk factors for Alzheimer's disease is the formation of free oxygen radicals (118). Findings that dietary antioxidants may be protective for cognitive impairment (119), and that antioxidants such as estrogens (120) and red wine (121) may be protective for AD are compatible with this hypothesis.

Studies in rats suggest that increased glucocorticoid levels, e.g., provoked by stress, are associated with early aging and damage to the hippocampus (122,123), and might thus be involved in the etiology of AD. Reports that psychological trauma in early life (124) and depression (125,126) might be associated with an increased incidence of AD are often linked to this theory.

Alzheimer's disease has recently been associated with hypertension (127,128), coronary heart disease (129,130,131), atrial fibrillation (132), diabetes mellitus (133,134), generalized atherosclerosis (135), and ischemic white matter lesions (136–138). Although these findings may reflect an overdiagnosis of AD in persons with cerebrovascular disease (139), or that cerebrovascular disease increases the possibility that individuals with AD lesions will express a dementia syndrome (140), vascular diseases may exacerbate the AD process, or similar mechanisms may be involved in the pathogenesis of both disorders (141).

Apoptosis is a form of cell death caused by an internally encoded suicide program (142), which may be activated by a number of stimuli related to AD, such as the β-amyloid peptide, free radicals, glucocorticoids, and ischemia (142). Estrogens, which are suggested to be protective for AD (120), inhibit apoptosis.

Diagnosis

Histopathology is often stated to be the "golden standard" for a diagnosis of AD. Neuropathological criteria for AD include the Khachaturian criteria (143) and the CERAD criteria (144), which are mainly based on age-dependent limits of the amount of SP in the neocortex (although the Khachaturian criteria require some presence of NFTs before age 75), and the Braak and Braak criteria (145), which are based on the pattern of NFT changes. However, the interrater reliability between neuropathologists is not always satisfactory (146,147), and all these changes may be found in persons who show no signs of dementia during life (148–151).

The most often used criteria for clinical diagnosis of AD are the NINCDS–ADRDA criteria (Table 12.3) (152), which mainly represent diagnosis by exclusion and do not specify how to diagnose patients with concomitant vascular diseases. The agreement between the NINCDS–ADRDA criteria and neuropathological diagnosis of AD has been reported to be 80–90% (153–156). However, these correlations emanate from specialized academic centers, and are based on patients followed for several years. The accuracy rate in the earlier stages of the disease and in epidemiological studies is not known. Other often-used criteria for AD are the DSM–IV (157), proposed by the American Psychiatric Association, and the ICD–10 (158), proposed by the WHO.

The dimensional rather than categorical character makes mild AD often difficult to separate from normal aging (159–161). Fairly small differences in criteria may have large effects on the prevalence rates (161). If a decline from a previously higher level can be shown (by obtaining information from key informants or by following the patients over time) the validity of mild AD may be higher (8).

A complete work-up in cases of suspected AD includes careful history-taking, neurological, psychiatric, and physical examinations, interview of a close inform-ant, brain imaging, a chest X-ray, and biochemical screening including vitamin

Table 12.3. Tne National Institute of Neurological and Communicative Disorders and Stroke and the Alzheimer's Disease and Related Disorders Association (NINCDS–ADRDA) Criteria for Alzheimer's disease

1. Clinical diagnosis of "probable Alzheimer's disease" include:

Dementia established by clinical examination, documented by brief mental testing confirmed by neuropsychological tests

Deficits in two or more areas of cognition

Progressive worsening of memory and other cognitive functions

No disturbance of consciousness

Onset between ages 40 and 90

Absence of systemic disorders or other diseases that in and of themselves could account for the progressive deficits in memory and cognition

2. Clinical diagnosis of "possible Alzheimer's disease":

May be made on the basis of the dementia syndrome, in the absence of other neurologic, psychiatric, or systemic disorders sufficient to cause dementia, and in the presence of variations in the onset, in the presentation, or in the clinical course

May be made in the presence of a second systemic or brain disorder sufficient to produce dementia, which is not considered to be the cause of the dementia

Should be used in research studies when a single, gradually progressive severe cognitive deficit is identified in the absence of other identifiable cause

Adapted from (152).

B12 level, a thyroid function test, and cerebrospinal fluid examinations (162). These procedures are necessary to exclude other causes of dementia (such as hypothyroidism, vitamin B12 deficiency, brain tumors, normal pressure hydrocephalus, subdural hematoma, or cerebrovascular disease) and have generally not been possible to perform in epidemiological studies. In general, the more examinations that are performed, the more other possible causes of dementia will be found.

The main diagnostic problem is to distinguish AD from vascular dementia (VAD). Depending on the criteria used, the proportion of demented individuals diagnosed as AD or VAD may differ considerably (139,163,164). AD may sometimes have a course suggestive of VAD, and VAD may have a course suggestive of AD (165,166). AD may be underdiagnosed in persons with cerebral infarcts as neither clinical nor pathological evidence of cerebrovascular disease means that it caused the dementia. However, AD may also be overdiagnosed as many infarctions are clinically silent and infarcts in cases of typical AD may be dismissed as being irrelevant. It was recently reported that concomitant cerebrovascular diseases increases the possibility that individuals with AD pathology will express a dementia syndrome (140).

There is a great need for diagnostic biological markers of AD. Regional cerebral blood flow (SPECT or PET) often shows reduced activity over affected brain areas (167,168), but its diagnostic value remains to be established. Similarly, the clinical utility of ApoE genotyping is debated, but in special evaluation units, where comprehensive examinations are performed, the presence of the apoE $\varepsilon4$ allele in patients with suspected AD increases the specificity against a neuropathologic diagnosis (169–171). In more unselected populations, the positive predictive value is probably considerably lower.

A markedly decreased cerebrospinal fluid (CSF) level of β-amyloid $A\beta_{(1-42)}$, thought to reflect β-amyloid metabolism and deposition in the brain, is reported in AD (172–175). The sensitivity and specificity of CSF-$A\beta_{(1-42)}$ have to be further evaluated.

An increased CSF-tau, believed to reflect neuronal and axonal degeneration or damage, is seen early in AD in both clinical (176–178) and population-based (179) samples. The sensitivity of CSF-tau in identifying AD is above 80% in clinical samples, and most patients with other dementias and chronic neurological or psychiatric disorders have normal values (176,178).

Prognosis

Survival is reduced in AD (180,181), and it is considered to be the fourth or fifth most common cause of death in Western society. Although the relative risk of death in dementia is reduced in advanced age (182,183), the influence of dementia on survival at high ages is substantial because of its high prevalence. Katzman et al. (183) reported a population attributable risk (PAR) for death in AD and VAD of 5% in the age group 65–74 years and 21% in those above age 75. In 85-year-olds, Aevarsson et al. (184) reported a PAR for death in Alzheimer's disease and vascular dementia of 31% in men and 50% in women.

AD is a chronic disorder. During the course of the disease, the patients' functions in daily living inevitably deteriorate. AD is therefore the most important cause of institutionalization in the very elderly (139,185).

Intervention

Symptomatic treatment with acetylcholine esterase inhibitors, which slightly improve dementia symptoms by preventing the breakdown of acetylcholine, in mild to moderate AD was approved in the United States in 1993 (tacrine), 1996 (donepezil) and 1998 (rivastigmine). Several compounds for treatment of AD are in clinical trials all over the world. Most of them act against the acetylcholine deficit, but some act directly against the neuronal damage in AD. A recent clinical trial suggested that treatment with antioxidants slows the progression of AD (186). The recent finding that treatment of isolated systolic hypertension with the long-acting calcium channel blocker nitrendipine reduces the incidence of dementia and AD suggested that hypertension is one possible target for prevention (187). There are clinical trials underway to test if intervention with estrogens, anti-inflammatory drugs and antihypertensives may prevent AD.

Implications for clinical practice

Epidemiology shows that AD is a major disease burden in the elderly, and that only a minority of cases are recognized by health and social service professionals. These findings have had an impact on the organization of health services and public awareness of the disorder. Population surveys have emphasized the need for precise and accurate diagnostic criteria of AD suitable for use in different settings (188,189), and have also tested the reliability of these criteria (190). They have completed the clinical picture of AD by identifying early symptoms, and have led to development of brief case-finding instruments to be used for early detection by, for instance, general practitioners, and tested the change over time in cognitive tests which is of value for treatment trials. Although risk factors and protective factors have been identified, with potential value for prevention, they have to be tested in clinical trials.

REFERENCES

1. Skoog I, Blennow K, Marcusson J. Dementia. In Birren JE (Ed.). *Encyclopedia of Gerontology. Volume 1.* San Diego: Academic Press, 1996: 383–403.
2. Lantos PL, Cairns NJ. The neuropathology of Alzheimer's disease. In Burns A, Levy R (Eds.). *Dementia.* London: Chapman and Hall, 1994:185–207.
3. Jorm AF, Korten AE, Henderson AS. The prevalence of dementia: a quantitative integration of the literature. *Acta Psychiatr Scand* 1987;76:465–79.
4. Fratiglioni L, Grut M, Forsell Y, et al. Prevalence of Alzheimer's disease and other dementias in an elderly urban population: relationship with age, sex and education. *Neurology* 1991;41:1886–92.
5. Ott A, Breteler MMB, van Harskamp F, et al. Prevalence of Alzheimer's disease and vascular dementia: association with education. The Rotterdam Study. *BMJ* 1995;310:970–3.
6. Rocca WA, Bonaiuto S, Lippi A, et al. Prevalence of clinically diagnosed Alzheimer's disease and other dementing disorders: a door-to-door survey in Appignano, Macerata Province, Italy. *Neurology* 1990;40:626–31.
7. O'Connor DW, Pollitt PA, Hyde JB, et al. The prevalence of dementia as measured by the Cambridge Mental Disorders of the Elderly Examination. *Acta Psychiat Scand* 1989;79: 190–8.

8. Aevarsson O, Skoog I. Dementia disorders in a birth cohort followed from age 85 to 88. The influence of mortality, non-response and diagnostic change on prevalence. *Int Psychogeriatrics* 1997;9:11–23.

9. Evans DK, Funkenstein H, Albert MS, et al. Prevalence of Alzheimer's disease in a community population of older persons. Higher than previously reported. *JAMA* 1989;262:2551–6.

10. Bachman DL, Wolf PA, Linn R, et al. Prevalence of dementia and probable senile dementia of the Alzheimer type in the Framingham study. *Neurology* 1992;42:115–19.

11. Ebly EM, Parhad IM, Hogan DB, Fung TS. Prevalence and types of dementia in the very old: results from the Canadian study of health and ageing. *Neurology* 1994;44:1593–600.

12. Hendrie HC, Osuntokun BO, Hall KS, et al. Prevalence of Alzheimer's disease and dementia in two communities: Nigerian Africans and African Americans. *Am J Psychiatry* 1995;152:1485–92.

13. Zhang M, Katzman R, Salmon D, et al. The prevalence of dementia and Alzheimer's disease in Shanghai, China: impact of age, gender, and education. *Ann Neurol* 1990;27:428–37.

14. Ueda K, Kawano H, Hasuo Y, Fujishima M. Prevalence and etiology of dementia in a Japanese community. *Stroke* 1992;23:798–803.

15. Shaji S, Promodu K, Abraham T, Roy KJ, Verghese A. An epidemiological study of dementia in a rural community in Kerala, India. *Br J Psychiatry* 1996;168:745–9.

16. White L, Petrovitch H, Ross GW, et al. Prevalence of dementia in older Japanese-American men in Hawaii. The Honolulu-Asia Aging Study. *JAMA* 1996;276:955–60.

17. Gao S, Hendrie HC, Hall KS, Hui S. The relationships between age, sex, and the incidence of dementia and Alzheimer disease: a meta-analysis. *Arch Gen Psychiatry* 1998;55:809–15.

18. Jorm AF, Jolley D. The incidence of dementia: a meta-analysis. *Neurology* 1998;51:728–33.

19. Fratiglioni L, Viitanen M, von Strauss E, Tontonati V, Herlitz A, Winblad B. Very old women at highest risk of dementia and Alzheimer's disease: Incidence data from the Kungsholmen Project, Stockholm. *Neurology* 1997;48:132–8.

20. Ott A, Breteler MMB, van Harskamp F, Stijnen T, Hofman A. Incidence and risk of dementia. The Rotterdam Study. *Am J Epidemiol* 1998;147:574–580.

21. Aevarsson O, Skoog I. A population-based study on the incidence of dementia disorders between 85 and 88 years of age. *J Am Geriatr Soc* 1996;44:1455–60.

22. Paykel ES, Brayne C, Huppert FA, et al. Incidence of dementia in a population older than 75 years in the United Kingdom. *Arch Gen Psychiatry* 1994;51:325–32.

23. Brayne C, Gill C, Huppert FA, et al. Incidence of clinically diagnosed subtypes of dementia in an elderly population. Cambridge Project of Later Life. *Br J Psychiatry* 1995;167:255–62.

24. Hebert LE, Scherr PA, Becket LA, et al. Age-specific incidence of Alzheimer's disease. *JAMA* 1995;273:1354–9.

25. Bachman DL, Wolf PA, Linn R, et al. Incidence of dementia and probable Alzheimer's disease in a general population: the Framingham study. *Neurology* 1993;43:515–19.

26. Aronson MK, Ooi WL, Geva DL, Masur D, Blau A, Frishman W. Dementia. Age-dependent incidence, prevalence and mortality in the old old. *Arch Intern Med* 1991;151:989–92.

27. Yoshitake T, Kiyohara Y, Kato I, et al. Incidence and risk factors of vascular dementia and Alzheimer's disease in a defined elderly Japanese population: the Hisayama Study. *Neurology* 1995;45:1161–8.

28. Hill GB, Forbes WF, Lindsay J. Life expectancy and dementia in Canada: the Canadian study of health and aging. *Chronic Dis Can* 1997;18:166–7.

29. Seshadri S, Wolf PA, Beiser A, et al. Lifetime risk of dementia and Alzheimer's disease. The impact of mortality on risk estimates in the Framingham Study. *Neurology* 1997;49:1498–504.

30. Masters CL, Simms G, Weinman NA, Multhaup G, McDonald BL, Beyreuther K. Amyloid plaque core protein in Alzheimer's disease and Down syndrome. *Proc Natl Acad Sci* 1985;82:4245–9.

31. Beyreuther K, Masters CL. Amyloid precursor protein (APP) and βA4 amyloid in the etiology of Alzheimer's disease: precursor-product relationships in the derangement of neuronal function. *Brain Pathol* 1991;1:241–51.

32. Hardy J, Allsop D. Amyloid deposition as the central event in the aetiology of Alzheimer's disease. *Trends Pharmacol Sci* 1991;12:383–8.

33. Joachim CL, Selkoe DJ. The seminal role of β-amyloid in the pathogenesis of Alzheimer's disease. *Alz Dis Assoc Disord* 1992;6:7–34.

34. Mann DMA. Association between Alzheimer disease and Down syndrome: neuropathological observations. In Berg JM, Karlinsky H, Holland AJ (Eds.). *Alzheimer Disease, Down Syndrome, and their Relationship.* Oxford: Oxford University Press, 1993:71–92.

35. van Duijn CM, Tanja TA, Haaxma R, et al. Head trauma and the risk of Alzheimer's disease. *Am J Epidemiol* 1992;135:775–82.

36. French LR, Schuman LM, Mortimer JA, Hutton JT, Boatman RA, Christians B. A case-control study of dementia of the Alzheimer type. *Am J Epidemiol* 1985;414–21.

37. Heyman A, Wilkinson WE, Stafford JA, Helms MJ, Sigmon AH, Weinberg T. Alzheimer's disease: a study of epidemiological aspects. *Ann Neurol* 1984;15:335–41.

38. Mortimer JA, van Duijn CM, Chandra V, et al. for the Eurodem Risk Factors Research Group. Head trauma as a risk factor for Alzheimer's disease: a collaborative re-analysis of case-control studies. *Int J Epidemiol* 1991;20(suppl2):S28–S35.

39. Henderson AS, Jorm AF, Korten AE, et al. Environmental risk factors for Alzheimer's disease: their relationship to age of onset and to familiar or sporadic types. *Psychol Med* 1992;22:429–36.

40. Roberts GW, Gentleman SM, Lynch A, Graham DI. Beta A4 amyloid protein deposition after head trauma. *Lancet* 1991;2:1422–3.

41. Roberts GW, Allsop D, Bruton C. The occult aftermath of boxing. *J Neurol Neurosurg Psychiatry* 1990;53:373–8.

42. Regland B, Gottfries CG. The role of amyloid β-protein in Alzheimer's disease. *Lancet* 1992;340:467–9.

43. Hoyer S. Sporadic dementia of Alzheimer's disease: role of amyloid in the etiology is challenged. *J Neural Transm (P-D Sect)* 1993;6:159–65.

44. Davies P. Neuronal abnormalities, not amyloid, are the cause of dementia in Alzheimer disease. In Terry RD, Katzman R, Bick KL (Eds.) *Alzheimer Disease.* New York: Raven Press, 1994:327–33.

45. Davies L, Wolska B, Hilbich C, et al. A4 amyloid protein deposition and the diagnosis of Alzheimer's disease: prevalence in aged brains determined by immunocytochemistry compared with conventional neuropathologic techniques. *Neurology* 1988;38:1688–93.

46. Delaère P, He Y, Fayet G, Duyckaerts C, Hauw JJ. βA4 deposits are constant in the brain of the oldest old: an immunocytochemical study of 20 French centenarians. *Neurobiol Aging* 1993;14:191–4.

47. Kosik KS, Greenberg SM. Tau protein and Alzheimer disease. In Terry RD, Katzman R, Bick KL. (Eds.) *Alzheimer Disease.* New York: Raven Press, 1994:335–44.

48. Grundke-Iqbal I, Iqbal K, Tung YC, Quinlan M, Wisniewski HM, Binder LI. Abnormal phosphorylation of the microtubule-associated protein τ (tau) in Alzheimer cytoskeletal pathology. *Proc Natl Acad Sci USA* 1986;83:4913–17.

49. Goedert M. Tau protein and the neurofibrillary pathology of Alzheimer's disease. *TINS* 1993;16:460–5.

50. Wisniewski K, George AJ, Moretz RC, Wisniewski HM. Alzheimer neurofibrillary tangles in diseases other than senile and presenile dementia. *Ann Neurol* 1979;5:288–94.

51. Tomlinson BE, Henderson G. Some quantitative cerebral findings in normal and demented old people. In Terry RD, Gershon S (Eds.). *Neurobiology of Aging.* New York: Raven Press, 1976:183–204.

52. Garver TD, Harris KA, Lehman RAW, Lee VMY, Trojanowski JQ, Billingsley ML. τ phosphorylation in human, primate, and rat brain: evidence that a pool of τ is highly phosphorylated in vivo and is rapidly dephosphorylated in vitro. *J Neurochem* 1994;63:2279–87.

53. DeKosky ST, Scheff SW. Synapse loss in frontal cortex biopsies in Alzheimer's disease: correlation with cognitive severity. *Ann Neurol* 1990;27:457–64.

54. Masliah E, Terry RD, DeTeresa RM, Hansen LA. Immunohistochemical quantification of the synapse-related protein synaptophysin in Alzheimer's disease. *Neurosci Lett* 1989;103:234–9.

55. Masliah E, Hansen L, Albright T, Mallory M, Terry RD. Immunoelectron microscopic study of synaptic pathology in Alzheimer's disease. *Acta Neuropathol* 1991;81:428–33.

56. Terry RD, Masliah E, Salmon DP, et al. Physical basis of cognitive alterations in Alzheimer's disease: synapse loss is the major correlate of cognitive impairment. *Ann Neurol* 1991;30:572–80.

57. Blennow K, Bogdanivich N, Alafuzoff I, Ekman R, Davidsson P. Synaptic pathology in Alzheimer's disease: relation to severity of dementia, but not to senile plaques, neurofibrillary tangles, or the ApoE4 allele. *J Neural Transm (P-D section)* 1996;103:603–18.

58. Davidsson P, Jahn R, Bergquist J, Ekman R, Blennow K. Synaptotagmin, a synaptic vesicle protein, is present in human cerebrospinal fluid: a new biochemical marker for synaptic pathology in Alzheimer's disease? *Mol Chem Neuropathol* 1996;27:195–210.

59. The Canadian Study of Health and Aging:Risk factors for Alzheimer's disease in Canada. *Neurology* 1994;44:2073–80.

60. Katzman R. Education and the prevalence of dementia and Alzheimer's disease. *Neurology* 1993;43:13–20.

61. Glenner GG. Congophilic microangiopathy in the pathogenesis of Alzheimer's syndrome (presenile dementia). *Med Hypoth* 1979;5:1231–6.

62. Vinters HV. Cerebral amyloid angiopathy: a critical review. *Stroke* 1987;18:311–24.

63. Kalaria RN, Hedera P. β-amyloid vasoactivity in Alzheimer's disease [letter]. *Lancet* 1996;347:1492–3.

64. Claudio L. Ultrastructural features of the blood-brain barrier in biopsy tissue from Alzheimer's disease patients. *Acta Neuropathol* 1996;91:6–14.

65. Wisniewski HM, Kozlowski PB. Evidence for blood–brain barrier changes in senile dementia of the Alzheimer type (SDAT). *Ann NY Acad Sci* 1982;396:119–31.

66. Mann DMA, Davies JS, Hawkes J, Yates PO. Immunohistochemical staining of senile plaques. *Neuropathol Appl Neurobiol* 1982;8:55–61.

67. Hardy J, Mann D, Wester P, Winblad B. An integrative hypothesis concerning the pathogenesis and progression of Alzheimer's disease. *Neurobiol Aging* 1986;7:489–502.

68. Skoog I, Wallin A, Fredman P, et al. A population-study on blood–brain barrier function in 85-year-olds. Relation to Alzheimer's disease and vascular dementia. *Neurology* 1998;50:966–71.

69. Perlmutter LS, Myers MA, Barrón E. Vascular basement membrane components and the lesions of Alzheimer's disease: light and electron microscopic analyses. *Microsc Res Tech* 1994;28:204–15.

70. Blennow K, Cowburn RF. The neurochemistry of Alzheimer's disease. *Acta Neurol Scand* (Suppl.) 1996;168:77–86.

71. Bierer LM, Haroutunian V, Gabriel S, et al. Neurochemical correlates of dementia severity in Alzheimer's disease: relative importance of the cholinergic deficits. *J Neurochem* 1995;64:749–60.

72. van Duijn CM, Hofman A. Relation between nicotine intake and Alzheimer's disease. *BMJ* 1991;302:1491–4.

73. Skoog I. Risk factors for vascular dementia. A review. *Dementia* 1994;5:137–44.

74. Ott A, Slooter AJ, Hofman A, et al. Smoking and risk of dementia and Alzheimer's disease in a population-based cohort study: the Rotterdam Study. *Lancet* 1998;351:1840–3.

75. Amaducci LA, Fratiglioni L, Rocca WA, et al. Risk factors for clinically diagnosed Alzheimer's disease: A case-control study of an Italian population. *Neurology* 1986;36:922–31.

76. Fratiglioni L, Ahlbom A, Viitanen M, Winblad B. Risk factors for late-onset Alzheimer's disease: a population-based, case-control study. *Ann Neurol* 1993;33:258–66.

77. Broe GA, Henderson AS, Creasey H, et al. A case-control study of Alzheimer's disease in Australia. *Neurology* 1990;40:1698–707.

78. Mendez MF, Underwood KL, Zander BA, Mastri AR, Sung JH, Frey II WH. Risk factors in Alzheimer's disease: a clinicopathologic study. *Neurology* 1992;42:770–5.

79. Borenstein Graves A, White E, Koepsell TD, et al. A case-control study of Alzheimer's disease. *Ann Neurol* 1990;28:766–74.

80. Lendon CL, Ashall F, Goate AM. Exploring the etiology of Alzheimer disease using molecular genetics. *JAMA* 1997;227:825–31.

81. Hardy J. Amyloid, the presenilins and Alzheimer's disease. *Trends Neurosci* 1997;20:154–9.

82. McGeer PL, Kawamata T, McGeer EG. Localization and possible functions of presenilins in brain. *Rev Neurosci* 1998;9:1–15.

83. Kovacs DM, Fausett HJ, Page KJ, et al. Alzheimer-associated presenilins 1 and 2: neuronal

expression in brain and localization to intracellular membranes in mammalian cells. *Nat Med* 1996;2:224–9.

84. Weidemann A, Paliga K, Durrwang U, et al. Formation of stable complexes between two Alzheimer's disease gene products: presenilin–2 and beta-amyloid precursor protein. *Nat Med* 1997;3:328–32.

85. Wolozin B, Iwasaki K, Vito P, et al. Participation of presenilin 2 in apoptosis: enhanced basal activity conferred by an Alzheimer mutation. *Science* 1996;274:1710–3.

86. Beyreuther K, Masters CL. Serpents on the road to dementia and death. Accumulating evidence from several studies points to the normal function of presenilin 1 and suggests how the mutant protein contributes to deposition of amyloid plaques in Alzheimer's disease. *Nat Med* 1997;3:723–5.

87. Corder EH, Saunders AM, Strittmatter WJ, et al. Gene dose of apolipoprotein E type 4 allele and the risk of Alzheimer's disease in late onset families. *Science* 1993;261:921–3.

88. Saunders AM, Strittmatter WJ, Schmechel D, et al. Association of apolipoprotein E allele ε4 with late-onset familial and sporadic Alzheimer's disease. *Neurology* 1993;43:1467–72.

89. Poirier J, Davignon J, Bouthillier D, Kogan S, Bertrand P, Gauthier S. Apolipoprotein E polymorphism and Alzheimer's disease. *Lancet* 1993;342:697–9.

90. Roses AD. Apolipoprotein E alleles as risk factors in Alzheimer's disease. *Annu Rev Med* 1996;47:387–400.

91. Kuusisto J, Koivisto K, Kervinen K, et al. Association of apolipoprotein E phenotypes with late onset Alzheimer's disease: population based study. *BMJ* 1994;309:636–8.

92. Stengård JH, Pekkanen J, Sulkava R, Ehnholm C, Erkinjuntti T, Nissinen A. Apolipoprotein E polymorphism, Alzheimer's disease and vascular dementia among elderly Finnish men. *Acta Neurol Scand* 1995;92:297–8.

93. Myers RH, Schaefer EJ, Wilson PWF, et al. Apolipoprotein E ε4 association with dementia in a population-based study: The Framingham Study. *Neurology* 1996;46:673–7.

94. Evans DA, Becket LA, Field TS, et al. Apolipoprotein E e4 and incidence of Alzheimer disease in a community population of older persons. *JAMA* 1997;277:822–4

95. Rebeck GW, Perls TT, West HL, Sodhi P, Lipsitz LA, Hyman BT. Reduced apolipoprotein ε4 allele frequency in the oldest old. Alzheimer's patients and cognitively normal individuals. *Neurology* 1994;44:1513–16.

96. Corder E, Basun H, Lannfelt L, Viitanen M, Winblad B. Apolipoprotein E-ε4 gene dose. *Lancet* 1995;346:967–8.

97. Sobel E, Louhija J, Sulkava R, et al. Lack of association of apolipoprotein E allele ε4 with late-onset Alzheimer's disease among Finnish centenarians. *Neurology* 1995;45:903–7.

98. Skoog I, Hesse C, Aevarsson O, et al. A population study of Apo E genotype at the age of 85: relation to dementia, cerebrovascular disease and mortality. *J Neurol Neurosurg Psychiatry* 1998;64:37–43.

99. Strittmatter WJ, Weisgraber KH, Huang DY, et al. Binding of human apolipoprotein E to synthetic amyloid β peptide: isoform-specific effects and implications for late-onset Alzheimer's disease. *Proc Natl Acad Sci USA* 1993;90:8098–102.

100. Wisniewski T, Frangione B. Apolipoprotein E: a pathological chaperone protein in patients with cerebral and systemic amyloid. *Neurosci Lett* 1992;135:235–8.

101. Strittmatter WJ, Weisgraber KH, Goedert M, et al. Hypothesis: microtubule instability and

paired helical filaments formation in the Alzheimer's disease brain are related to apolipoprotein E genotype. *Exp Neurol* 1994;125:163–71.

102. Poirier J. Apolipoprotein E in animal models of CNS injury and in Alzheimer's disease. *TINS* 1994;17:525–30.

103. Blacker D, Wilcox MA, Laird NM, et al. Alpha-2 macroglobulin is genetically associated with Alzheimer disease. *Nat Genet* 1998;19:357–60.

104. Rebeck GW, Harr SD, Strickland DK, Hyman BT. Multiple, diverse senile plaque-associated proteins are ligands of an apolipoprotein E receptor, the alpha 2-macroglobulin receptor/low-density-lipoprotein receptor-related protein. *Ann Neurol* 1995;37:211–17.

105. Du Y, Bales KR, Dodel RC, et al. Alpha2-macroglobulin attenuates beta-amyloid peptide 1–40 fibril formation and associated neurotoxicity of cultured fetal rat cortical neurons. *J Neurochem* 1998;70:1182–8.

106. Qiu WQ, Borth W, Ye Z, Haass C, Teplow DB, Selkoe DJ. Degradation of amyloid beta-protein by a serine protease-alpha2-macroglobulin complex. *J Biol Chem* 1996;271:8443–51.

107. Narita M, Holtzman DM, Schwartz AL, Bu G. Alpha2-macroglobulin complexes with and mediates the endocytosis of beta-amyloid peptide via cell surface low-density lipoprotein receptor-related protein. *J Neurochem* 1997;69:1904–11.

108. McGeer PL, McGeer EG. The inflammatory response system of the brain: implications for therapy of Alzheimer and other neurodegenerative diseases. *Brain Res Rev* 1995;21:195–218.

109. McGeer PL, Schulzer M, McGeer EG. Arthritis and anti-inflammatory agents as possible protective factors for Alzheimer's disease: a review of 17 epidemiologic studies. *Neurology* 1996;47:425–32.

110. Andersen K, Launer LJ, Ott A, Hoes AW, Breteler MMB, Hofman A. Do nonsteroidal anti-inflammatory drugs decrease the risk for Alzheimer's disease? The Rotterdam Study. *Neurology* 1995;45:1441–5.

111. Breitner JCS, Gau, BA, Welsh KA, et al. Inverse association of anti-inflammatory treatments and Alzheimer's disease: initial results of a co-twin control study. *Neurology* 1994;44:227–32.

112. Breitner JCS, Welsh KA, Helms MJ, et al. Delayed onset of Alzheimer's disease with non-steroidal anti-inflammatory and histamine H2 blocking drugs. *Neurobiol Aging* 1995;16:523–30.

113. Lethem R, Orrell M. Antioxidants and dementia. *Lancet* 1997;349:1189–90.

114. Smith MA, Sayre LM, Monnier VM, Perry G. Radical AGEing in Alzheimer's disease. *Trends Neurosci* 1995;18:172–6.

115. El Khoury J, Hickman SE, Thomas CA, Cao L, Silverstein SC, Loike JD. Scavenger receptor-mediated adhesion of microglia to β-amyloid fibrils. *Nature* 1996;382:716–19.

116. Yan SD, Chen X, Fu J, et al. RAGE and amyloid-β peptide neurotoxicity in Alzheimer's disease. *Nature* 1996;382:685–91.

117. Thomas T, Thomas G, McLendon C, Sutton T, Mullan M. β-amyloid-mediated vasoactivity and vascular endothelial damage. *Nature* 1996;380:168–71.

118. Henderson AS. The risk factors for Alzheimer's disease: a review and a hypothesis. *Acta Psychiatr Scand* 1988;78:257–75.

119. Warsama Jama J, Launer LJ, et al. Dietary antioxidants and cognitive function in a population-based sample of older persons. The Rotterdam Study. *Am J Epidemiol* 1996;144:275–80.

120. Tang M-X, Jacobs D, Stern Y, et al. Effect of oestrogen during menopause on risk and age at onset of Alzheimer's disease. *Lancet* 1996;348:429–32.

121. Orgogozo J-M, Dartigues J-F, Lafont S, Letenneur L, Commenges D, Salamon R, Renaud S, et al. Wine consumption and dementia in the elderly: a prospective community study in the Bordeaux area. *Rev Neurol (Paris)* 1997;153:185–92.

122. Meaney MJ, Aitken DH, van Berkel C, Bhatnagar S, Sapolsky RM. Effect of neonatal handling on age-related impairments associated with the hippocampus. *Science* 1988;239:766–8.

123. Sapolsky R, Armanini M, Packan D, Tombaugh G. Stress and glucocorticoids in aging. *Endocrinol Metab Clin Clin North Am* 1987;16:965–80.

124. Persson G, Skoog I. A prospective population study of psychosocial risk factors for late-onset dementia. *Int J Geriatric Psychiatry* 1996;11:15–22.

125. Speck CE, Kukull W.A., Brenner DE, et al. History of depression as a risk factor for Alzheimer's disease. *Epidemiology* 1995;6:366–9.

126. Devanand DP, Sano M, Tang M-X, et al. Depressed mood and the incidence of Alzheimer's disease in the elderly living in the community. *Arch Gen Psych* 1996;53:175–82.

127. Skoog I, Lernfelt B, Landahl S, et al. A 15-year longitudinal study on blood pressure and dementia. *Lancet* 1996;347:1141–5.

128. Sparks DL, Scheff SW, Liu H, Landers TM, Coyne CM, Hunsaker III JC. Increased incidence of neurofibrillary tangles (NFT) in non-demented individuals with hypertension. *J Neurol Sci* 1995;131:162–9.

129. Aronson MK, Ooi WL, Morgenstern H, et al. Women, myocardial infarction, and dementia in the very old. *Neurology* 1990;40:1102–6.

130. Soneira CF, Scott TM. Severe cardiovascular disease and Alzheimer's disease: senile plaque formation in cortical areas. *Clin Anat* 1996;9:118–27.

131. Sparks DL, Hunsaker III JC, Scheff SW, Kryscio RJ, Henson JL, Markesbery WR. Cortical senile plaques in coronary artery disease, aging and Alzheimer's disease. *Neurobiol Aging* 1990;11:601–7.

132. Ott A, Breteler MMB, de Bruyne MC, van Harskamp F, Grobbee DE, Hofman A. Atrial fibrillation and dementia in a population-based study. The Rotterdam Study. *Stroke* 1997;28:316–21.

133. Ott A, Stolk RP, Hofman A, van Harskamp F, Grobbee DE, Breteler MMB. Association of diabetes mellitus and dementia: The Rotterdam Study. *Diabetologia* 1996;39:1392–7.

134. Leibson CL, Rocca WA, Hanson VA, et al. Risk of dementia among persons with diabetes mellitus: a population-based cohort study. *Am J Epidemiol* 1997;145:301–8.

135. Hofman A, Ott A, Breteler MMB, et al. Atherosclerosis, apolipoprotein E, and the prevalence of dementia and Alzheimer's disease in the Rotterdam Study. *Lancet* 1997;349:151–4.

136. Brun A, Englund E. A white matter disorder in dementia of the Alzheimer type: a pathoanatomical study. *Ann Neurol* 1986;19:253–62.

137. De la Monte SM. Quantitation of cerebral atrophy in preclinical and end-stage Alzheimer's disease. *Ann Neurol* 1989;25:450–9.

138. Skoog I, Palmertz B, Andreasson L-A. The prevalence of white matter lesions on computed tomography of the brain in demented and non-demented 85-year-olds. *J Geriatr Psychiatry Neurol* 1994;7:169–75.

139. Skoog I, Nilsson L, Palmertz B, Andreasson L-A, Svanborg A. A population-based study of dementia in 85-year-olds. *N Engl J Med* 1993;328:153–8.

140. Snowdon DA, Greiner LH, Mortimer JA, Riley KP, Greiner PA, Markesbery WR. Brain infarction and the clinical expression of Alzheimer disease. The Nun Study. *JAMA* 1997;277:813–17.

141. Skoog I. Arterial hypertension and Alzheimer's disease. In Leys D, Pasquier F, Scheltens P (Eds.). *Stroke and Alzheimer's Disease*. Holland Academic Graphics. The Hague 1998:89–100.

142. Thompson CB. Apoptosis in the pathogenesis and treatment of disease. *Science* 1995;267:1456–62.

143. Khachaturian ZS. Diagnosis of Alzheimer's disease. *Arch Neurol* 1985;42:1097–105.

144. Mirra SS, Heyman A, McKeel D, et al. The Consortium to Establish a Registry for Alzheimer's Disease (CERAD). Part II. Standardization of the neuropathologic assessment of Alzheimer's disease. *Neurology* 1991;41:479–86.

145. Braak H, Braak E. Neuropathologic staging of Alzheimer-related changes. *Acta Neuropathol (Berlin)* 1991;82:239–59.

146. Wisniewski HM, Rabe A, Zigman W, Silverman W. Neuropathological diagnosis of Alzheimer's disease. *J Neuropathol Exp Neurol* 1989;48:606–9.

147. Duyckaerts C, Delaère P, Hauw J-J, et al. Rating of the lesions in senile dementia of the Alzheimer type: concordance between laboratories. A European multicenter study under the auspices of EURAGE. *J Neurol Sci* 1990;97:295–323.

148. Tomlinson BE, Blessed G, Roth M. Observations on the brains of demented old people. *J Neurol Sci* 1970;11:205–42.

149. Arriagada P, Marzloff K, Hyman B. Distribution of Alzheimer-type pathologic changes in nondemented elderly individuals matches the pattern in Alzheimer's disease. *Neurology* 1992;42:1681–8.

150. Tomlinson BE. The neuropathology of Alzheimer's disease – issues in need of resolution. *Neuropathol Appl Neurobiol* 1989;15:491–512.

151. Geddes JW, Tekirian TL, Soultanian NS, Ashford JW, Davis DG, Markesbery WR. Comparison of neuropathologic criteria for the diagnosis of Alzheimer's disease. *Neurobiol Aging* 1997;18(suppl4):S99–S105.

152. McKhann G, Drachman D, Folstein M, Katzman R, Price D, Stadlan EM. Clinical diagnosis of Alzheimer's disease: report of the NINCDS–ADRDA Work Group under the auspices of department of health and human services task force on Alzheimer's disease. *Neurology* 1984;34:939–44.

153. Jellinger K, Danielczyk W, Fischer P, Gabriel E. Clinicopathological analysis of dementia disorders in the elderly. *J Neurol Sci* 1990;95:239–58.

154. Wade JP, Mirsen TR, Hachinski VC, Fisman M, Lau C, Merskey H. The clinical diagnosis of Alzheimer's disease. *Arch Neurol* 1987;44:24–9.

155. Mendez MF, Mastri AR, Sung JH, Frey WH. Clinically diagnosed Alzheimer disease: neuropathologic findings in 650 cases. *Alzheimer Dis Assoc Disord* 1992;6:35–43.

156. Jellinger KA. Diagnostic accuracy of Alzheimer's disease: a clinicopathological study. *Acta Neuropathol* 1996;91:219–20.

157. American Psychiatric Association. *Diagnostic and Statistical Manual of Mental Disorders.* (Fourth Edition) (DSM–IV). Washington, DC: American Psychiatric Association, 1994.

158. World Health Organization. *The ICD–10 Classification of Mental and Behavioural Disorders: Diagnostic Criteria for Research.* Geneva: WHO, 1993.

159. Brayne C, Calloway P. An epidemiological study of dementia in a rural population of elderly women. *Br J Psychiatry* 1989;155:214–19.

160. Henderson AS, Huppert FA. The problem of mild dementia. *Psychol Med* 1984;14:5–11.

161. Mowry BJ, Burvill PW. A study of mild dementia in the community using a wide range of diagnostic criteria. *Br J Psychiatry* 1988;153:328–34.

162. Katzman R. Alzheimer's disease. *N Engl J Med* 1986;314:964–73.

163. Amar K., Wilcock GK, Scott M. The diagnosis of vascular dementia in the light of the new criteria. *Age Ageing* 1996;25:51–5.

164. Wetterling T, Kanitz R-D, Borgis K-J. Comparison of different diagnostic criteria for vascular dementia (ADDTC, DSM–IV, ICD–10, NINDS–AIREN). *Stroke* 1996;27:30–6.

165. Erkinjuntti T, Sulkava R. Diagnosis of multi-infarct dementia. *Alzheimer Dis Assoc Disord* 1991;5:112–21.

166. Fischer P, Gatterer G, Marterer A, Simanyi M, Danielczyk W. Course characteristics in the differentiation of dementia of the Alzheimer type and multi-infarct dementia. *Acta Psychiatr Scand* 1990;81:551–3.

167. Geaney DP. Single photon emission tomography. In Burns A, Levy R (Eds.). *Dementia.* London: Chapman and Hall, 1994:437–56.

168. McKeith IG, Bartholomew PH, Irvine EM, Cook J, Adams R, Simpson AES. Single photon emission computerised tomography in elderly patients with Alzheimer's disease and multi-infarct dementia. Regional uptake of technetium-labelled HMPAO related to clinical measurements. *Br J Psychiatry* 1993;163:597–603.

169. Saunders AM, Hulette O, Welsh-Bohmer KA, et al. Specificity, sensitivity, and predictive value of apolipoprotein-E genotyping for sporadic Alzheimer's disease. *Lancet* 1996;348:90–3.

170. Welshbohmer KA, Gearing M, Saunders AM, Roses AD, Mirra S. Apolipoprotein E genotypes in a neuropathological series from the consortium to establish a registry for Alzheimer's disease. *Ann Neurol* 1997;42:319–25.

171. Mayeux R, Saunders AM, Shea S, et al. Utility of the apolipoprotein E genotype in the diagnosis of Alzheimer's disease. Alzheimer's Disease Centers Consortium on Apolipoprotein E and Alzheimer's Disease. *N Engl J Med* 1998;338:506–11.

172. Motter R, Vigo-Pelfrey C, Kholodenko D, et al. Reduction of β-amyloid peptide$_{42}$ in the cerebrospinal fluid of patients with Alzheimer's disease. *Ann Neurol* 1995;38:643–8.

173. Blennow K, Vanmechelen E. Combination of the different biological markers for increasing specificity of in vivo Alzheimer's testing. *J Neural Transm Suppl* 1998;53:223–35.

174. Ida N, Hartmann T, Pantel J, et al. Analysis of heterogeneous A4 peptides in human

cerebrospinal fluid and blood by a newly developed sensitive Western blot assay. *J Biol Chem* 1996; 271:22908–14.

175. Tamaoka A, Sawamura N, Fukushima T, et al. Amyloid beta protein 42(43) in cerebrospinal fluid of patients with Alzheimer's disease. *J Neurol Sci* 1997;148:41–5.

176. Blennow K, Vanmechelen E, Wallin A. Tau protein in cerebrospinal fluid: a biochemical diagnostic marker for axonal degeneration in Alzheimer's disease? *Mol Chem Neuropathology* 1995;26:231–45.

177. Riemenschneider M, Buch K, Schmolke M, Kurz A, Guder WG. Cerebrospinal protein tau is elevated in early Alzheimer's disease. *Neurosci Lett* 1996;212:209–11.

178. Andreasen N, Vanmechelen E, Van de Voorde A, et al. Cerebrospinal fluid tau protein as a biochemical marker for Alzheimer's disease: a community-based follow-up study. *J Neurol Neurosurg Psychiatry* 1998;64:298–305.

179. Skoog I, Vanmechelen E, Andreasson L-A, et al. A population-based study of tau protein and ubiquitin in cerebrospinal fluid in 85-year-olds: relation to severity of dementia and cerebral atrophy, but not to the apolipoprotein E4 allele. *Neurodegeneration* 1995;4:433–42.

180. Schoenberg BS, Okazaki H, Kokmen E. Reduced survival in patients with dementia: a population study. *Trans Am Neurol Assoc* 1981;106:306–8.

181. Bowen JD, Malter AD, Sheppard L, et al. Predictors of mortality in patients diagnosed with probable Alzheimer's disease. *Neurology* 1996;47:433–9.

182. van Dijk PTM, van de Sande HJ, Dippel DWJ, Habbema JDF. The nature of excess mortality in nursing home patients with dementia. *J Gerontol* 1992;47:28–34.

183. Katzman R, Hill LR, Yu ESH, et al. The malignancy of dementia. Predictors of mortality in clinically diagnosed dementia in a population survey of Shanghai, China. *Arch Neurol* 1994;51:1220–5.

184. Aevarsson O, Svanborg A, Skoog I. Seven-year survival after age 85 years. Relation to Alzheimer disease and vascular dementia. *Arch Neurol* 1998;55:1226–32.

185. Fratiglioni L, Forsell Y, Torres HA, Winblad B. Severity of dementia and institutionalization in the elderly: prevalence data from an urban area in Sweden. *Neuroepidemiology* 1994;13:79–88.

186. Sano M, Ernesto C, Thomas RG, et al. A controlled trial of selegiline, alpha-tocopherol, or both as treatment for Alzheimer's disease. *N Engl J Med* 1997;336:1216–22.

187. Forette F, Scux M-L, Staessen JA, et al. Prevention of dementia in randomised double-blind placebo-controlled systolic hypertension in Europe (syst-Eur) trial. *Lancet* 1998;352:1347–51.

188. Henderson AS. The epidemiology of Alzheimer's disease. *Br Med Bull* 1986;42:3–10.

189. Fratiglioni L. Epidemiology of Alzheimer's disease and current possibilities for prevention. *Acta Neurol Scand* 1996;(suppl165):33–40.

190. Fratiglioni L, Grut M, Forsell Y, Viitanen M, Winblad B. Clinical diagnosis of Alzheimer's disease and other dementias in a population survey. Agreement and causes of disagreement in applying *Diagnostic and Statistical Manual of Mental Disorders. Revised Third Edition*, criteria. Arch Neurol 1992;49:927–32.

13

Parkinson's disease

Maarten C. de Rijk and Monique M. B. Breteler

Parkinson's disease (PD) is one of the most frequent progressive neuro-degenerative diseases in the elderly. In spite of extensive research, the etiology of PD is still unknown. Relatively little epidemiologic research has been conducted on PD. In this chapter, recent developments in epidemiologic research of PD will be reviewed. We will successively discuss risk factors, diagnosis, disease frequency, prognosis, intervention, and implications for clinical practice.

Etiology

Numerous studies on risk factors for PD have been published, but the causes of the dopaminergic cell loss have not been settled yet. Most studies were based on register-based prevalent cases which have some well-known methodologic draw-backs as discussed in Chapter 1. In this section, we will mainly focus either on the few prospective studies in which the exposure was measured before the onset of the disease, or on large cross-sectional studies. Notwithstanding the ample potential for bias in case-control studies based on prevalent cases, we included results from some of the larger case-control studies as well. The results from these studies should however be interpreted with caution. The associations between most putative determinants and PD still have to be confirmed in cohort studies, ideally in a community-based setting.

Age

Age is the most important risk factor for PD. Under the age of 45 years PD is very uncommon. Reported age-specific prevalence and incidence figures varied widely (1), which might be due to differences in case-finding procedures, diagnostic criteria, and response rates across studies. Case-finding methods that are based on existing medical records will miss patients who did not seek medical attention for their parkinsonism and will tend to underestimate prevalence and incidence. Through an in-person screening of all subjects within a defined population these PD patients may be included (2–4); their proportion varies from 24 to 42%

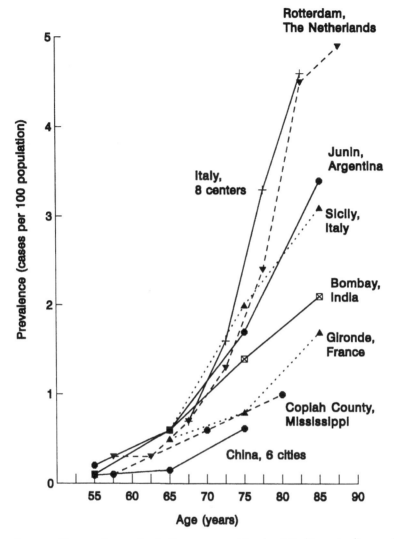

Figure 13.1 Age-specific prevalence, for both sexes combined, of Parkinson's disease from several community-based surveys with an in-person screening to detect Parkinson's disease.

(2,3,5–7). Apart from case-finding methods, different diagnostic criteria may also have their impact on frequency estimates (6,8).

Prevalence

In many register-based studies, it was found that the prevalence of PD increased with age till a certain age after which it declines (1,9–12). However, all community-based prevalence surveys with an in-person screening showed an increase in the prevalence of PD or parkinsonism with age, even in the highest age categories

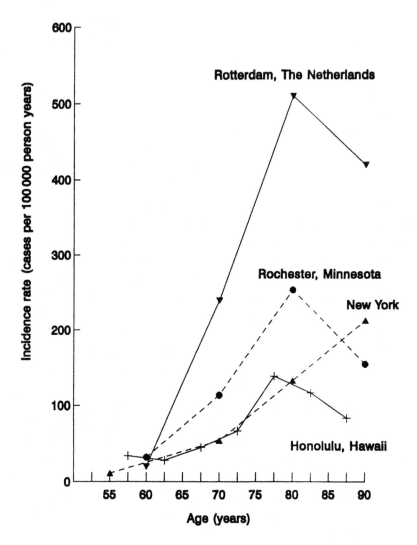

Figure 13.2 Age-specific incidence rates of Parkinson's disease from several community-based surveys.

(Figure 13.1) (2–7,13–15). A European study suggested remarkably similar prevalences across European countries if similar methodologies and diagnostic criteria were used; overall, the prevalence estimates ranged from 0.6% for those aged 65 to 69 years to 3.5% for those aged 85 to 89 years, with an overall prevalence of 1.6% for subjects aged 65 years or older (7). The Washington Heights Study from New York City suggested lower prevalence figures for Blacks than for Whites and Hispanics (11). However, selective mortality or delay in diagnosis due to limited access to appropriate health services could not be excluded as possible explanations (11).

Incidence

Incidence rates provide better estimates of occurrence of PD, but studies on incidence of PD are scarce. Only few studies provide age- and sex-specific estimates (11,16–19). The Rotterdam study was the only study to administer a screening instrument for PD to each individual, both at baseline and follow-up (19). The incidence per 100 000 person years varies around 250 for the age group 75 to 84 years (Figure 13.2) (11,16,19,20). More incidence estimates provided by community surveys with an in-person screening at both baseline and follow-up have to be awaited to establish the true incidence and pattern of incidence of PD.

Gender

Higher prevalences of PD for men (10–12) or for women (9,21) have been reported in register-based studies, while in most community surveys with an in-person screening no significant differences in the prevalence of PD between men and women were found (2–5,7,13). In incidence studies on PD with age- and sex-specific estimates, no differences between sexes were reported (16–18,22), except in two (11,12). These findings suggest that gender differences may have resulted from survival or diagnosis bias.

Smoking

Smoking is one of the determinants of PD that has been studied most frequently. Since Dorn first reported an inverse association between smoking and PD (23), this finding has been confirmed in most other studies (24–29), but not in all (30,31). Most studies that found an inverse association were based on prevalent cases and the inverse association was disputed with various arguments like biased results due to confounding, selective mortality, cause-effect bias, symptom suppression, or diagnostic competition (24). To date, few prospective studies exist (23,27,27,32–35), of which two were community based with an in-person screening (27,28). In all these studies, an on average two- to three-fold reduction of the risk of PD among smokers was found. Among the speculations regarding the biologic mechanisms that may explain the protective effect are: (1) reduced monoamino oxidase B (MAO B) levels in the substantia nigra of smokers (36); (2) reduced MAO B mediated oxidation of protoxins to neurotoxins (37,38); (3) smoking induced other enzymatic processes that are involved in the metabolism of xenobiotics (39); or (4) persons who get PD may have a genetic make-up or a (premorbid) personality that predelicts them to restrain from smoking (24,40–42).

In general, one could argue for the existence of a true inverse association of smoking with PD, because of consistent, biologically plausible, findings in epidemiologic studies that have been confirmed in prospective community-based studies.

Table 13.1. The associations* between potentially toxic environmental factors and Parkinson's disease from selected case-control studies

Investigator	Number of patients	Rural living	Farming	Well water drinking	Pesticides use	Industrial toxins
Ho et al. (179)	35	2.2 (1.0–5.0)[†]	1.7 (0.8–3.8)	—	3.6 (1.0–12.9)	—
Tanner et al. (180)	100	0.6 (0.2–1.0)	0.4 (0.2–0.8)[‡]	0.7 (0.4–1.3)	—	2.4 (1.3–4.3)
Koller et al. (181)	150	1.9 (1.2–3.0)[§]	1.3 (0.9–2.1)	1.7 (1.0–2.7)	1.1 (0.7–1.7)	—
Golbe et al. (48)	106	2.0 (1.1–3.7)[§]	1.3 (0.7–2.6)	1.1 (0.6–2.3)	7.0 (2.0–25.0)	—
Wong et al. (182)	38	4.3 (1.4–13.7)[§]	2.7 (0.7–9.5)	2.8 (0.9–8.2)	1.0	—
Stern et al. (183)	149	1.7 (0.9–3.1)	—	0.8 (0.5–1.6)	0.9 (0.6–1.5)[ǁ]	—
Semchuk et al. (184–186)[¶]	130	0.8 (0.5–1.2)	1.9 (1.1–3.3)	1.1 (0.6–2.0)	2.3 (1.3–4.0)	n.s.[#]
Marder et al. (58)	89	n.s.[#]	n.s.[#]	1.8 (1.0–3.1)[‡‡]	—	—
Seidler et al. (26)**	380	1.0 (0.7–1.4)	0.8 (0.6–1.1)	0.8 (0.6–1.2)	1.6 (1.1–2.4)	1.0 (0.7–1.4)[††]

*Odds ratios (OR) with 95% confidence intervals (95% CI) in parentheses.

[†]In original paper, 95% CI was not presented. We reconstructed the 95% CI.

[‡]Wheat growing.

[§]In original paper, 95% CI was not presented. We reconstructed the 95% CI by using the McNemar test for matched pairs.

[ǁ]Herbicide use, the OR for insecticide use was 0.5 (0.2–1.1).

[¶]Exposure in first 45 years of life.

[#]Nonsignificant, OR was not provided in article.

**In original paper, exposures were categorized. The overall ORs for exposure versus no exposure were kindly provided by the investigators.

[††]Exposure to anorganic compounds, assessed through job exposure matrix. Data were kindly provided by the investigators.

[‡‡]Unfiltered drinking water.

Antioxidants

Increased free radical production and an inadequate antioxidant defense system may play a role in the etiology of PD (43–45). It has been speculated that high intake of antioxidants, either through diet or supplements, may decrease the risk of PD or slow down its progression. The few studies on dietary antioxidant intake and the association with PD yielded equivocal results (46–52). Two recent large case-control studies based on prevalent cases found no protective effect of dietary antioxidants on PD (46,52), but potential biases could not be excluded (52). A recent case-control study, nested in a prospective study, suggested a significant inverse association between PD and consumption of foods containing vitamin E (legumes) more than 25 years before (odds ratio of 0.28 per at least one serving per day) (51). In persons who have already developed PD, vitamin E supplements are probably ineffective (53). Theoretically, β-carotene (54) and vitamin C could have an antioxidative effect in the brain as well, but in studies on PD such effects have not been found (46,50,52). Considering the currently existing evidence, vitamin E may be a dietary antioxidant that protects against the development of Parkinson's disease before the disease becomes apparent, but this needs further investigation in prospective studies.

Toxins

Renewed interest in neurotoxins that may cause PD was raised when it was observed that through intravenous injection the chemical 1-methyl-4-phenyl-1,2,3,6-tetrahydropyridine (MPTP) causes a parkinsonian syndrome strikingly resembling PD, both clinically and pathologically (55). Much research was focused on the relation between PD and direct or indirect exposure to potentially toxic compounds such as MPTP (and its metabolite MPP and analogues) containing pesticides, especially herbicides (56). Pesticide use, rural living, farming, well water drinking (all reflecting possible exposure to compounds of pesticides), and industrial environments seem to increase the risk of PD (Table 13.1) (57). Marder et al. showed that within the same community the risk estimates for various factors may vary across ethnic groups (58). As all case-control studies were retrospective and register-based, the results have to be interpreted with caution. Information bias may have occurred, especially when the notion exists that inhalation of toxic compounds could cause some brain damage. Moreover, almost exclusively the associations have been established indirectly without direct measurement of the true exposure.

To date, it is not clear whether environmental neurotoxins are potentiated by genetic defects in detoxification systems in the brain (59,60), but involvement of polymorphisms of such susceptibility genes in the etiology of PD have been suggested (61–64).

Table 13.2. The associations* between risk factors and Parkinson's disease from follow-up and selected case-control studies

Study	Type of study	Head trauma (any)	Head trauma (with loss of consciousness)	Family history of PD	Family history of dementia
Stern (187)	Case-control	2.9 (1.5–5.8)	—	—	—
Williams et al. (72)	Retrospective follow-up	0.9 (0.4–1.9)	—	—	—
Factor and Weiner (188)	Case-control	2.3 (1.0–4.9)[†]	3.1 (1.1–8.7)[†]	—	—
Semchuk et al. (186)	Case-control	4.0 (1.9–8.3)	—	5.1 (2.2–11.9)	—
Breteler et al. (67)	Case-control	0.8 (0.5–1.2)	1.3 (0.7–2.3)	2.9 (1.4–6.1)	1.0 (0.6–1.5)
De Michele et al. (25)	Case-control	2.3 (1.0–5.6)	—	14.6 (7.2–29.6)	—
Seidler et al. (26)	Case-control	1.3 (0.8–2.0)[‡]	—	12.6 (4.4–36.1)	8.2 (1.7–39.0)[§]
Marder et al. (75)	Case-control	—	—	2.3 (1.3–4.0)[¶]	—
de Rijk et al. (73)	Prospective follow-up	0.7 (0.3–1.7)	0.6 (0.1–2.5)	2.5 (0.9–7.3)[‖]	1.4 (0.7–3.0)[‖]

*Odds ratios (OR) with 95% confidence intervals (95% CI) in parentheses.
[†]In original paper, 95% CI was not presented. We reconstructed the 95% CI.
[‡]In original paper, exposure was categorized. The overall OR for exposure versus no exposure was kindly provided by the investigators.
[§]In original paper, data were not presented. Data were kindly provided by the investigators.
[‖]Unpublished data.
[¶]Risk of Parkinson's disease among first degree relatives of Parkinson's disease patients.

Head trauma

The notion that multiple or severe head injury can cause parkinsonism (65,66) led to the hypothesis that PD and head trauma may be etiologically related. Neither in most recent case-control studies (25,26,67–71) nor in follow-up studies from Rochester, Minnesota (72), and Rotterdam, the Netherlands (73) the relation between head trauma and the occurrence of PD could be confirmed (Table 13.2). These observations in follow-up studies make an etiologic relation between PD and head trauma unlikely.

Genetics

It has long been considered that hereditary factors may play an important role in the etiology of Parkinson's disease. Recent studies showed family aggregation, with a relative risk of around 3 for subjects with first-degree relatives with Parkinson (67,74,75), but some showed a more elevated risk (Table 13.2) (25,26). However, several twin studies initially reported very low concordance rates in twins and no differences in concordance rates between monozygotic and dizygotic twins (76–78); reappraisal of these studies showed that they were methodologically limited and far from conclusive, and their results compatible with autosomal dominant inheritance with reduced penetrance, heterogeneity, or a multifactorial etiology (79). At present, a considerable number of studies have been published describing families in which several members were affected with PD (80–84). The segregation ratios in most of these families suggest autosomal dominant inheritance with reduced penetrance.

In 1996, in one of these families linkage was shown with chromosome 4 (4q21–23) (85), and in 1997 in this and three other families a mutation in the alpha-synuclein gene was found (86). The mutation seems rare, though (87–89). A genetic heterogeneity became clear as linkage with several other genetic loci (e.g., 2p13 and 6q25.2–27) has been described recently (90,91). Several genes that on biochemical or pathophysiological grounds might be involved in PD have been evaluated in association studies. Most of these studies showed no allelic associations with PD and candidate gene polymorphisms (92–97), but associations with gene polymorphisms of monoamino oxidase B and A (MAO B, MAO A) (98,99), cytochrome P450 (CYP2D6) (62,63,100,101), N-acetyltransferase 2 (96), and the alpha-ketoglutarate dehydrogenase complex (102) have been reported. However, the most likely hypotheses regarding the etiology of Parkinson's disease at the moment are that the disease results from a genetically determined susceptibility for exogeneous toxins, from a genetically determined defect that leads to overproduction of endogeneous neurotoxins or a decreased clearing of toxic substances that normally appear in the brain, or an inherited mitochondrial dysfunction (39,61,96,103). Yet, studies on the etiology of PD exploring this interaction between genetic and environmental factors have not been performed.

Diagnosis

Neuropathologically, PD is defined by selective and excessive degeneration of pigmented neurons of the pars compacta of the substantia nigra and other brainstem ganglia, with cytoplasmic inclusions, called Lewy bodies, in the surviving neurons as the hallmark (104–106). These lesions lead to a deficiency of striatal dopamine. For the diagnosis of PD, the postmortem neuropathologic examination of the brain is generally considered to be the gold standard. For the clinical diagnosis of PD, the generally accepted prerequisite is assessment of the presence of parkinsonism, based on a combination of four typical clinical features, referred to as cardinal signs, i.e., resting tremor, bradykinesia, rigidity, and impaired postural reflexes. Various combinations of these cardinal signs have been proposed for ascertainment of the presence of parkinsonism (8,107–110), sometimes with additional requirements related to duration of symptoms, asymmetry of signs, or responsiveness to levodopa treatment. The diagnosis of PD requires that other causes of parkinsonism be excluded, such as dementia, Lewy body disease, multiple system atrophy, progressive supranuclear palsy, drug-induced parkinsonism, and vascular parkinsonism.

Prognosis

Progression

In PD, extrapyramidal signs only become clinically overt after dopaminergic cell loss of approximately 50% (41,106,111,112), and endogeneous dopamine is depleted by 80% at that moment (41,106,113). For long, the prevailing idea has been that the duration of the preclinical phase in PD is probably more than 20 years (41,60,114,115). New evidence, however, in part based on positron emission tomography scanning studies correlating in vivo the proportion of functional dopaminergic neurons with the disease duration, advocates a much shorter presymptomatic period of approximately 5 years (113,116). The rate of deterioration of nigral cells is probably most prominent and curvilinear in the preclinical or very early phase of Parkinson's disease (106,113,114,116,117). A more rapid decline may be associated with a later age of onset (118,119) (not observed by others) (120,121) with more severe symptoms at onset, especially bradykinesia and gait disturbances (119,121), and with cognitive dysfunction (121,122).

Comorbidity

A large percentage of PD patients will encounter a depression during the course of their disease. Most estimates vary around 45% (123–127), which is much higher than in the general population. Reduced serotonin in the brain of PD patients has been implicated in the etiology of depression (128,129). Low serotonin levels in PD patients could partly be attributed to concurrent neurodegeneration of serotonin pathways as a result of PD alterations in the brain (125,126,130).

Dementia, also, appears in a high frequency (around 35%) in PD patients during the course of their disease (10,131,132). In nondemented PD patients, mild cognitive changes such as visuospatial deficits, impaired executive functions, and verbal fluency may occur as well (133,134), and the latter might predict incident dementia (134). In most studies it was shown that PD patients have a two- to three-fold increased risk of dementia when compared with nonparkinsonian persons (70,131,135,136). The etiology of dementia in PD remains unsettled. PD dementia may be caused by neuropathologic lesions located in the middle part of the substantia nigra (130,137), or cortex (138,139) but concurrent Alzheimer's disease pathology may, in some instances, attribute to the dementia in PD as well (130,140–142). Neuropathologic studies on dementia in PD were small and some were possibly subject to selection bias.

Other concurrent diseases in PD, like cancer, cerebrovascular diseases, and ischemic heart diseases, have been less well established and results from studies are conflicting (132,143–148). When comparisons were made between a relatively unselected PD population and population controls, Ben-Shlomo and Marmot observed among PD patients a higher adjusted risk of dying from ischemic heart disease, cerebrovascular disease, and respiratory disease (hazard ratios were 2.3, 3.6, and 3.7, respectively) (146). Prospective follow-up studies in which the occurrence of disease is closely measured, preferably in a community-based setting, are needed to provide more evidence.

Mortality

It could be expected that the burden of concurrent diseases, like dementia and depression, will reduce the life expectancy of PD patients. Indeed, without exception a standardized mortality ratio higher than 1 was observed (16,146,148–150), ranging from 1.6 (16) to 3.4 (150). Since the beginning of the 1970s, a shift in PD mortality rates has occurred towards the older ages suggesting an increase in survival of PD patients (151–153). It still remains unclear whether this is due to levodopa treatment or better general management of PD patients. On the other hand, many studies, all based on death certificates, reported an increase in age-adjusted PD mortality rate in the last decades (151,152,154,155). These observations, however, could be readily explained by improved accuracy of death certificates or changes in certification (153), changes in diagnostic criteria, improved diagnosis, and increased awareness of PD as a prominent neurodegenerative disease in the higher ages.

Intervention

Despite several options for successful symptomatic therapy in PD, no therapy exists that can stop or reverse the neurodegenerative process that leads to PD. The initial decision in the treatment of PD is whether or not to start pharmacotherapy in the early phase of the disease. In the early 1990s, the emphasis in treatment in the early stages of the disease had shifted from symptomatic to neuroprotective drugs as the preliminary results from the DATATOP study that investigated whether in Parkinson's disease patients treatment with selegiline (an MAO B inhibitor) slowed down the progression of the disease, were promising (156). Later reports, however, suggested that it probably was not the neuroprotective effect but the symptomatic effect of selegiline that had caused the beneficial effect of selegiline (157–159). Moreover, the use of selegiline was further discredited by a report that levodopa treatment in combination with selegiline seemed to confer a higher mortality than levodopa treatment alone (160,161). Currently, selegiline's role in the treament of PD is debatable (162).

At present, levodopa is the most effective symptomatic option available. Unfortunately, it bears the risk of troublesome long-term side-effects, such as wearing-off, response fluctuations (163,164), and dyskinesias (164), which may be promoted by various factors (165,166). As low doses of levodopa and delaying the introduction of levodopa may postpone the adverse reactions to levodopa, often anticholinergic drugs, amantadine, or dopamine agonists are used for initial symptomatic treatment (164). New adjuncts, such as Catechol-o-Methyl transferase (COMT) inhibitors that increase the absorption and decrease the metabolism of levodopa, thereby stabilizing levodopa plasma levels, are promising (167–169). Longer follow-up is needed to evaluate the long-term efficacy of these drugs. Another relatively novel treatment strategy to obtain stable levodopa concentrations is continuous subcutaneous infusion of an antiparkinsonian drug (e.g., dopamine agonist) (170). However, the compliance of patients may be troublesome.

In the early 1990s, stereotactic one-sided lesions of the globus pallidus (to reduce rigidity, dykinesia, and hypokinesia), or thalamus (to reduce tremor) gained new interest when it became clear that in many parkinsonian patients in later stages of the disease the effectiveness of levodopa treatment diminishes and dyskinesia occurs. In a recent study, the latter symptom was considerably reduced in all patients who underwent posteroventral pallidotomy (171). Also, a considerable reduction of levodopa response fluctuation can be established by pallidotomy resulting in less frequent off-periods, and a 30–65% reduction of rigidity and hypokinesia (172,173). Thalamotomy has the potential to abolish the resting tremor (174). However, as the disease becomes bilateral, the contralateral side will eventually have to be lesioned as well (either thalamotomy or pallidotomy) which bears the risk of serious adverse effects such as dysarthria, impaired balance, and hemianopsy. Chronic thalamic and subthalamic stimulation by electrodes in the brain may circumvent these undesirable complications, and experience with these techniques is now accumulating (175,176).

Whether fetal dopaminergic tissue implantation (177,178) or gene therapy will be options for therapy is to be awaited.

Implications for clinical practice

Parkinson's disease is a frequent neurodegenerative disorder. Its frequency is higher than commonly thought, in particular at high age. Physicians have to be aware that the symptoms that accompany an early parkinsonian syndrome may mimic normal aging.

The disease is heterogeneous. Apart from age, smoking, and possibly also exposure to pesticides and other toxins, no distinct risk factors have been identified. Also studies on genetic factors in PD showed ambiguous results. Apart from some multiply affected families where the disease is clearly inherited as an autsomal dominant trait, it seems likely that in the majority of cases it is not only genetic factors or only environmental factors, but the interplay between genetically determined susceptibility and specific environmental factors that can lead to PD. Therefore, studies on the interaction between candidate genes and environmental factors might be more promising.

Factors that are linked to progression of the disease, and that can be avoided or modified, should be recognized and managed in a PD patient.

Eventually, insight into the etiology of PD could give clues to neuroprotective treatment and may result in effective measures to prevent this devastating disease in the elderly.

REFERENCES

1. Zhang ZX, Roman GC. Worldwide occurrence of Parkinson's disease: an updated review. *Neuroepidemiology* 1993;12:195–208.

2. Schoenberg BS, Anderson DW, Haerer AF. Prevalence of Parkinson's disease in the biracial population of Copiah County, Mississippi. *Neurology* 1985;35:841–5.

3. Morgante L, Rocca WA, Di Rosa AE, et al. Prevalence of Parkinson's disease and other types of parkinsonism: a door-to-door survey in three Sicilian municipalities. The Sicilian Neuro-

Epidemiologic Study (SNES) Group. *Neurology* 1992;42:1901–7.

4. de Rijk MC, Breteler MMB, Graveland GA, et al. Prevalence of Parkinson's disease in the elderly: the Rotterdam Study. *Neurology* 1995;45:2143–6.

5. Tison F, Dartigues JF, Dubes L, Zuber M, Alperovitch A, Henry P. Prevalence of Parkinson's disease in the elderly: a population study in Gironde, France. *Acta Neurol Scand* 1994;90:111–15.

6. Melcon MO, Anderson DW, Vergara RH, Rocca WA. Prevalence of Parkinson's disease in Junín, Buenos Aires, Argentina. *Mov Disord* 1997;12:197–205.

7. de Rijk MC, Tzourio C, Breteler MMB, et al. Prevalence of parkinsonism and Parkinson's disease in Europe: the EUROPARKINSON collaborative study. *J Neurol Neurosurg Psychiatry* 1997;62:10–15.

8. de Rijk MC, Rocca WA, Anderson DW, Melcon MO, Breteler MMB, Maraganore DM. A population perspective on diagnostic criteria for Parkinson's disease. *Neurology* 1997;48:1277–81.

9. Okada K, Kobayashi S, Tsunematsu T. Prevalence of Parkinson's disease in Izumo City, Japan. *Gerontology* 1990;36:340–4.

10. Mayeux R, Denaro J, Hemenegildo N, et al. A population-based investigation of Parkinson's disease with and without dementia. Relationship to age and gender. *Arch Neurol* 1992;49:492–7.

11. Mayeux R, Marder K, Cote LJ, et al. The frequency of idiopathic Parkinson's disease by age, ethnic group, and sex in northern Manhattan, 1988–1993. *Am J Epidemiol* 1995;142:820–7.

12. Fall PA, Axelson O, Frederiksson M, et al. Age-standardized incidence and prevalence of Parkinson's disease in a Swedish community. *J Clin Epidemiol* 1996;49:637–41.

13. Bharucha NE, Bharucha EP, Bharucha AE, Bhise AV, Schoenberg BS. Prevalence of Parkinson's disease in the Parsi community of Bombay, India. *Arch Neurol* 1988;45:1321–3.

14. Li SC, Schoenberg BS, Wang CC, et al. A prevalence survey of Parkinson's disease and other movement disorders in the People's Republic of China. *Arch Neurol* 1985;42:655–7.

15. Bennett DA, Beckett LA, Murray AM, et al. Prevalence of parkinsonian signs and associated mortality in a community population of older people. *N Engl J Med* 1996;334:71–6.

16. Rajput AH, Offord KP, Beard CM, Kurland LT. Epidemiology of parkinsonism: incidence, classification, and mortality. *Ann Neurol* 1984;16:278–82.

17. Marttila RJ, Rinne UK. Epidemiology of Parkinson's disease in Finland. *Acta Neurol Scand* 1976;53:81–102.

18. Granieri E, Carreras M, Casetta I, et al. Parkinson's disease in Ferrara, Italy, 1967 through 1987. *Arch Neurol* 1991;48:854–7.

19. de Rijk MC, Breteler MMB, Ott A, Graveland GA, van der Meché FGA, Hofman A. Incidence of Parkinson's disease in a population-based study: the Rotterdam Study [abstract]. *Neurology* 1996;46(suppl.2):A332.

20. Morens DM, Davis JW, Grandinetti A, Ross GW, Popper JS, White LR. Epidemiologic observations on Parkinson's disease: incidence and mortality in a prospective study of middle-aged men. *Neurology* 1996;46:1044–50.

21. Harada H, Nishikawa S, Takahashi K. Epidemiology of Parkinson's disease in a Japanese city. *Arch Neurol* 1983;40:151–4.

22. Gudmundsson KR. A clinical survey of parkinsonism in Iceland. *Acta Neurol Scand* 1967;33:1–61.

23. Dorn HF. Tobacco consumption and mortality from cancer and other diseases. *Public Health Rep* 1959;74:581–93.

24. Morens DM, Grandinetti A, Reed D, White LR, Ross GW. Cigarette smoking and protection from Parkinson's disease: false association or etiologic clue? *Neurology* 1995;45:1041–51.

25. De Michele G, Filla A, Volpe G, et al. Environmental and genetic risk factors in Parkinson's disease: a case-control study in southern Italy. *Mov Disord* 1996;11:17–23.

26. Seidler A, Hellenbrand W, Robra BP, et al. Possible environmental, occupational, and other etiologic factors for Parkinson's disease: a case-control study in Germany. *Neurology* 1996;46:1275–84.

27. Morens DW, Grandinetti A, Davis JW, Ross GW, White LR, Reed D. Evidence against the operation of selective mortality in explaining the association between cigarette smoking and reduced occurrence of idiopathic Parkinson's disease. *Am J Epidemiol* 1996;144:400–4.

28. de Rijk MC, Breteler MMB, van der Meché FGA, Hofman A. Smoking and the risk of Parkinson's disease: the Rotterdam Study [abstract]. *Mov Disord* 1996;11(suppl.1):156.

29. Hellenbrand W, Seidler A, Robra B-P, et al. Smoking and Parkinson's disease: results of a case-control study in Germany. *Int J Epidemiol* 1997;26:328–39.

30. Golbe LI, Cody RA, Duvoisin RC. Smoking and Parkinson's disease. Search for a dose-response relationship. *Arch Neurol* 1986;43:774–8.

31. Mayeux R, Tang MX, Marder K, Cote LJ, Stern Y. Smoking and Parkinson's disease. *Mov Disord* 1994;9:207–12.

32. Kahn HA. The Dorn study of smoking and mortality among U.S. veterans: report on eight and one-half years of observation. *Natl Cancer Inst Monogr* 1966;19:1–125.

33. Hammond EC. Smoking in relation to the death rates of one million men and women. *Natl Cancer Inst Monogr* 1966;19:127–204.

34. Doll R, Peto R. Mortality in relation to smoking: 20 years' observations on male British doctors. *BMJ* 1976;2:1525–36.

35. Doll R, Peto R, Wheatley K, Gray R, Sutherland I. Mortality in relation to smoking: 40 years' observations on male British doctors. *BMJ* 1994;309:901–11.

36. Fowler JS, Volkow ND, Wang GJ, et al. Inhibition of monoamine oxidase B in the brains of smokers. *Nature* 1996;379:733–6.

37. Langston JW, Irwin I, Langston EB, Forno LS. 1-Methyl–4-phenylpyridinium ion (MPP +): identification of a metabolite of MPTP, a toxin selective to the substantia nigra. *Neurosci Lett* 1984;48:87–92.

38. Janson AM, Fuxe K, Goldstein M. Differential effects of acute and chronic nicotine treatment on MPTP-(1-methyl-4-phenyl-1,2,3,6-tetrahydropyridine) induced degeneration of nigrostriatal dopamine neurons in the black mouse. *Clin Investig* 1992;70:232–8.

39. Landi MT, Ceroni M, Martignoni E, Bertazzi PA, Caporaso NE, Nappi G. Gene-environment interaction in parkinson's disease. The case of CYP2D6 gene polymorphism. *Adv Neurol* 1996;69:61–72.

40. Bharucha NE, Stokes L, Schoenberg BS, et al. A case-control study of twin pairs discordant

for Parkinson's disease: a search for environmental risk factors. *Neurology* 1986;36:284–8.

41. Marsden CD. Parkinson's disease. *Lancet* 1990;335:948–52.

42. Hubble JP, Koller WC. The parkinsonian personality. *Adv Neurol* 1995;65:43–8.

43. Fahn S, Cohen G. The oxidant stress hypothesis in Parkinson's disease: evidence supporting it. *Ann Neurol* 1992;32:804–12.

44. Jenner P, Dexter DT, Sian J, Schapira AH, Marsden CD. Oxidative stress as a cause of nigral cell death in Parkinson's disease and incidental Lewy body disease. *Ann Neurol* 1992;32(suppl.):S82–S87.

45. Jenner P. Oxidative damage in neurodegenerative disease. *Lancet* 1994;344:796–8.

46. Logroscino G, Marder K, Cote L, Tang M-X, Shea S, Mayeux R. Dietary lipids and antioxidants in Parkinson's disease: a population-based, case-control study. *Ann Neurol* 1996;39:89–94.

47. Golbe LI, Farrell TM, Davis PH. Case-control study of early life dietary factors in Parkinson's disease. *Arch Neurol* 1988;45:1350–3.

48. Golbe LI, Farrell TM, Davis PH. Follow-up study of early-life protective and risk factors in Parkinson's disease. *Mov Disord* 1990;5:66–70.

49. King D, Playfer JR, Roberts NB. Concentrations of vitamins A, C and E in elderly patients with Parkinson's disease. *Postgrad Med J* 1992;68:634–7.

50. de Rijk MC, Breteler MMB, den Breeijen JH, Laumer LJ, van der Meché FGA, Hofman A. Dietary antioxidants and Parkinson's disease: the Rotterdam study. *Arch Neurol* 1997;54:782–5.

51. Morens DM, Grandinetti A, Waslien CI, Park CB, Ross GW, White LR. Case-control study of idiopathic Parkinson's disease and dietary vitamin E intake. *Neurology* 1996;46:1270–4.

52. Hellenbrand W, Seidler A, Boeing H, et al. Diet and Parkinson's disease II: a possible role for the past intake of specific nutrients. Results from a self-administered food-frequency questionnaire in a case-control study. *Neurology* 1996;47:644–50.

53. The Parkinson Study Group. Effects of tocopherol and deprenyl on the progression of disability in early Parkinson's disease. The Parkinson Study Group. *N Engl J Med* 1993;328:176–83.

54. Burton GW, Ingold KU. Beta-carotene: an unusual type of lipid antioxidant. *Science* 1984;224:569–73.

55. Langston JW, Ballard P, Tetrud JW, Irwin I. Chronic Parkinsonism in humans due to a product of meperidine-analog synthesis. *Science* 1983;219:979–80.

56. Tanner CM, Langston JW. Do environmental toxins cause Parkinson's disease? A critical review. *Neurology* 1990;40:17–30.

57. Barbeau A, Roy M, Langston JW. Neurological consequence of industrial exposure to 1-methyl-4-phenyl-1,2,3,6-tetrahydropyridine [letter]. *Lancet* 1985;1:747.

58. Marder K, Logroscino G, Alfaro B, et al. Environmental risk factors for Parkinson's disease in an urban multiethnic community. *Neurology* 1998;50:279–81.

59. Langston JW, Koller WC. The next frontier in Parkinson's disease: presymptomatic detection. *Neurology* 1991;41:5–7.

60. Calne DB. Is idiopathic parkinsonism the consequence of an event or a process? *Neurology* 1994;44:5–10.

61. Barbeau A, Cloutier T, Roy M, Plasse L, Paris S, Poirier J. Ecogenetics of Parkinson's disease: 4-hydroxylation of debrisoquine. *Lancet* 1985;2:1213–16.

62. Armstrong M, Daly AK, Cholerton S, Bateman DN, Idle JR. Mutant debrisoquine hydroxylation genes in Parkinson's disease. *Lancet* 1992;339:1017–18.

63. Smith CA, Gough AC, Leigh PN, et al. Debrisoquine hydroxylase gene polymorphism and susceptibility to Parkinson's disease. *Lancet* 1992;339:1375–7.

64. DiDonato S, Zeviani M, Giovannini P, et al. Respiratory chain and mitochondrial DNA in muscle and brain in Parkinson's disease patients. *Neurology* 1993;43:2262–8.

65. Nayernouri T. Posttraumatic parkinsonism. *Surg Neurol* 1985;24:263–4.

66. Krauss JK, Wakhloo AK, Nobbe F, Trankle R, Mundinger F, Seeger W. Lesion of dentatothalamic pathways in severe post-traumatic tremor. *Neurol Res* 1995;17:409–16.

67. Breteler MMB, Tzourio C, Manubens-Bertran JM, et al. Risk factors for Parkinson's disease: a population-based case-control study (Europarkinson). *Neurology* 1995;45(suppl 4):A214.

68. Hubble JP, Cao T, Hassanein RE, Neuberger JS, Koller WC. Risk factors for Parkinson's disease. *Neurology* 1993;43:1693–7.

69. Factor SA, Sanchez-Ramos J, Weiner WJ. Trauma as an etiology of parkinsonism: a historical review of the concept. *Mov Disord* 1988;3:30–6.

70. Hofman A, Collette HJ, Bartelds AI. Incidence and risk factors of Parkinson's disease in The Netherlands. *Neuroepidemiology* 1989;8:296–9.

71. Krauss JK, Tränkle R, Kopp K-H. Post-traumatic movement disorders in survivors of severe head injury. *Neurology* 1996;47:1488–1492.

72. Williams DB, Annegers JF, Kokmen E, O'Brien PC, Kurland LT. Brain injury and neurologic sequelae: a cohort study of dementia, parkinsonism, and amyotrophic lateral sclerosis. *Neurology* 1991;41:1554–7.

73. de Rijk MC, Breteler MMB, Ott A, van der Meché FGA, Hofman A. Risk factors for Parkinson's disease: the Rotterdam Study [abstract]. *J Neurol* 1996;243(suppl.2):S8.

74. Payami H, Larsen K, Bernard S, Nutt J. Increased risk of Parkinson's disease in parents and siblings of patients. *Ann Neurol* 1994;36:659–61.

75. Marder K, Tang MX, Mejia H, et al. Risk of Parkinson's disease among first-degree relatives: a community-based study. *Neurology* 1996;47:155–60.

76. Ward CD, Duvoisin RC, Ince SE, Nutt JD, Eldridge R, Calne DB. Parkinson's disease in 65 pairs of twins and in a set of quadruplets. *Neurology* 1983;33:815–24.

77. Marsden CD. Parkinson's disease in twins [letter]. *J Neurol Neurosurg Psychiatry* 1987;50:105–6.

78. Marttila RJ, Kaprio J, Koskenvuo M, Rinne UK. Parkinson's disease in a nationwide twin cohort. *Neurology* 1988;38:1217–19.

79. Johnson WG, Hodge SE, Duvoisin R. Twin studies and the genetics of Parkinson's disease – a reappraisal. *Mov Disord* 1990;5:187–94.

80. Maraganore DM, Harding AE, Marsden CD. A clinical and genetic study of familial Parkinson's disease. *Mov Disord* 1991;6:205–11.

81. Lazzarini AM, Myers RH, Zimmerman T, Jr., et al. A clinical genetic study of Parkinson's disease: evidence for dominant transmission. *Neurology* 1994;44:499–506.

82. Golbe LI, Di Iorio G, Bonavita V, Miller DC, Duvoisin RC. A large kindred with autosomal dominant Parkinson's disease. *Ann Neurol* 1990;27:276–82.

83. Waters CH, Miller CA. Autosomal dominant Lewy body parkinsonism in a four-generation family. *Ann Neurol* 1994;35:59–64.

84. Wszolek ZK, Pfeiffer B, Fulgham JR, et al. Western Nebraska family (family D) with autosomal dominant parkinsonism. *Neurology* 1995;45:502–5.

85. Polymeropoulos MH, Higgins JJ, Golbe LI, et al. Mapping of a gene for Parkinson's disease to chromosome 4q21-q23. *Science* 1996;274:1197–9.

86. Polymeropoulos MH, Lavedan C, Leroy E, et al. Mutation in the alpha-synuclein gene identified in families with Parkinson's disease. *Science* 1997;276:2045–7.

87. Munoz E, Oliva R, Obach V, et al. Identification of Spanish familial Parkinson's disease and screening for the Ala53Thr mutation of the alpha-synuclein gene in early onset patients. *Neurosci Lett* 1997;235:57–60.

88. Chan P, Tanner CM, Jiang X, Langston JW. Failure to find the alpha-synuclein gene missense mutation (G209A) in 100 patients with younger onset Parkinson's disease. *Neurology* 1998;50:513–4.

89. Vaughan JR, Farrer MJ, Wszolek ZK, et al. Sequencing of the a-synuclein gene in a large series of cases of familial Parkinson's disease fails to reveal any further mutations. *Hum Mol Genet* 1998;7:751–753.

90. Gasser T, Muller-Myhsok B, Wszolek ZK, et al. A susceptibility locus for Parkinson's disease maps to chromosome2p13. *Nat Genet* 1998;18:262–5.

91. Matsumine H, Saito M, Shimoda-Matsubayashi S, et al. Localization of a gene for an autosomal recessive form of juvenile Parkinsonism to chromosome 6q25.2-27. *Am J Hum Genet* 1997;60:588–96.

92. Nanko S, Ueki A, Hattori M, et al. No allelic association between Parkinson's disease and dopamine D2, D3, and D4 receptor gene polymorphisms. *Am J Med Genet* 1994;54:361–4.

93. Gasser T, Wszolek ZK, Trofatter J, et al. Genetic linkage studies in autosomal dominant parkinsonism: evaluation of seven candidate genes. *Ann Neurol* 1994;36:387–96.

94. Ho SL, Kapadi AL, Ramsden DB, Williams AC. An allelic association study of monoamine oxidase B in Parkinson's disease. *Ann Neurol* 1995;37:403–5.

95. Gasser T, Müller-Myhsok B, Supala A, et al. The CYP2D6B allele is not overrepresented in a population of German patients with idiopathic Parkinson's disease. *J Neurol Neurosurg Psychiatry* 1996.

96. Bandmann O, Vaughan J, Holmans P, Marsden CD, Wood NW. Association of slow acetylator genotype for N-acetyltransferase 2 with familial Parkinson's disease. *Lancet* 1997;350:1136–9.

97. Wilhelmsen K, Mirel D, Marder K, et al. Is there a genetic susceptibility locus for Parkinson's disease on chromosome 22q13? *Ann Neurol* 1997;41:813–17.

98. Kurth JH, Kurth MC, Poduslo SE, Schwankhaus JD. Association of a monoamine oxidase B allele with Parkinson's disease. *Ann Neurol* 1993;33:368–72.

99. Hotamisligil GS, Girmen AS, Fink JS, et al. Hereditary variations in monoamine oxidase as a risk factor for Parkinson's disease. *Mov Disord* 1994;9:305–10.

100. Plante-Bordeneuve V, Taussig D, Thomas F, Ziegler M, Said G. A clinical and genetic study

of familial cases of Parkinson's disease. J Neurol Sci 1995;133:164–72.

101. Mazzetti P, Le Guern E, Bonnet AM, Vidailhet M, Brice A, Agid Y. Familial Parkinson's disease and polymorphism at the CYP2D6 locus [letter]. *J Neurol Neurosurg Psychiatry* 1994;57:871–2.

102. Kobayashi T, Matsumine H, Matuda S, Mizuno Y. Association between the gene encoding the E2 subunit of the alpha-ketoglutarate dehydrogenase complex and Parkinson's disease. *Ann Neurol* 1998;43:120–3.

103. Jenner P, Schapira AH, Marsden CD. New insights into the cause of Parkinson's disease. *Neurology* 1992;42:2241–50.

104. Hornykiewicz O, Kish SJ. Biochemical pathophysiology of Parkinson's disease. *Adv Neurol* 1987;45:19–34.

105. Gibb WR, Lees AJ. The relevance of the Lewy body to the pathogenesis of idiopathic Parkinson's disease. *J Neurol Neurosurg Psychiatry* 1988;51:745–52.

106. Fearnley JM, Lees AJ. Ageing and Parkinson's disease: substantia nigra regional selectivity. *Brain* 1991;114:2283–301.

107. Hughes AJ, Ben-Shlomo Y, Daniel SE, Lees AJ. What features improve the accuracy of clinical diagnosis in Parkinson's disease: a clinicopathologic study. *Neurology* 1992;42:1142–6.

108. Calne DB, Snow BJ, Lee C. Criteria for diagnosing Parkinson's disease. *Ann Neurol* 1992;32:S125–7.

109. Koller WC. How accurately can Parkinson's disease be diagnosed? *Neurology* 1992;42:6–16.

110. Rajput AH, Rozdilsky B, Rajput A. Accuracy of clinical diagnosis in parkinsonism – a prospective study. *Can J Neurol Sci* 1991;18:275–8.

111. Leenders KL, Salmon EP, Tyrrell P, et al. The nigrostriatal dopaminergic system assessed in vivo by positron emission tomography in healthy volunteer subjects and patients with Parkinson's disease. *Arch Neurol* 1990;47:1290–8.

112. Morrish PK, Sawle GV, Brooks DJ. The rate of progression of Parkinson's disease. A longitudinal [18F]DOPA PET study. *Adv Neurol* 1996;69:427–31.

113. Morrish PK, Sawle GV, Brooks DJ. Clinical and [18F] dopa PET findings in early Parkinson's disease. *J Neurol Neurosurg Psychiatry* 1995;59:597–600.

114. Scherman D, Desnos C, Darchen F, Pollak P, Javoy-Agid F, Agid Y. Striatal dopamine deficiency in Parkinson's disease: role of aging. *Ann Neurol* 1989;26:551–7.

115. Koller WC. When does Parkinson's disease begin? *Neurology* 1992;42:27–31.

116. Leenders KL, Antonini A. PET ^{18}F-fluorodopa uptake and disease progression in Parkinson's disease [abstract]. *Neurology* 1995;45(suppl.4):A220.

117. Lee CS, Schulzer M, Mak EK, et al. Clinical observations on the rate of progression of idiopathic parkinsonism. *Brain* 1994;117:501–7.

118. Goetz CG, Tanner CM, Stebbins GT, Buchman AS. Risk factors for progression in Parkinson's disease. *Neurology* 1988;38:1841–4.

119. Jankovic J, McDermott M, Carter J, et al. Variable expression of Parkinson's disease: a base-line analysis of the DATATOP cohort. The Parkinson Study Group. *Neurology* 1990;40:1529–34.

120. Gibb WR, Lees AJ. A comparison of clinical and pathological features of young- and old-onset Parkinson's disease. *Neurology* 1988;38:1402–6.

121. McDermott MP, Jankovic J, Carter J, et al. Factors predictive of the need for levodopa therapy in early, untreated Parkinson's disease. The Parkinson Study Group. *Arch Neurol* 1995;52:565–70.

122. Uitti RJ, Rajput AH, Ahlskog JE, et al. Amantadine treatment is an independent predictor of improved survival in Parkinson's disease. *Neurology* 1996;46:1551–6.

123. Santamaria J, Tolosa E, Valles A. Parkinson's disease with depression: a possible subgroup of idiopathic parkinsonism. *Neurology* 1986;36:1130–3.

124. Mayeux R, Stern Y, Williams JB, Cote L, Frantz A, Dyrenfurth I. Clinical and biochemical features of depression in Parkinson's disease. *Am J Psychiatry* 1986;143:756–9.

125. Mayeux R. Depression in the patient with Parkinson's disease. *J Clin Psychiatry* 1990.

126. Cummings JL. Depression and Parkinson's disease: a review. *Am J Psychiatry* 1992;149:443–54.

127. Dooneief G, Mirabello E, Bell K, Marder K, Stern Y, Mayeux R. An estimate of the incidence of depression in idiopathic Parkinson's disease. *Arch Neurol* 1992;49:305–7.

128. Mayeux R, Stern Y, Cote L, Williams JB. Altered serotonin metabolism in depressed patients with parkinson's disease. *Neurology* 1984;34:642–6.

129. McCance KE, Marek KL, Price LH. Serotonergic dysfunction in depression associated with Parkinson's disease. *Neurology* 1992;42:1813–4.

130. Paulus W, Jellinger K. The neuropathologic basis of different clinical subgroups of Parkinson's disease. *J Neuropathol Exp Neurol* 1991;50:743–55.

131. Marder K, Tang MX, Cote L, Stern Y, Mayeux R. The frequency and associated risk factors for dementia in patients with Parkinson's disease. *Arch Neurol* 1995;52:695–701.

132. Di Rocco A, Molinari SP, Kollmeier B, Yahr MD. Parkinson's disease: progression and mortality in the L-DOPA era. *Adv Neurol* 1996;69:3–11.

133. Stern Y, Richards M, Sano M, Mayeux R. Comparison of cognitive changes in patients with Alzheimer's and Parkinson's disease. *Arch Neurol* 1993;50:1040–5.

134. Jacobs DM, Marder K, Cote LJ, Sano M, Stern Y, Mayeux R. Neuropsychological characteristics of preclinical dementia in Parkinson's disease. *Neurology* 1995;45:1691–6.

135. Mayeux R, Stern Y, Rosenstein R, et al. An estimate of the prevalence of dementia in idiopathic Parkinson's disease. *Arch Neurol* 1988;45:260–2.

136. Breteler MM, de Groot RR, van Romunde LK, Hofman A. Risk of dementia in patients with Parkinson's disease, epilepsy, and severe head trauma: a register-based follow-up study. *Am J Epidemiol* 1995;142:1300–5.

137. Rinne JO, Rummukainen J, Paljarvi L, Rinne UK. Dementia in Parkinson's disease is related to neuronal loss in the medial substantia nigra. *Ann Neurol* 1989;26:47–50.

138. Jellinger K, Braak H, Braak E, Fischer P. Alzheimer lesions in the entorhinal region and isocortex in Parkinson's and Alzheimer's diseases. *Ann N Y Acad Sci* 1991;640:203–9.

139. Vermersch P, Delacourte A, Javoy-Agid F, Hauw JJ, Agid Y. Dementia in Parkinson's disease: biochemical evidence for cortical involvement using the immunodetection of abnormal Tau proteins. *Ann Neurol* 1993;33:445–50.

140. Boller F, Mizutani T, Roessmann U, Gambetti P. Parkinson disease, dementia, and Alzheimer disease: clinicopathological correlations. *Ann Neurol* 1980;7:329–35.

141. Whitehouse PJ, Hedreen JC, White CD, Price DL. Basal forebrain neurons in the dementia of Parkinson disease. *Ann Neurol* 1983;13:243–8.

142. Bancher C, Braak H, Fischer P, Jellinger KA. Neuropathological staging of Alzheimer lesions and intellectual status in Alzheimer's and Parkinson's disease patients. *Neurosci Lett* 1993;162:179–82.

143. Jansson B, Jankovic J. Low cancer rates among patients with Parkinson's disease. *Ann Neurol* 1985;17:505–9.

144. Barbeau A, Roy M, Cloutier T. Smoking, cancer, and Parkinson's disease. *Ann Neurol* 1986;20:105–6.

145. Gorell JM, Johnson CC, Rybicki BA. Parkinson's disease and its comorbid disorders: an analysis of Michigan mortality data, 1970 to 1990. *Neurology* 1994;44:1865–8.

146. Ben-Shlomo Y, Marmot MG. Survival and cause of death in a cohort of patients with parkinsonism: possible clues to aetiology? *J Neurol Neurosurg Psychiatry* 1995;58:293–9.

147. Struck LK, Rodnitzky RL, Dobson JK. Stroke and its modification in Parkinson's disease. *Stroke* 1990;21:1395–9.

148. Wermuth L, Stenager EN, Stenager E, Boldsen J. Mortality in patients with Parkinson's disease. *Acta Neurol Scand* 1995;92:55–8.

149. Diamond SG, Markham CH, Hoehn MM, McDowell FH, Muenter MD. An examination of male-female differences in progression and mortality of Parkinson's disease. *Neurology* 1990;40:763–6.

150. Tison F, Letenneur L, Djossou F, Dartigues JF. Further evidence of increased risk of mortality of Parkinson's disease [letter]. *J Neurol Neurosurg Psychiatry* 1996;60:592–3.

151. Kurtzke JF, Murphy FM. The changing patterns of death rates in parkinsonism. Neurology 1990;40:42–9.

152. Chio A, Magnani C, Tolardo G, Schiffer D. Parkinson's disease mortality in Italy, 1951 through 1987. Analysis of an increasing trend. *Arch Neurol* 1993;50:149–53.

153. Clarke CE. Mortality from Parkinson's disease in England and Wales 1921–89. *J Neurol Neurosurg Psychiatry* 1993;56:690–3.

154. Vanacore N, Bonifati V, Bellatreccia A, Edito F, Meco G. Mortality rates for Parkinson's disease and parkinsonism in Italy (1969–1987). *Neuroepidemiology* 1992;11:65–73.

155. Chio A, Magnani C, Schiffer D. The increase of Parkinson's disease mortality could be due to a cohort effect. *Acta Neurol Scand* 1995;92:113–5.

156. The Parkinson Study Group. Effect of deprenyl on the progression of disability in early Parkinson's disease. The Parkinson Study Group. *N Engl J Med* 1989;321:1364–71.

157. Ward CD. Does selegiline delay progression of Parkinson's disease? A critical re-evaluation of the DATATOP study. *J Neurol Neurosurg Psychiatry* 1994;57:217–20.

158. Brannan T, Yahr MD. Comparative study of selegiline plus l-dopa-carbidopa versus l-dopa-carbidopa alone in the treatment of parkinson's disease. *Ann Neurol* 1995;37:95–98.

159. Calne DB. Selegiline in Parkinson's disease [editorial]. *BMJ* 1995;311:1583–4.

160. Lees AJ. Comparison of therapeutic effects and mortality data of levodopa and levodopa combined with selegiline in patients with early, mild Parkinson's disease. Parkinson's Disease Research Group of the United Kingdom. *BMJ* 1995;311:1602–7.

161. Ben-Shlomo Y, Churchyard A, Head J, et al. Investigation by Parkinson's disease Research Group of United Kingdom into excess mortality seen with combined levodopa selegiline treatment in patients with early, mild Parkinson's disease: further results of randomised trial and confidential inquiry. *BMJ* 1998;316:1191–6.

162. Breteler MMB. Selegiline, or the problem of early termination of clinical trials. *BMJ* 1998;316:1182–3.

163. Roos RA, Vredevoogd CB, van der Velde EA. Response fluctuations in Parkinson's disease. *Neurology* 1990;40:1344–6.

164. Marsden CD. Parkinson's disease. *J Neurol Neurosurg Psychiatry* 1994;57:672–81.

165. Horstink MW, Zijlmans JC, Pasman JW, Berger HJ, Korten JJ, van 't Hof MA. Which risk factors predict the levodopa response in fluctuating Parkinson's disease? *Ann Neurol* 1990;27:537–43.

166. Horstink MW, Zijlmans JC, Pasman JW, Berger HJ, van't Hof MA. Severity of Parkinson's disease is a risk factor for peak-dose dyskinesia. *J Neurol Neurosurg Psychiatry* 1990;53:224–6.

167. Kurth MC, Adler CH, Hilaire MS, et al. Tolcapone improves motor function and reduces levodopa requirement in patients with Parkinson's disease experiencing motor fluctuations: a multicenter, double-blind, randomized, placebo-controlled trial. Tolcapone Fluctuator Study Group I. *Neurology* 1997;48:81–7.

168. Ruottinen HM, Rinne UK. A double-blind pharmacokinetic and clinical dose-response study of entacapone as an adjuvant to levodopa therapy in advanced Parkinson's disease. *Clin Neuropharmacol* 1996;19:283–96.

169. Waters CH, Kurth M, Bailey P, et al. Tolcapone in stable Parkinson's disease: efficacy and safety of long-term treatment. The Tolcapone Stable Study Group. *Neurology* 1997;49:665–71.

170. Baronti F, Mouradian MM, Davis TL, et al. Continuous lisuride effects on central dopaminergic mechanisms in Parkinson's disease. *Ann Neurol* 1992;32:776–81.

171. Johansson F, Malm J, Nordh E, Hariz M. Usefulness of pallidotomy in advanced Parkinson's disease. *J Neurol Neurosurg Psychiatry* 1997;62:125–32.

172. Lozano AM, Lang AE, Galvez-Jimenez N, et al. Effect of GPi pallidotomy on motor function in Parkinson's disease. *Lancet* 1995;346:1383–7.

173. Dogali M, Fazzini E, Kolodny E, et al. Stereotactic ventral pallidotomy for Parkinson's disease. *Neurology* 1995;45:753–61.

174. Jankovic J, Cardoso F, Grossman RG, Hamilton WJ. Outcome after stereotactic thalamotomy for parkinsonian, essential, and other types of tremor. *Neurosurgery* 1995;37:680–6.

175. Benabid AL, Pollak P, Gervason C, et al. Long-term suppression of tremor by chronic stimulation of the ventral intermediate thalamic nucleus. *Lancet* 1991;337:403–6.

176. Limousin P, Pollak P, Benazzouz A, et al. Effect of parkinsonian signs and symptoms of bilateral subthalamic nucleus stimulation. *Lancet* 1995;345:91–5.

177. Madrazo I, Leon V, Torres C, et al. Transplantation of fetal substantia nigra and adrenal medulla to the caudate nucleus in two patients with Parkinson's disease [letter]. *N Engl J Med* 1988;318:51.

178. Lindvall O, Rehncrona S, Brundin P, et al. Human fetal dopamine neurons grafted into the striatum in two patients with severe Parkinson's disease. A detailed account of methodology and a 6-month follow-up. *Arch Neurol* 1989;46:615–31.

179. Ho SC, Woo J, Lee CM. Epidemiologic study of Parkinson's disease in Hong Kong. *Neurology* 1989;39:1314–8.

180. Tanner CM, Chen B, Wang W, et al. Environmental factors and Parkinson's disease: a case-control study in China. *Neurology* 1989;39:660–4.

181. Koller W, Vetere-Overfield B, Gray C, et al. Environmental risk factors in Parkinson's disease. *Neurology* 1990;40:1218–21.

182. Wong GF, Gray CS, Hassanein RS, Koller WC. Environmental risk factors in siblings with Parkinson's disease. *Arch Neurol* 1991;48:287–9.

183. Stern M, Dulaney E, Gruber SB, et al. The epidemiology of Parkinson's disease. A case-control study of young-onset and old-onset patients. *Arch Neurol* 1991;48:903–7.

184. Semchuk KM, Love EJ, Lee RG. Parkinson's disease and exposure to rural environmental factors: a population based case-control study. *Can J Neurol Sci* 1991;18:279–86.

185. Semchuk KM, Love EJ, Lee RG. Parkinson's disease and exposure to agricultural work and pesticide chemicals. *Neurology* 1992;42:1328–35.

186. Semchuk KM, Love EJ, Lee RG. Parkinson's disease: a test of the multifactorial etiologic hypothesis. *Neurology* 1993;43:1173–80.

187. Stern MB. Head trauma as a risk factor for Parkinson's disease. *Mov Disord* 1991;6:95–7.

188. Factor SA, Weiner WJ. Prior history of head trauma in Parkinson's disease. *Mov Disord* 1991;6:225–9.

14

Multiple sclerosis

A. Alpérovitch

Introduction

A large part of neurological disabilities of the young adult population of developed countries is due to multiple sclerosis. The number of persons affected by MS is at least 250 000 in the United States (1) and of the same order in the European Union, this latter estimate being based on numerous studies conducted in individual European countries (2). With few exceptions, onset of MS occurs between 15 and 50 years, with a marked peak between 25 and 35 years (3). The disease is more frequent in women than in men; the female/male ratio ranges from 1.5 to 2.0.

Macroscopically, the pathology of MS is characterized by lesions widely distributed in the white matter of the brain and spinal cord. Microscopic examination of the lesions shows the typical breakdown of the myelin sheath. The MS lesions have a perivenous distribution. They contain macrophages and lymphocytes, and small amounts of myelin basic protein.

All neurological functions are affected by MS; subsequent disabilities include assistance required for walking, bladder dysfunction, loss of visual acuity. Until now, no treatment has a definitively established durable effect on disease course.

This short chapter will not be an extensive review on MS. It will focus on the most prominent features of the etiology, natural history, and treatment of the disease.

Etiology

There is strong evidence that MS is an immune disease, but its cause and pathogenesis are unknown. However, hundreds of epidemiological studies on MS prevalence which have been conducted throughout the world (approximately 200 were recorded as early as 1980) (4) provide evidence that the disease involves the interplay of genetic susceptibility factors and environmental exposures, possibly to infectious agents.

Studies show geographical differences in MS frequency, the disease being more common in northern Europe, North America and Australia than in Asia (including Japan), Africa and South America. Prevalence of MS is higher than 40 cases per 100 000 in most of the former countries (reaching 120 cases per 100 000 in some northern European areas) and lower than 20 in the latter ones. The overall geographical distribution of MS suggests a latitudinal north–south gradient from the equator. However, different prevalences have been reported in regions at similar latitudes. So, MS prevalence is higher in Italy or Sardinia than in Spain, and also higher in Orkney and Shetlands than in north-east Scotland (see (5) for review).

The geographical pattern of MS prevalence can be explained by either genetic background, or by environment, or by their synergy. Two types of study, migrant studies and twin studies, are particularly appropriate for investigating this issue. Studies have been conducted in migrants to South Africa (6), to Israel (7), to the UK (8) and within the United States (9). They suggested that younger migrants tend to adopt the MS frequency of the indigenous population. This trend has been reported for migration to and from both high and low MS prevalence countries. Studies suggested also that age at migration modulated the risk of MS, older migrants keeping the risk of their native country. However, migrant studies were based on small numbers and had important methodological weaknesses (10) which made their results not very reliable.

Studies of concordance for MS in twins conducted in Canadian (11,12) and in British (13) populations showed a significantly higher clinical concordance rate in monozygotic (25% of concordant pairs) compared with dizygotic twins (3%). In contrast, a French study found similar concordance rates in monozygotic and dizygotic pairs (5%) (14). Concordance rates were higher, both in monozygotic and dizygotic pairs, when magnetic resonance imaging was used to assess disease status (14,15). Thus, twin studies indicated that genetic background plays a significant role in MS etiology. However, they indicated also that having the susceptible genetic background does not automatically lead to MS development. About 75% of monozygotic cotwins remain unaffected, suggesting that environmental exposures are required for disease development.

In summary, there is almost no doubt that an interplay between environmental exposures and genetic background is involved in MS pathogenesis. But two schools of thought disagree about the nature – environmental or genetic – of the primary etiological determinant (16). This controversy will probably continue as long as the search for definite environmental or genetic causative factor(s) remains unsuccessful.

Concerning environment, epidemiologic and clinical studies provide support for the possible role of infections, particularly of viral infections. Adams and Imigawa (17) were the first to report that measles antibody titres were higher in the sera of MS patients compared with controls (17). Since then, numerous case-control studies have established that MS patients tend to have elevated antibody titres for a wide variety of viruses (18). Interestingly, high antibody titres against measles virus and canine distemper virus, two viruses belonging to the same subgroup of the paramyxoviruses, have been frequently reported compared to other types of virus. On the other hand, age of infections in childhood is somewhat older in MS patients than in controls. These findings, among others, support the appealing but unproved hypothesis that MS may be an age-dependent host-immune response to childhood infections (19). This hypothesis is compatible with the geographic pattern of MS frequency (MS is rare where childhood infections occur at an early age) and with the findings of migrant studies. Basic research on maturation of the immune system and on experimental allergic encephalomyelitis, which is an animal model for studying demyelinating diseases of the CNS, provides biological arguments for an age-dependent immune mechanism.

In addition to studies on common classical viruses, the possible role of a retrovirus in MS has been investigated by several groups; recent observations have given renewal to this hypothesis (20). The role of an infectious agent might also explain the occurrence of foci, clusters, or epidemics of MS which have been reported from time to time, in the past and very recently (21,22). Even if some of these clusters were real (5), none has so far substantially contributed to a better understanding of the etiology of MS.

Concerning genetic susceptibility, attempts to identify the relevant genetic loci have been disappointing so far. Numerous case-control studies have shown HLA class II associations with MS. This association was found both in early studies using HLA serological specificities and later ones using DNA-based typing methods (23). In most populations, in particular in northern European populations and in those of northern European ancestry (24), the relative risk of MS is higher (× 4) in individuals with a common caucasian DR2 haplotype. The increased risk of HLA-DR2 individuals might contribute to explain the north–south gradient of MS in Europe. Other HLA class II associations with MS are controversial and studies detecting no association suffer from methodological weaknesses (25). DNA sequencing showed no abnormality of HLA class II alleles of MS patients compared with controls (26). At the present time, there are still two indistinguishable explanations for the association between HLA class II and MS: either the HLA-class region contains a disease susceptibility gene, or this putative gene is a non-HLA gene linked to the DR2 haplotype. Studies on the association between T-cell receptor genes, immunoglobulin genes or myelin basic protein genes and MS led to negative or conflicting results (25).

In addition to association studies, linkage studies in multiplex families have been conducted to identify genetic loci involved in susceptibility to MS. About 10 to 15% of MS patients report a family history of MS and studies show that first-degree relatives of MS patients have a 3–5 times increased risk of developing the disease (27). Linkage genome screening has been completed in three samples of multiplex families. The three genome screens have confirmed the importance of the HLA region but have not provided convincing evidence that any other region is involved in susceptibility to MS (28).

Diagnosis

Up to now, there is no diagnostic test for MS and the diagnosis remains mainly based on clinical data. In neurological practice, the MS diagnostic investigation aims to establish that the patient has at least two separate central nervous system lesions and that he or she has presented two separate episodes of worsening (dissemination in space and time). The different sets of criteria that have been proposed for research purposes are built from the same diagnostic approach of MS as that used in clinical practice. But diagnostic guidelines distinguish different levels of evidence for dissemination in space and time, allowing to define diagnostic categories with different levels of certainty (definite MS, probable MS, risk of or possible MS). The diagnostic criteria that have been proposed by Schumacher et al. (29) and Poser et al. (30) have been used extensively in epidemiological studies and clinical trials. More stringent diagnostic criteria have been proposed for genetic studies on MS, in particular for research involving multiply affected families (31).

The presence of signs or symptoms reflecting two separate CNS lesions is mainly elicited from neurological examination, anamnestic investigation and, in many instances, follow-up. Supportive data can also be obtained by MRI, evoked potentials, or cerebrospinal fluid examination. Magnetic resonance imaging and evoked potentials can be used to document a second lesion when only one abnormality has been found by clinical examination. Cerebrospinal fluid examination shows increased IgG synthesis and oligoclonal banding. Cerebrospinal fluid abnormalities are required to meet the Poser's criteria for laboratory-supported definite MS (2), while they have very little weight in the most recent diagnostic guidelines (31).

Criteria for defining different levels of evidence for MS from MRI are also available (32). Follow-up studies of patients in whom MS was suspected show that about 50% of those with MRI strongly suggestive of MS developed clinically definite MS within 2 years, as compared with 40% when MS is supported from other paraclinical tests (33).

The diagnosis of MS is considered as difficult to make. As compared with autopsy, about 90% of MS diagnoses made by neurologists are accurate (34), the diagnostic accuracy rate reaching 95% for clinically definite MS (35). It is likely that these rates are higher than accuracy of MS diagnosis in prevalence studies in which diagnosis cannot rely on follow-up data.

Natural history and prognosis

There are two main types of MS course, relapsing–remitting MS and progressive MS (the latter course being either primary progressive from onset or secondary progressive) which have been described in many studies (see (36) and (37) for review). More than 75% of MS are relapsing–remitting at onset, this type of course being significantly more frequent in women than in men. The Expanded Disability Status Scale (EDSS) which was devised by Kurtzke (38) to evaluate neurological impairment in MS is widely used to describe disease progression in MS patients. The EDSS ranges from 0 (no impairment) to 9 (death due to MS). From EDSS step 5, disability is severe enough to impair full daily activities and assistance to walk is required from step 6. Cross-sectional studies of prevalent MS cases indicate that 50 to 60% of MS patients are fairly disabled (EDSS <5) (38).

All studies on the natural history of MS show that the type of course at onset is the most important prognostic factor. In a recent cohort study, the median time to reach EDSS 6 was approximately 6 years for patients with primary progressive MS and 20 years for those with relapsing–remitting MS. At 25 years from onset, a high proportion of MS patients (<60%) have progressive MS (37). But it is likely that patients with active MS are overrepresented and that patients with stable state are underrepresented in most of the available studies which have been conducted in hospital or clinics.

Apart from the type of MS course, other clinical or biological factors are of little prognostic value. Most studies conclude that male gender, older age at disease onset, and incomplete remission after the first bout are associated with a poorer prognosis. The prognostic significance of the type of symptoms at onset is controversial, but many studies have found that patients with optic neuritis have a better prognosis. Overall, these factors explain only a small part of the variability of MS course, which remains unpredictable at the individual level.

The effect of pregnancy on MS course has been discussed. It is now well established that the relapse rate decreases during pregnancy and increases in the first three months after delivery. But, overall, pregnancy does not appear to influence subsequent disease progression (39).

All studies on life expectancy of patients with MS have major methodological weaknesses. Early studies suggested that survival after MS onset (mean age at onset: 30 years) was in the order of 30 to 40 years (40,41). In a more recent

Canadian study comparing a sample of patients attending MS clinics with an insured population, the overall life expectancy of MS patients was reduced by 6 to 7 years (42).

Intervention

Interventions in MS aim to reduce duration and severity of exacerbations, to alter the natural history of the disease, mainly by reducing the relapse rate, or to treat the consequences of neurological disorders including spasticity, chronic pain, or bowel and bladder dysfunction. These symptomatic treatments are of major importance for improving quality of life of MS patients, but very few have been rigorously evaluated. ACTH and corticosteroids are frequently used for treating MS attacks. It has been shown that these drugs reduce duration of exacerbations (43) but it has not definitively been shown, however, that they have a significant effect on the degree of recovery (see (44) for review).

Clinical trials aiming to alter MS progression involve a number of specific methodological difficulties, in addition to those encountered in other therapies (45). Specific difficulties relate to unpredictable disease course and to the absence of any intermediate marker of the disease process strongly correlated to the clinical course. The therapeutic effect is generally assessed by comparing changes in EDSS and/or number of attacks in the placebo group and the treated group. In other clinical trials, the time required for a one step increase on the EDSS, or the time free of attack are used as the main endpoints. Recent therapeutic trials include MRI at entry and exit. Rate of formation of new lesions, or overall measurement of the area of abnormalities, are used as additional criteria for assessing the effects of treatment (46). All these measurements are subject to errors or biases which may affect the power and the reliability of the trial (47).

Most of the therapies which have been investigated for altering the natural progression of MS were directed toward an immunological process (48). Overall, there is currently no treatment for which it is established that benefits are durable and long-term outweigh side-effects. This applies to classical treatment such as azathioprine (49) and to more recent therapeutic approaches with interferon beta (50,51).

Implications for clinical practice

Although MS is one of the main causes of neurological disabilities of young adults living in developed countries, the absolute frequency of the disease is low. Hence, general practitioners follow very few MS patients; even a neurologist, apart from those working in MS clinics, would have in charge a small number of MS patients.

In an emotional context, practitioners are confronted by patients' questions and fears about prognosis, treatment, pregnancy, and risk for offspring.

Although the possible severity of the disease cannot be hidden from patients, epidemiological studies allow some cheering information to be given. MS has no major effect on life expectancy. A large proportion of MS patients have a moderately severe disease course, the majority of those with relapsing–remitting MS being able to maintain full daily life activities for many years. Pregnancy does not influence disease course. The absolute risk of MS in offspring is very low, except in rare multiplex families.

It is distressing for patients to know that no treatment has a definitively established durable effect on MS course. This has two major implications for clinical practice. First, practitioners should warn patients against false claims of cure based on inadequate studies and discourage patients from participating in nonrandomized, nonblinded, nonplacebo controlled studies (17). They should however encourage patients to enter in well designed trials which are the only way to establish whether a therapy is effective in MS.

REFERENCES

1. Anderson DW, Ellenberg JH, Leventhal CM, Reingold SC, Rodriguez M, Silberberg DH. Revised estimate of the prevalence of multiple sclerosis in the United States. *Ann Neurol* 1992;31:333–6.

2. Acheson ED. The epidemiology of multiple sclerosis. In Matthews WB (Ed.). *McAlpine's Multiple Sclerosis.* Edinburgh: Churchill Livingstone, 1985:3–46.

3. Weinshenker BG, Ebers GC. The natural history of multiple sclerosis. *Can J Neurol Sci* 1987;14:255–61.

4. Kurtzke JF. Epidemiologic contributions to multiple sclerosis: an overview. *Neurology* 1980;30:61–79.

5. Sadovnick AD, Ebers GC. Epidemiology of multiple sclerosis: a critical overview. *Can J Neurol Sci* 1993;20:17–29.

6. Dean G, Kurtzke JF. On the risk of multiple sclerosis according to age at immigration to South Africa. *BMJ* 1971;3:725–9.

7. Alter M, Kahana E, Loewenson R. Migration and risk of multiple sclerosis. *Neurology* 1978;28:1089–93.

8. Elian M, Nightingale S, Dean G. Multiple sclerosis among United Kingdom-born children of immigrants from the Indian subcontinent, Africa and the West Indies. *J Neurol Neurosurg Psychiatry* 1990;53:906–11.

9. Detels R, Visscher BR, Haile RW, Malmgren RM, Dudley JP, Coulson AH. Multiple sclerosis and age at migration. *Am J Epid* 1978;108:386–93.

10. Delasnerie-Lauprêtre N, Alpérovitch A. Migration and age at onset of multiple sclerosis: some pitfalls of migrant studies. *Acta Neurol Scand* 1992;85:408–11.

11. Ebers GC, Bulman DE, Sadovnick AD, et al. A population-based study of multiple sclerosis in twins. *N Engl J Med* 1986;315:1638–42.

12. Sadovnick AD, Armstrong H, Rice GPA, et al. A population-based study of multiple sclerosis in twins: update. *Ann Neurol* 1992;33:281–5.

13. Mumford C, Wood N, Kellar-Wood H, et al. The British Isles survey of multiple sclerosis in twins. *Neurology* 1994;44:11–15.

14. French Research Group on Multiple Sclerosis. Multiple sclerosis in 54 twinships: concordance rate is independent of zygosity. *Ann Neurol* 1992;32:724–7.

15. Thorpe J, Mumford CJ, Miller DH, et al. The British Isles study of multiple sclerosis in twins; magnetic resonance imaging. *J Neurol Neurosurg Psychiatry* 1994;57:491–6.

16. Weinshenker BG. Seeking the cause of multiple sclerosis. *Epidemiology* 1993;4:393–4.

17. Adams JM, Imagawa DT. Measles antibodies in multiple sclerosis. *Proc Soc Exp Biol Med* 1962;3:562–6.

18. Cook SD, Dowling PC. Multiple sclerosis and viruses: an overview. *Neurology* 1980;30:80–91.

19. Alter M, Zhen-xin Z, Davanipour Z, Sobel E, et al. Multiple sclerosis and childhood infections. *Neurology* 1986;36:1386–9.

20. Rudge P. Does a retrovirally encoded superantigen cause multiple sclerosis? *J Neurol Neurosurg Psychiatry* 1991;54:853–5.

21. Kurtzke JF, Hyllested K. Validity of the epidemics of multiple sclerosis in the Faröe Islands. *Neuroepidemiology* 1988:190–227.

22. Haahr S, Munch M, Christensen T, Moller-Larsen A, Hvas J. Cluster of multiple sclerosis patients from a Danish community. *Lancet* 1997;349:923.

23. Compson A, Sadovnick AD. Epidemiology and genetics of multiple sclerosis. *Curr Opin Neurol Neurosurg* 1992;5:175–81.

24. Page WF, Kurtzke JF, Murphy FM, Norman JE. Epidemiology of multiple sclerosis in U.S. veterans: V. Ancestry and the risk of multiple sclerosis. *Ann Neurol* 1993;33:632–9.

25. Haegert DG, Marrosu MG. Genetic susceptibility to multiple sclerosis. *Ann Neurol* 1994;36(S2):S204–S210.

26. Cowan EP, Pierce ML, McFarland HF, McFarlin DE. HLA-DR and DQ allelic sequences in multiple sclerosis patients are identical to those found in the general population. *Hum Immunol* 1991;32:203–10.

27. Sadovnick AD, Baird PA, Ward RA. Multiple sclerosis: updated risks for relatives. *Am J Med Genet* 1988;29:533–41.

28. Sawcer S, Goodfellow PN, Compston A. The genetic analysis of multiple sclerosis. *Trends Genet* 1997;13:234–9.

29. Schumacher GA, Beebe GW, Kibler RF, et al. Problems of experimental trials of therapy in multiple sclerosis. *Ann NY Acad Sci* 1965;122:552–68.

30. Poser CM, Paty DW, Scheinberg L, et al. New diagnostic criteria for multiple sclerosis: guidelines for research protocols. *Ann Neurol* 1983;13:227–31.

31. Goodkin DE, Doolittle TH, Hauser SS, Ransohoff RM, Roses AD, Rudick RA. Diagnostic criteria for multiple sclerosis research involving multiply affected families. *Arch Neurol* 1991;48:805–7.

32. Paty DW, Asbury AK, Herndon RM, et al. Use of magnetic resonance imaging in the diagnosis of multiple sclerosis: policy statement. *Neurology* 1986;36:1575.

33. Lee KH, Hashimoto SA, Hooge JP, et al. Magnetic resonance imaging of the head in the diagnosis of multiple sclerosis: a prospective 2-year follow-up with comparison of clinical evaluation, evoked potentials, oligoclonal banding, and CT. *Neurology* 1991;41:657–60.

34. Herndon RM, Brooks B. Misdiagnosis of multiple sclerosis. *Semin Neurol* 1985;5:94–8.

35. Kurtzke JF. Multiple sclerosis: what's in a name? *Neurology* 1988;38:309–14.

36. Swanson JW. Multiple sclerosis: update in diagnosis and review of prognostic factors. *Mayo Clin Proc* 1989;64:577–86.

37. Runmaker B, Andersen O. Prognostic factors in a multiple sclerosis incidence cohort with twenty-five years of follow-up. *Brain* 1993;116:117–34.

38. Kurtzke JF. Rating neurologic impairment in multiple sclerosis: an expanded disability status scale (EDSS). *Neurology* 1983;33:1444–52.

39. Roullet E, Verdier-Taillefer MH, Amarenco P, Gharbi G, Alpérovitch A, Marteau R. Pregnancy and multiple sclerosis: a longitudinal study of 125 remittent patients. *J Neurol Neurosurg Psychiatry* 1993;56:1062–5.

40. Percy AK, Nobrega F, Okazaki H, Glattre E, Kurland LT. Multiple sclerosis in Rochester, Minnesota: a 60-year appraisal. *Arch Neurol* 1971;25:105–11.

41. Kurtzke JF, Beebe GW, Nagler B, Nefzger MD, Auth TL, Kurland LT. Studies on the natural history of multiple sclerosis. V. Long-term survival in young men. *Arch Neurol* 1970;22:215–25.

42. Sadovnick AD, Ebers GC, Wilson RW, Paty DW. Life expectancy in patients attending multiple sclerosis clinics. *Neurology* 1992;42:991–4.

43. Troiano R, Cook SD, Dowling PC. Steroid therapy in multiple sclerosis. Point of view. *Arch Neurol* 1987;44:803–7.

44. Noseworthy JH. Therapeutics of multiple sclerosis. *Clin Neuropharm* 1991;14:49–61.

45. Goodin DS. The use of immunosuppressive agents in the treatment of multiple sclerosis: a critical review. *Neurology* 1991;41:980–5.

46. Paty DW. Multiple sclerosis: assessment of disease progression and effects of treatment. *Can J Neuro Sci* 1987;14:518–20.

47. Verdier-Taillefer MH, Zuber M, Lyon-Caen O, et al. Observer disagreement in rating neurologic impairment in multiple sclerosis: facts and consequences. *Eur Neurol* 1991;31:117–19.

48. Rationale for immunomodulating therapies of multiple sclerosis. *Neurology* 1988;38:Suppl. 2.

49. Yudkin PL, Ellison GW, Ghezzi A, et al. Overview of azathioprine treatment in multiple sclerosis. *Lancet* 1991;338:1051–5.

50. IFBN Multiple Sclerosis Study Group. Interferon beta 1b is effective in relapsing remitting multiple sclerosis. I – Clinical results of a multicenter randomized double blind placebo controlled trial. *Neurology* 1993;43:655–61.

51. Paty DW, Li DKB, The UBC/MRI Study Group and the IFBN Multiple Sclerosis Study Group. Interferon beta 1b is effective in relapsing remitting multiple sclerosis. II–MRI analysis results of a multicenter, randomized, double blind, placebo-controlled trial. *Neurology* 1993;43:662–7.

15

Myasthenia gravis

Therese A. Treves

Myasthenia gravis (MG) is characterized by fluctuating weakness of striated muscles and is due to a neuromuscular transmission defect secondary to an autoimmune response toward the acetylcholine receptors (AchR) at the neuro-muscular junction (NMJ). It is a heterogeneous disorder that can be classified upon the age at onset: as pediatric or adult forms (10% and 90%, respectively) (1), or upon the distribution of the muscles involved, as suggested by Osserman (2). The milder form is localized ocular myasthenia (I), that may progress within 1–2 years to generalized myasthenia that can be mild (IIA), moderately severe (IIB), acute fulminating with bulbar involvement (III) or late severe MG (IV) (2,3). Involvement of bulbar function may lead to acute respiratory failure which is the hallmark of myasthenic crisis and is still life-threatening (4). MG is a rare disease, even though its incidence and prevalence rates are growing: for example, its prevalence was 7.8–14.2 per 100 000 population in the 1970s and 1980s (5,6) while it was 2.5–6.4 per 100 000 in the 1960s (7). These increases are probably due to improvement in the diagnosis and longer survival of patients requiring respiratory care (4,8–10). Its case-fatality rate is 2–4% (11,12). MG is associated with other autoimmune diseases in 9–14% of the cases (13); as in such disease, it has a bimodal age at onset, especially in women, at the 3rd–4th and at the 8th decade (14,15).

Etiology

It is the pathogenesis rather than the etiology of MG that has been established. The evidence that MG results from an autoimmune disorder is based on: the presence of antibodies (Ab) directed to the nicotinic acetylcholine receptor (AchR-Ab) in the sera and at the NMJ of myasthenic patients, the induction of experimental MG in animals injected with AchR, and the passive immune transfer of the disease. But how this immune response is induced is not known. The AchR-Ab are assumed to cause pharmacologic blockade of the cholinergic sites and play a role in the destruction of the AchR: the antibodies bound to the receptors activate complement reactions which damage the postsynaptic membrane and change the ion channel properties of the receptors (16–19). MG is associated with a reduction of the postsynaptic nicotinic receptors and flattened postsynaptic folds (19–22).

The immune dysfunction involves the thymus in which immunologic self-tolerance is generated through maturation of T cells that mediate immune protection without promoting autoimmune response. The thymus also contains B cells that secrete AchR-Ab, while their production is regulated by CD4 + helper T cells that recognize AchR (23–25).

The AchR-Ab, which are mostly IgG, are detected in up to 85–90% of MG patients (26–28). "Seronegative" MG may have antibodies (e.g., IgM) to other neuromuscular determinants that interfere with AchR function (29).

Hyperplasia of the thymus, with germinal centers, is found in 70% of myasthenic patients, 10% of patients with thymoma and 20% with thymic atrophy (25); however, higher frequencies of thymoma have been reported (9,30). Thymic hyperplasia is more frequent in young onset MG (before the age of 40 years), while thymoma is more commonly found in older patients (age of onset > 30 years) (29).

Persons at risk

Transient neonatal myasthenia occurs in 8–14% of births to myasthenic mothers (31). It is due to transplacental transfer of maternal antibodies; the absence of fetal symptoms of MG, and the delayed onset of neonatal MG may be due to high fetal levels of alpha-fetoprotein, which inhibits the binding of AchR-Ab, and its decline after birth (32–34). This form of acquired myasthenia differs from congenital MG which accounts for 1% or MG and in which AchR-Ab are absent (35).

Secondary cases of MG have been found in 3–7% of families of myasthenic patients (36,37). It seems that familial MG occurs at an earlier age and tends to have a benign course (36). Abnormal AchR-Ab levels and impaired neuromuscular transmission may be found in asymptomatic relatives of MG patients, which suggests genetic susceptibility to MG (38).

In Caucasians, HLA haplotypes B8 and DR3 have been found to be associated with early onset, generalized myasthenia, seropositive, female MG with thymic hyperplasia while HLA-A3, B7 and DR2 are more frequent in older, seronegative MG (37,39–41) and HLA-DR1 with ocular MG (41). Patients with thymoma had no particular relationship with HLA antigens (40,41). In American Blacks HLA-A1, B8 and DR5 are associated with MG (40). HLA-DR3 allele is also associated with the presence of additional autoimmune disorders (41), which are relatively frequently associated with MG (13,41,42).

Myasthenia was also found to be relatively frequently associated with malignancy (43,44).

MG can be induced by D-penicillamine which subsides when the drug is discontinued (45). It may also occur after bone marrow transplantation (46) and magnesium administration (47).

Triggers

Viral infections, inflammatory episodes, delivery and miscarriage, or emotional burden may precipitate the occurrence of MG (48,49).

Diagnosis

The diagnosis of MG is based on the clinical findings of weakness and fatigue in muscle group(s), aggravated by exercise and relieved by rest. It is confirmed by pharmacologic and laboratory test findings: AchR-Ab, repetitive nerve stimulation, single fiber electromyogram (SFEMG).

Edrophonium (Tensilon) is a very short-acting anticholinesterase drug used as a diagnostic probe. Tensilon test is positive in 86–95% of ocular myasthenia while the effect is clearer in ptosis than in diplopia (50,51), and in 95% of generalized MG (50).

AchR-Ab are found in 83–87% of generalized MG and 50% of ocular myasthenia (9,26,52).

Electromyogram with repetitive stimulation shows decrement, exceeding 10%, in 32–46% of ocular myasthenia and 55–76% of mild generalized MG patients, depending whether the stimulated muscle is distal or proximal, and in all severe cases (5,53). SFEMG measures jitter, which is the variability in time intervals between consecutive discharges of two action potentials belonging to the same motor unit (54). The yield of SFEMG is high in cases without decrement on repetitive stimulation, abnormal SFEMG were observed in 80% of ocular forms and 94% of mild generalized MG (55). This test is also more sensitive than AchR-Ab assay which was abnormal in 70% of MG patients with ocular form and in 80% of patients with severe generalized MG, while, in these patients SFEMG was abnormal in 80% and 100%, respectively (55).

The ice test remains of occasional use only, for differentiating ocular MG from nonmyasthenic blepharoptosis, which does not improve by cooling (56,57).

Computed tomography of the mediastinum detects 85% of thymomas with a specificity of 99% (58).

Prognosis

The prognosis of MG depends upon the age of the patient at onset of the disease, the clinical stage, and the presence or absence of thymoma.

Transient neonatal myasthenia lasts between 5 days and 2 months (59). Infants with transient neonatal myasthenia do not develop MG in later life (59). Intermittent anticholinesterase medication may be required to overcome feeding or respiratory difficulties, although exchange transfusion may be required for the latter (60). AchR-Ab may be elevated in asymptomatic, as well as in symptomatic newborns (61).

Restricted ocular MG occurs in 71% of juvenile onset cases (62). In adult patients, ocular symptoms are the most frequent at presentation but more than 80% of them progress to generalized weakness (63). The maximum severity of symptoms was reported to occur within the first year in 83% of the patients (3). In a more recent work, the maximum severity was usually seen during the first 3 years, while the disease has a remitting–relapsing course in half of the patients (11).

Respiratory insufficiency is more likely to occur in patients with thymomas (53% vs. 14% in patients without thymoma) (64). The mortality in crisis was 3% during the 1970s (4).

Myasthenic crisis or exacerbation of MG can be precipitated by drugs such as anticonvulsants (e.g., dilantin, barbiturates), antibiotics (e.g., aminoglycosides), amantadine, amitriptyline, haloperidol and morphine (1,65,66).

There is no correlation between the severity of symptoms and the level of AchR-Ab (67). Seronegativity is more frequent among MG patients with ocular MG than among those with generalized involvement; however, absence of AchR-Ab does not preclude favorable response to thymectomy or plasmapheresis (52).

Five years after MG was diagnosed, the probability of achieving complete remission (not requiring treatment) reaches 13% while 33% achieve pharmacological remission, i.e., symptom-free while under treatment (12). Remission does not imply recovery since patients are liable to exacerbations (e.g., after anesthesia) and relapsing–remitting course occurs in 48% (11) while EMG or AchR-Ab levels may remain abnormal in clinically asymptomatic patients (26,68). After about 10 years, the survival curve tends to stabilize at 77% (69).

As a whole, the evolution of MG comprises three stages. During the first phase, which lasts a few years, the patients present remissions and exacerbations and the response to thymectomy is satisfactory. However, this is also the stage of relatively higher mortality. At a later stage, which lasts about 10 years, the disease is more stable but the response to thymectomy is less favorable. The third stage is the "burnt out" one, during which patients are unresponsive to thymectomy or acetylcholinesterase inhibitors. At this stage only immunomodulators may help (70).

Intervention

The objective of the treatment of MG is to improve NMJ function and to alter the course of the disease by achieving prolonged remissions. Remission is defined as no need for treatment for at least 6 months (71) or one year (12); remission rate can be used as an efficacy measure.

The therapy of MG has two basic strategies: symptomatic relief and immunomodulation. The aim of immunomodulation is to increase the self-tolerance to the AchR that has been lost and to decrease the anti-AchR Ab. The mechanisms of action of the different treatment modalities have been compiled in Verma and Oger's review (72).

Acetylcholinesterase inhibitors allow increase of acetylcholine concentrations at the NMJ by slowing its hydrolysis. Anticholinesterase drug therapy is the first treatment used in MG. Pyridostigmine is most commonly used because it is longer acting. Overtreatment may induce cholinergic weakness or even crisis.

Thymectomy is indicated when thymoma is suspected, in young adults rather than in juvenile forms, or in severe MG refractory to medical treatment (63,73). After thymectomy, there is improvement in the clinical stage of most of the patients, increase in pharmacological and complete remission rates, decrease in the use of acetylcholinesterase inhibitors and no further need for plasmapheresis, while it is more with steroids and azathioprine that patients are treated. Globally, treatment requirement was decreased in 65% and increased in 13% of the patients who underwent thymectomy (63). The peak effect of thymectomy is observed after 3 years (72). Thymectomy improves survival of MG patients (30,74,75), particularly in those without thymoma (30). Patients with thymoma may show initial exacerbation following thymectomy (76). Post-thymectomy mortality is affected by the presence of thymoma, severity of the symptoms, older age of the patients and a transthoracic approach (30). Earlier remissions and better prognosis are related to shorter duration of MG before thymectomy, younger age at onset of disease, lower severity, and early thymectomy (12,30). Patients may clinically deteriorate for the first 24–96 hours after surgery (73).

Although rare, late recurrences of thymoma were reported (77), probably reflecting incomplete removal of the tumor. Therefore, wide excision might be preferred to limited approaches (77). However, it has been shown that video-assisted thoracoscopic thymectomy (VAT) is associated with less morbidity than other techniques, although conversion to sternotomy may be required during VAT (78).

Remissions are more frequent when thymectomy is associated with perioperative prednisone therapy (79).

Corticosteroids

Marked improvement or remission was observed in 63–94% of the adult MG patients who received prednisone for 2–4 years, with better response among older patients (80–83). An initial worsening that lasts for a few days may be observed (81), especially with high daily doses (81). Acute exacerbations are less frequent if corticosteroids are initiated with progressively increasing daily doses up to the optimal dose and then switched to an alternate-day regimen (72,84). Clinical stabilization is observed after 2 months (81). As rapid decrease of steroids dose may induce exacerbations, tapering down of 5 mg per month is recommended (85,86).

Azathioprine

After prednisone, azathioprine is the most frequently used immunosuppressant in MG because of its relatively few side-effects (87). When steroids are required, azathioprine reduces their need down to 0–10 mg per day (86,88). It is given as a long-term regimen and at a dose of 2 mg/kg per day. The effect is obtained after 6 months, and is maximal after 1 year.

Improvement was observed in most myasthenic patients who took azathioprine; relapse occurred within a few months if the drug was discontinued (88–90). In a randomized clinical trial in which the effect of azathioprine was compared to that of prednisone, after 3 years of treatment, patients under prednisone tended to be less responsive (91). In an open study, no significant difference in the therapeutic response was observed when azathioprine was compared to steroids alone or in combination with azathioprine. However, it was suggested that although azathioprine may not be more effective than prednisone, it is an agent for sparing corticosteroid therapy, which has a relatively high frequency of side-effects (81–83,92).

Azathioprine has more favorable effects in patients with older age at onset (>36 years), shorter duration of myasthenia (<10 years), associated thymoma and high levels of AchR-Ab (87). The drug should be avoided during reproductive age (93).

Plasmapheresis

Plasmapheresis, or plasma exchange (PE), removes circulating macromolecules, including IgG (72). PE induces a decrease of the AchR-Ab by 25–60% (94), with rapid clinical remissions. Because its cessation may induce AchR-Ab rebound, patients should also receive immunosuppressive drugs concomitantly (94). Azathioprine increases the interval between PE treatments (96,97). The therapy regimen suggested is by courses of 3–4 PE/week or five daily exchanges (95). Clinical improvement starts 1–3 days after the first exchange, the peak effect is observed 3 days after the last exchange, and the effect lasts for up to 5 weeks

(95,98). Beneficial effect is obtained in 63–75% (95,96), while poor or absent response are observed in 10% (95).

Plasma exchange is indicated in severe generalized MG refractory to other treatments, acute relapses, exacerbations before or during corticosteroid therapy or before thymectomy (93,96,98,99). PE has better effects in patients with shorter disease duration (96) and may also benefit patients without detectable AchR-Ab (100).

Extracorporeal plasma immunoadsorption of the AchR-Ab has the same indications as PE. It is preferred because protein replacement is not required (101–103). AchR-Ab are decreased by 70–75% (103,104), but the original levels are reached within 1–3 weeks (104).

Intravenous immunoglobulin

It is possible that intravenous immunoglobulin (IVIg) contains globulin that may increase the effect of T-suppressor cells and/or inhibit the AchR-Ab, by binding to them (105,106). They do not induce change in serum levels of AchR-Ab (107). Their use allows decrease of corticosteroids dose from 70 mg/day to 30 mg/day (107). Conventional treatment is of 400 mg/day for 5 consecutive days (107). They may induce transitory worsening for about 3 days in 30% of cases. The response begins after 4 days and the maximum effect is observed after 9 days, and the benefit is retained for about 2 months. Favorable effect is kept with repeated use (107).

Intravenous immunoglobulin and plasma exchange are equally expensive.

Implications

The introduction of new therapeutic modalities did not eclipse the older ones, but decreased the number of patients refractory to any treatment. However, the use of IVIg and PE may be limited by their high cost. In the absence of controlled studies, the therapeutic approach is based on the experience gained from well documented series that indicate that in older patients, immunosuppressant therapy is particularly indicated and that PE has its place as treatment of acute exacerbations. Development of drugs that inhibit further T-cell responses could improve further the management of myasthenic patients (108).

REFERENCES

1. Osserman KE, Genkis G. Studies in myasthenia gravis: review of a twenty-year experience in over 1200 patients. *Mount Sinai J Med* 1971;38:497–537.
2. Osserman KE. *Myasthenia Gravis.* New York: Grune & Stratton, 1958.

3. Grob D, Brunner NG, Namba T. The natural course of myasthenia gravis and effect of therapeutic measures. *Ann NY Acad Sci* 1981;377:652–69.

4. Cohen MS, Younger D. Aspects of the natural history of myasthenia gravis: crisis and death. *Ann NY Acad Sci* 1981;377:670–7.

5. Christensen PB, Jensen TS, Tsiropulos I, et al. Incidence and prevalence of myasthenia gravis in western Denmark: 1975 to 1989. *Neurology* 1993;43:1779–83.

6. Phillips LH, Torner JC, Anderson MS, Cox GM. The epidemiology of myasthenia gravis in central and western Virginia. *Neurology* 1992;42:1888–93.

7. Kurtzke J. Epidemiology of myasthenia gravis. *Adv Neurol* 1978;19:545–66.

8. Grob D, Arsura EL, Brunner NG, Namba T. The course of myasthenia gravis and therapies affecting outcome. *Ann NY Acad Sci* 1987;505:472–99.

9. Oosterhuis HJ. The natural course of myasthenia gravis: a long term follow up study. *J Neurol Neurosurg Psychiatry* 1989;52:1121–7.

10. Phillips LH, Torner JC. Epidemiologic evidence for a changing natural history of myasthenia gravis. *Neurology* 1996;47:1233–8.

11. Mantegazza R, Beghi E, Pareyson D, et al. A multicenter follow-up study of 1152 patients with myasthenia gravis in Italy. *J Neurol* 1990;237:339–44.

12. Beghi E, Antozzi C, Batocchi AP, et al. Prognosis of myasthenia gravis: a multicenter follow-up study of 844 patients. *J Neurol Sci* 1991;106:213–20.

13. Christensen PB, Jensen TS, Tsiropoulos I, et al. Associated autoimmune diseases in myasthenia gravis. *Acta Neurol Scand* 1995;91:192–5.

14. Somnier FE, Keiding N, Paulson OB. Epidemiology of myasthenia gravis in Denmark. A longitudinal and comprehensive population survey. *Arch Neurol* 1991;48:733–9.

15. Ferrari G, Lovaste MG. Epidemiology of myasthenia gravis in the province of Trento (Northern Italy). *Neuroepidemiology* 1992;11:135–42.

16. Stanley EF, Drachman DB. Effect of myasthenic immunoglobulin on acetylcholine receptors of intact mammalian neuromuscular junctions. *Science* 1978;200:1285–7.

17. Engel AG. Myasthenia gravis and myasthenic syndromes. *Ann Neurol* 1984;16:519–34.

18. Richman DP, Agius MA. Acquired myasthenia gravis. Immunopathology. *Neurol Clin North Am* 1994;12:273–84.

19. Penn AS, Rowland LP. Disorders of the neuromuscular junction. In Rowland LP (Ed.). *Merritt's Textbook of Neurology*. 9th Edition. Baltimore: Williams & Wilkins, 1995:754–65.

20. Engel AG. Morphologic and immunopathologic findings in myasthenia gravis and in congenital myasthenic syndromes. *J Neurol Neurosurg Psychiatry* 1980;43:577–89.

21. Pestronk A, Drachman DB, Self SG. Measurement of junctional acetylcholine receptors in myasthenia gravis: clinical correlates. *Muscle Nerve* 1985;8:245–51.

22. Juhn MS. Myasthenia gravis. Diagnostic methods and control measures for a chronic disease. *Postgrad Med* 1993;94:161–74.

23. Shah A, Lisak R. Immunopharmacologic therapy in myasthenia gravis. *Clin Neuropharmacol* 1993;16:97–103.

24. Sprent J. T lymphocytes and the thymus. In Paul WE (Ed.). *Fundamental Immunology*. 3rd Edition. New York: Raven Press, 1993:75–109.

25. Hohlfeld R, Wekerle H. The thymus in myasthenia gravis. *Neurol Clin North Am* 1994;12:331–42.

26. Lindstrom JM, Seybold ME, Lennon VA, Whittingham S, Duane DD. Antibody to acetylcholine receptor in myasthenia gravis: prevalence, clinical correlates, and diagnostic value. *Neurology* 1976;16:1054–9.

27. Brenner T, Abramsky O, Lisak RP, Zweiman B, Tarrab-Hazdai R, Fuchs S. Radioimmunoassay of antibodies to acetylcholine receptor in serum of myasthenia gravis patients. *Isr J Med Sci* 1978;14:986–9.

28. Drachman DB, De Silva S, Ramsay D, Pestronk A. Humoral pathogenesis of myasthenia gravis. *Ann NY Acad Sci* 1987;505:90–105.

29. Vincent A. Aetiological factors in development of myasthenia gravis. *Adv Neuroimmunol* 1994;4:355–71.

30. Papatestas AE, Genkins G, Kornfeld P, et al. Effects of thymectomy in myasthenia gravis. *Ann Surg* 1987;206:79–88.

31. Hokkanen E. Myasthenia gravis. A clinical analysis of the total material from Finland with specific reference to endocrinological and neurological disorders. *Ann Clin Res* 1969;1:94–108.

32. Abramsky O, Brenner T, Lisak RP, Zeidman A, Beyth Y. Significance in neonatal myasthenia gravis of inhibitory effect of amniotic fluid on binding of antibodies to acetylcholine receptor. *Lancet* 1979;ii:1333–5.

33. Brenner T, Beyth Y, Abramsky O. Inhibitory effect of alpha-fetoprotein on the binding of myasthenia gravis antibody to acetylcholine receptor. *Proc Natl Acad Sci* 1980;77:3635–9.

34. Donaldson JO, Penn AS, Lisak RP, Abramsky O, Brenner T, Schotland DL. Antiacetylcholine receptor antibody in neonatal myasthenia gravis. *Am J Dis Child* 1981;135:222–6.

35. Vincent A, Newsom-Davis J. Absence of anti-acetylcholine receptor antibodies in congenital myasthenia gravis. *Lancet* 1979;i:441–2.

36. Namba T, Brunner NG, Brown SB, Muguruma M, Grob D. Familial myasthenia gravis. *Arch Neurol* 1971;25:61–72.

37. Pirskanen R. Genetic aspects of myasthenia gravis. A family study of 264 Finnish patients. *Acta Neurol Scand* 1977;56:365–88.

38. Pirskanen R, Bergstrom K, Hammarstrom L. Neuromuscular safety margin: genetical, immunological, and electrophysiological determinants in relatives of myasthenic patients: a preliminary report. *Ann NY Acad Sci* 1981;377:606–13.

39. Pirskanen R. Genetic associations between myasthenia gravis and the HL-A system. *J Neurol Neurosurg Psychiatry* 1976;39:23–33.

40. Compston DA, Vincent A, Newsom-Davis J, Batchelor JR. Clinical, HLA antigen and immunological evidence for disease heterogeneity in myasthenia gravis. *Brain* 1980;103:579–601.

41. Tola MR, Caniatti LM, Casseta I, et al. Immunogenetic heterogeneity and associated autoimmune disorders in myasthenia gravis: a population-based survey in the province of Ferarra, northern Italy. *Acta Neurol Scand* 1994;90:318–23.

42. Oosterhuis HJ, De Haas WHD. Rheumatic diseases in patients with myasthenia gravis. *Acta Neurol Scand* 1968;44:219–27.

43. Levo Y, Kott E, Atsmon A. Association between myasthenia gravis and malignant lymphoma. *Eur Neurol* 1975;13:245–50.

44. Monden Y, Uyama T, Kimura S, Taniki T. Extrathymic malignancy in patients with myasthenia gravis. *Eur J Cancer* 1991;27:745–7.

45. Godley PJ, Morton TA, Karboski JA, Tami JA. Procainamide-induced myasthenic crisis. *Ther Drug Monit* 1990;12:411–14.

46. Grau JM, Casademont J, Monforte R, et al. Myasthenia gravis after allogeneic bone marrow transplantation: report of a new case and pathogenetic considerations. *Bone Marrow Transplant* 1990;5:435–7.

47. Bashuk RG, Krendel DA. Myasthenia gravis presenting as weakness after magnesium administration. *Muscle Nerve* 1990;13:708–12.

48. Korn IL, Abramsky O. Myasthenia gravis following viral infection. *Eur Neurol* 1981;20:435–9.

49. Giagheddu M, Puggioni G, Sanna G, et al. Epidemiological study of myasthenia gravis in Sardinia, Italy (1958–1986). *Acta Neurol Scand* 1989;79:326–33.

50. Phillips LH, Melnick PA. Diagnosis of myasthenia gravis in the 1990s. *Semin Neurol* 1990;10:62–9.

51. Evoli A, Tonali P, Bartoccioni E, Lo Monaco M. Ocular myasthenia: diagnostic and therapeutic problems. *Acta Neurol Scand* 1988;77:31–5.

52. Soliven BC, Lange DJ, Penn AS, et al. Seronegative myasthenia gravis. *Neurology* 1988;38:514–17.

53. Horowitz SH, Genkins G, Kornfeld P, Papatestas AE. Electrophysiologic diagnosis of myasthenia gravis and the regional curare test. *Neurology* 1976;26:410–17.

54. Gilchrist JM, Sanders DB. Double-step repetitive stimulation in myasthenia gravis. *Muscle Nerve* 1987;10:233–7.

55. Oh SJ, Kim DE, Kuruoglu R, Bradley RJ, Dwyer D. Diagnostic sensitivity of the laboratory tests in myasthenia gravis. *Muscle Nerve* 1992;15:720–4.

56. Sethi KD, Rivner MH, Swift TR. Ice pack test for myasthenia gravis. *Neurology* 1987;37:1383–5.

57. Ertas M, Arac N, Kumral K, Tuncbay T. Ice test as a simple diagnostic aid for myasthenia gravis. *Acta Neurol Scand* 1994;89:227–9.

58. Ellis K, Austin JH, Jaretzki A. Radiologic detection of thymoma in patients with myasthenia gravis. *Am J Radiol* 1988;151:873–81.

59. Fenichel GM. Myasthenia gravis. *Pediatr Ann* 1989;18:432–9.

60. Pasternak JF, Hageman J, Adams MA, Philip AGS, Gardner TH. Exchange transfusion in neonatal myasthenia. *J Pediatr* 1981;99:644–6.

61. Lefvert AK, Osterman PO. Newborn infants to myasthenic mothers: a clinical study and an investigation of acetylcholine receptor antibodies in 17 children. *Neurology* 1983;33:133–8.

62. Wong V, Hawkins BR, Yu YL. Myasthenia gravis in Hong Kong Chinese. 2. Paediatric disease. *Acta Neurol Scand* 1992;86:68–72.

63. Blossom GB, Ernstoff RM, Howells GA, Bendick PJ, Glover JL. Thymectomy for myasthenia gravis. *Arch Surg* 1993;128:855–62.

64. Oosterhuis HJ. Observations of the natural history of myasthenia gravis and the effect of thymectomy. *Ann NY Acad Sci* 1981;377:678–90.

65. Argov Z, Mastaglia FL. Disorders of neuromuscular transmission caused by drugs. *N Engl J Med* 1979;301:409–13.

66. Adams SL, Mathews J, Grammer LC. Drugs that may exacerbate myasthenia gravis. *Ann Emerg Med* 1984;13:532–8.

67. Roses AD, Olanow CW, McAdams MW, Lane RJM. There is no direct correlation between the serum anti-acetylcholine receptor antibody levels and the clinical status of individual patients with myasthenia gravis. *Neurology* 1981;31:220–4.

68. Scoppetta C, Bartocconi E, David P, et al. When is there a full recovery for myasthenia gravis patient? *J Neurol* 1982;227:61–5.

69. Treves TA, Rocca WA, Meneghini F. Epidemiology of myasthenia gravis. In Anderson DW, Schoenberg DG (Eds.). *Neuroepidemiology: A Tribute to Bruce Schoenberg.* Boston: CRC Press, 1991:297–309.

70. Simpson JA, Thomaides T. Treatment of myasthenia gravis: an audit. *QJM* 1987;64:693–704.

71. Perez MC, Buot WL, Mercado-Danguilan C, Bagabaldo Z, Renale LD. Stable remissions in myasthenia gravis. *Eur Neurol* 1981;31:32–7.

72. Verma P, Oger J. Treatment of acquired autoimmune myasthenia gravis: a topic review. *Can J Neurol Sci* 1992;19:360–75.

73. Galdi AP. Essentials in the management of myasthenia gravis. *Am Fam Physician* 1978;17:95–102.

74. Papatestas AE, Pozner J, Genkis G, Kornfeld P, Matta RJ. Prognosis in occult thymomas in myasthenia gravis following transcervical thymectomy. *Arch Surg* 1987;122:1352–6.

75. Palmisani MT, Evoli A, Batocchi AP, Provenzano C, Tonali P. Myasthenia gravis associated with thymoma: clinical characteristics and long-term outcome. *Eur Neurol* 1993;34:78–82.

76. Somnier FE. Exacerbation of myasthenia gravis after removal of thymomas. *Acta Neurol Scand* 1994;90:56–66.

77. Gotti G, Paladini P, Haid MM, et al. Late recurrence of thymoma and myasthenia gravis. Case report. *Scand J Thor Cardiovasc Surg* 1995;29:37–8.

78. Sabbagh MN, Garza JS, Patten B. Thoracoscopic thymectomy in patients with myasthenia gravis. *Muscle Nerve* 1995;18:1475–7.

79. Heiser JC, Rutherford RB, Ringel SP. Thymectomy for myasthenia gravis. A changing perspective. *Arch Surg* 1982;117:533–7.

80. Pascuzzi RM, Coslett HB, Johns TR. Long-term corticosteroid treatment of myasthenia gravis: report of 116 patients. *Ann Neurol* 1984;15:291–8.

81. Sghirlanzoni A, Peluchetti D, Mantegazza R, Fiacchino F, Cornelio F. Myasthenia gravis: prolonged treatment with steroids. *Neurology* 1984;34:170–4.

82. Cosi V, Citterio A, Lombardi M, Piccolo G, Romani A, Erbetta A. Effectiveness of steroid treatment in myasthenia gravis: a retrospective study. *Acta Neurol Scand* 1991;84:33–9.

83. Evoli A, Batocchi AP, Palmisani MT, Lo Monaco M, Tonali P. Long-term results of corticosteroid therapy in patients with myasthenia gravis. *Eur Neurol* 1992;32:37–43.

84. Sanders DB, Scoppetta C. The treatment of patients with myasthenia gravis. *Neurol Clin North Am* 1994;12:343–68.

85. Arsura E, Brunner N, Namba T, Grob D. High-dose intravenous methylprednisolone in myasthenia gravis. *Arch Neurol* 1985;42:1149–53.

86. Miano MA, Bosley TM, Heiman-Patterson TD, et al. Factors influencing outcome of prednisone dose reduction in myasthenia gravis. *Neurology* 1991;41:919–21.

87. Matell G. Immunosuppressive drugs: azathioprine in the treatment of myasthenia gravis. *Ann NY Acad Sci* 1987;505:588–94.

88. Witte AS, Cornblath DR, Parry GJ, Lisak RP, Schatz NJ. Azathioprine in the treatment of myasthenia gravis. *Ann Neurol* 1984;15:602–5.

89. Hohlfeld R, Toyka KV, Besinger UA, Gerhold B, Heininger K. Myasthenia gravis: reactivation of clinical disease and of autoimmune factors after discontinuation of long-term azathioprine. *Ann Neurol* 1985;17:238–42.

90. Niakan E, Harati Y, Rolak LA. Immunosuppressive drug therapy in myasthenia gravis. *Arch Neurol* 1986;43:155–6.

91. Myasthenia Gravis Clinical Study Group. A randomised clinical trial comparing prednisone and azathioprine in myasthenia gravis. Results of the second interim analysis. *J Neurol Neurosurg Psychiatry* 1993;56:1157–63.

92. Mantegazza R, Antozzi C, Peluchetti D, Sghirlanzoni A, Cornelio F. Azathioprine as a single drug or in combination with steroids in the treatment of myasthenia gravis. *J Neurol* 1988;235:449–53.

93. Lisak RP. Myasthenia gravis: mechanisms and management. *Hosp Pract* 1983;18:101–9.

94. Thorlacius S, Lefvert AK, Aarli JA, et al. Plasma exchange in myasthenia gravis: effect on anti-AChR antibodies and other autoantibodies. *Acta Neurol Scand* 1986;74:486–90.

95. Newsom-Davis J. Plasmapheresis in myasthenia gravis. In NIH Consensus Development Conference. The Utility of Therapeutic Plasmapheresis for Neurological Disorders. June 2–4, 1986.

96. Kornfeld P, Ambinder E, Mittag T, et al. Plasmapheresis in refractory generalized myasthenia gravis. *Arch Neurol* 1981;38:478–81.

97. Rodnitzky RL, Bosch EP. Chronic long-interval plasma exchange in myasthenia gravis. *Arch Neurol* 1984;41:715–17.

98. Pinching AJ, Peters DK, Newsom-Davis J. Remission of myasthenia gravis following plasma-exchange. *Lancet* 1976;ii:1373–6.

99. Stricker RB, Kwiatkowska BJ, Habis JA, Kiprov DD. Myasthenic crisis. Response to plasmapheresis following failure of intravenous gamma-globulin. *Arch Neurol* 1993;50:837–40.

100. Thorlacius S, Mollnes TE, Garred P, et al. Plasma exchange in myasthenia gravis: changes in serum complement and immunoglobulins. *Acta Neurol Scand* 1988;78:221–7.

101. Somnier FE, Langvad E. Plasma exchange with selective immunoadsorption of anti-acetylcholine receptor antibodies. *J Neuroimmunol* 1989;22:123–7.

102. Ichikawa M, Koh C-S, Hata Y, Tohyama M, Tsuno T, Komiyama A. Immunoadsorption plasmapheresis for severe generalized myasthenia gravis. *Arch Dis Child* 1993;69:236–8.

103. Berta E, Confalonieri P, Simoncini O, et al. Removal of antiacetylcholine receptor antibodies by protein-A immunoadsorption in myasthenia gravis. *Int J Artif Organs* 1994;17:603–8.

104. Grob D, Simpson D, Mitsumoto H, et al. Treatment of myasthenia gravis by immunoadsorption of plasma. *Neurology* 1995;45:338–44.

105. Antel JP, Medof ME, Oger J, Kuo HH, Arnason BGW. Generation of suppressor cells by aggregated human globulin. *Clin Exp Immunol* 1981;43:351–6.

106. Liblau R, Gajdos Ph, Bustarret FA, El Habib R, Bach JF, Morel E. Intravenous τ-globulin in myasthenia gravis: interaction with anti-acetylcholine receptor autoantibodies. *J Clin Immunol* 1991;11:128–31.

107. Arsura EL, Bick A, Brunner NG, Namba T, Grob D. High-dose intravenous immuno-globulin in the management of myasthenia gravis. *Arch Intern Med* 1986;146:1365–8.

108. Zisman E, Katz-Levy Y, Dayan M, et al. Peptide analogs to pathogenic epitopes of the human acetylcholine receptor alpha subunit as potential modulators of myasthenia gravis. *Proc Natl Acad Sci USA* 1996;93:4492–7.

16

Guillain–Barré syndrome

F. G. A. van der Meché and R. van Koningsveld

Etiology

Introduction and incidence

The Guillain–Barré syndrome (GBS) is a subacute immune-mediated disorder of the peripheral nerves. The diagnosis is primarily clinical, the essential features being a more or less symmetrical paresis, decrease of myotatic reflexes and a typical time course (1,2). In addition, other causes for polyneuropathy should be excluded. The paresis reaches its nadir by definition within 4 weeks, but usually it is seen within 2 weeks. In 20–30% of the patients the muscle weakness is so severe that artificial respiration is needed. Based upon clinical and laboratory arguments subpatterns or variants have been described. They will be discussed in more detail below.

Several studies have been published reporting incidence rates (IR) from 0.4 to 2.2 cases per 100 000 persons per year (Table 16.1). The variation in the reported IR may be more related to differences in methodology than to true differences in incidence. The data suggest that the occurrence of the disease does not change consistently over time and is not restricted to specific areas nor related to factors as race, standard of living or climate. GBS affects people from all ages but a clear increase in incidence with age has been reported in most studies (3–6). Some studies show a bimodal age distribution with a peak around 20–30 years (7–10). In most studies men are more frequently affected than women, but in only three studies was this difference statistically significant (3,6,11).

Two-thirds of GBS patients suffer from an infection approximately one to three weeks before the onset of weakness. These infections mostly involve the upper-respiratory and the gastrointestinal tract (12,13). Although some of these infections tend to show a seasonal preponderance, there is hardly ever a significant difference between seasons reported in the occurrence of GBS. From the studies reporting on the seasonal occurrence of GBS, there appears to be a slight lean towards autumn and early winter (3,5,14–16). Related to this, a typical observation has been made in northern China. McKhann et al. (17) described a group

Table 16.1. Reported incidence of Guillain–Barré syndrome

Study population (Reference)	Period of study	Number of patients	Incidence crude	Incidence age adjusted	NINCDS criteria
Carlisle, England (69)	1955–1961	3	0.6	—	No
Guam (70)	1960–1966	5	1.9	—	No
Iceland (71)	1954–1963	13	0.7	—	No
Olmsted County, USA (72)	1935–1976	40	1.7	—	No
Israel (73)	1969–1972	89	0.75	0.8	No
San Joaquin County, USA (74)	1972–1976	18	1.2	1.4	No
Campania, Italy (75)	1971–1980	46	0.16	—	No
Olmsted County, USA (6)	1935–1980	48	1.7	1.9	Yes
Hordaland, Norway (3)	1957–1982	109	1.1	1.2	Yes
Larimer County, USA (76)	1975–1983	29	2.2	—	No
Ringkobin County, Denmark (7)	1965–1982	51	1.1	1.1	No
Benghazi, Libya (14)	1983–1985	27	1.7	1.7	Yes
Perth, Australia (8)	1980–1985	109	1.4	1.4	Yes
Copenhagen County, Denmark (9)	1977–1984	34	2.0	—	Yes
Nairobi, Kenya (77)	1974–1981	54	—	—	No
Sardinia, Italy (78)	1961–1980	120	0.4	—	No
Uusimaa District, Finland (20)	1981–1986	71	1.0	—	No
Uusimaa County, Southern Finland (79)	1981–1985	62	1.1	—	Yes
Oxfordshire, England (5)	1974–1986	72	1.1	1.2	Yes
Ferrera, Italy (15)	1981–1987	16	1.3	1.1	Yes
Vermont, USA (80)	1980–1985	51	1.6	—	Yes
Ontario and Quebec, Canada (81)					
Ontario	1983–1989	1302	2.07	2.02	No
Quebec	1983–1989	1031	2.25	2.30	No
Alcoi, Spain (82)	1987–1991	5	0.9	—	Yes
Tanzania (83)	1984–1992	59	0.83	—	Yes
South-West Stockholm County, Sweden (16)	1973–1991	84	1.49	1.56	Yes
Cantabria, Spain (10)	1975–1988	69	0.95	0.86	Yes
Emilia-Romagna region, Italy (4)	1992–1993	94	1.20	—	Yes
South-east England (84)	1993–1994	79	1.20	—	Yes
South-west Netherlands (11)	1987–1996	476	1.18	1.14	Yes

of patients with remarkable epidemiological features. This group mainly consists of children in rural areas who are predominantly affected during late summer. Another noteworthy fact is that most of these patients suffered from the subtype "motor axonal form of neuropathy".

Antecedent factors

Many factors have been described preceding GBS with the suggestion that they play a role in the etiology of the disease. Convincing are the associations with certain viruses and bacteria (18,19). Also extensively described is the relationship with specific vaccines or drugs but most observations are, however, anecdotal (20–25). Little doubt is left about the relationship of GBS with the swine-flu vaccination in 1976 and the use of the antidepressive drug, Zimeldine (21,22). Finally, cases have been outlined where GBS followed pregnancy, surgery, and malignancies (26–28). Here again, no cause-and-effect relationship has been established so far.

Campylobacter jejuni, Cytomegalovirus, Epstein–Barr virus and *Mycoplasma pneumonia* are micro-organisms most frequently reported as preceding agents (12, 29–31). Recently, most attention has been drawn by *Campylobacter jejuni*. In 1984, Kaldor and Speed reported a preceding infection with this Gram-negative flagellated rod in 38% of their GBS patients (29). This relationship has been confirmed extensively and much effort has been made to further investigate this association (12,18,32–36). This has led to the definition of a *C. jejuni*-related subgroup which is associated with a pure motor form, a more severe clinical course, and anti-GM1 antibodies (18,37,38). Similarly, an association has been demonstrated between CMV infection and a more severe course of the disease (30).

The underlying pathophysiologic mechanism, by which antecedent factors may trigger GBS, is not fully understood. The theory of molecular mimicry has been given more support since cross-reacting antibodies have been demonstrated between lipopolysaccharides of certain strains of *C. jejuni* and anti-GM1 or anti-GQ1b antibodies. Furthermore, certain *C. jejuni* strains have been demonstrated to contain ganglioside-like structures (39–42).

Summary

GBS occurs sporadically, it extends worldwide and affects people of all ages and races. Although the pathogenesis has not yet been fully understood, recent findings point in the direction of molecular mimicry based on the cross-reactivity between lipopolysaccharides of certain strains of bacteria and anti-ganglioside antibodies.

Table 16.2. Causes of acute motor weakness

Myelitis transversa
Infarct of the pons
Poliomyelitis
Guillain–Barré syndrome
Toxins
Myasthenia gravis
Botulism
Lambert–Eaton
Polymyositis
Rhabdomyolysis

Diagnosis

Criteria

In 1978 diagnostic criteria for GBS were published (43). Consensus exists to define GBS clinically, according to simple diagnostic criteria, and subsequently add further characteristics. This may result in subgroups within the broad clinical definition. Before reaching the diagnosis of GBS, other causes of an acute motor weakness should be considered (Table 16.2).

Subgroups

As described above, much effort has been paid to define specific subgroups. Nowadays more laboratory parameters are available with respect to antecedent infections, auto-antibodies and electrophysiological changes. Therefore a subdivision of the syndrome, incorporating these parameters has been proposed. Table 16.3 gives an overview of the possible subgroups. In this table, among others one can find a division based upon pathological findings. These findings mostly derive from Chinese patients. This classification is difficult to use in the Western world where pathology is rarely available and electrophysiological techniques are not able to discriminate between primary or secondary axonal degeneration (44–48).

Some of the clinical variants are associated with specific antibodies against gangliosides. Anti-GM1 antibodies have been associated with acute or chronic motor neuropathy (49–51). Anti-GQ1b antibodies are specifically seen in GBS patients with ophthalmoplegia, either in the context of Miller Fisher syndrome, in patients with pure ophthalmoplegia or in classical GBS patients with severe oculomotor involvement (40,52). The implications of these associations are not yet fully understood but as mentioned above, molecular mimicry may play a role.

Table 16.3. Guillain–Barré syndrome, patterns within the clinical concept

Clinical patterns	Terminology based upon pathology	Related infections	Related antibody
Classically ascending			
Pure motor			
demyelinating*		C. jejuni	GM1
axonal*	Acute motor axonal neuropathy (AMAN)	C. jejuni	GM1
Sensory motor			
demyelinating*	Acute inflammatory demyelinating polyneuropathy (AIDP)	CMV	GM2
axonal*	Acute motor sensory axonal neuropathy (AMSAN)		
Cranial nerve variants			
Oculo motor nerves (Miller Fisher syndrome)		C. jejuni	GQ1b
Lower bulbar nerves (Pharyngo-brachial variant)			

*Pure demyelination and pure (primary) axonal patterns are not distinguishable in the clinical setting.

Prognosis

In about 28% of GBS patients the disease runs a mild course and these patients will remain ambulant during the course of the disease (11). In the other patients the disease progresses and finally, artificial respiration is necessary in 20–30% of the patients (53–55). After a period of progression a plateau phase follows, which may take several weeks. Subsequently recovery starts. For those who are not able to walk independently, the median time towards walking takes about 85 days without therapy (53).

De Jager et al. studied long-term outcome in 57 patients. With a follow-up time between 2 and 24 years, they found that 35% of the patients were fully recovered, in 35% of the patients a mild handicap was left, and 30% of the patients suffered from a severe handicap (56).

Outcome may be predicted in an early stage of disease using prognostic indicators, identified in a variety of studies. Most studies show that older age, need for ventilatory support, a rapidly progressive course, and low compound muscle

Table 16.4. The following need monitoring and supportive care

Respiratory complications
Thromboembolic complications
Cardiovascular instability
Compression neuropathies
Pain, primarily due to the neuropathy and secondary to lying paralysed
Contractures
Urinary tract infections
Obstipation/ileus
Decubitus
Psychological decompensation

action potentials after distal nerve stimulation (EMG) are predictors of poor outcome (53,57–61). In the Dutch trial, where treatment with intravenous immunoglobulin (IVIg) and plasmapheresis (PE) were compared, a multivariate analysis of the collected data of 147 GBS patients was performed in order to study prognostic factors (62). The importance of older age, a rapid onset and severity of weakness were confirmed. The most powerful predictor in this study was, however, an antecedent episode of diarrhea. A similar outcome was found by Rees et al. (1995) where a preceding infection with *C. jejuni*, the commonest recognized cause of diarrhea, was shown to be an important prognostic factor (36). The Italian Guillain–Barré study group also reported an antecedent gastroenteritis as a predictor of worse outcome (63). Interestingly, in the Dutch trial, diarrhea was only important in the patients treated with PE and not in patients treated with IVIg (38,62).

Intervention

Supportive treatment

Although at present specific treatment is available, general care is still of utmost importance for the GBS patient (Table 16.4). Because of the risk of autonomous dysfunction and the unpredictable course of the disease, the patient should be carefully monitored from the beginning. In doing so, one should be aware of the possibility of respiratory distress, aspiration, and cardiovascular problems. The latter expresses itself as wide fluctuations of pulse or blood pressure and asystoly. Pain often is a great burden to the patient. Although special mattresses and frequent repositioning may be helpful, epidural morphine application may be necessary (64).

Specific treatment

The efficacy of plasma exchange (PE) has been demonstrated in two large clinical trials (65,66). In both studies, improvement started earlier and artificial respiration was significantly decreased in patients treated with PE. After 6 and 12 months the difference was still observed. This reflects not only considerable decrease of morbidity, but also a considerable degree of economic savings. Drawbacks of PE treatment are its contraindications and treatment failures during administration. As an alternative to PE, IVIg has been investigated as a more practical alternative. In the Netherlands, a study was conducted comparing IVIg with PE in 150 GBS patients (54). This study showed that IVIg was at least as effective as PE. In addition, an international study has been published including 383 patients (67). Here, treatment with PE and IVIg resulted in similar improvement. Based upon these findings, IVIg can now be regarded as the most practical treatment and is in general preferable. Based on the promising result of a preliminary study on the additional effect of methylprednisolone on standard treatment with IVIg, the Dutch GBS study group has performed a large-scale randomized trial (68). The results of this study are not yet available.

Implications for clinical practice

The variety of clinical expression of GBS may cause diagnostic confusion. Therefore, as pointed out above, it is important to define GBS according to the basic clinical diagnostic criteria and subsequently add further characteristics in order to classify, if possible, the patient into a specific subgroup.

The classification into subgroups may have consequences for daily practice, for example in the choice of therapy. It has been demonstrated that IVIg treatment was more effective in patients with preceding *C. jejuni* and CMV infections in comparison to PE treatment (30,37,38,62). Further, prognostic evaluation is of importance in informing the patient and their family about the course and outcome of the illness. Finally, it should be stated that it is important that experienced care is given. With the introduction of IVIg, it is now possible to treat patients in small centers. This should not prevent one from referring high-risk patients to centers with dedicated neuro-intensive care facilities. Supportive care in experienced hands still remains most valuable in GBS patients.

REFERENCES

1. Ad Hoc Committee WHO-AIREN. *Acute Onset Flaccid Paralysis.* Geneva: World Health Organization, 1993.
2. van der Meché FGA, Van Doorn PA. Guillain–Barré syndrome and chronic inflammatory

demyelinating polyneuropathy; immune mechanisms and update on current therapies. *Ann Neurol* 1995;37(S1):S14–S31.

3. Larsen JP, Kvale G, Nyland H. Epidemiology of the Guillain–Barré syndrome in the county of Hordaland, western Norway. *Acta Neurol Scand* 1985;71:43–7.

4. Emilia-Romagna Study Group on Clinical and Epidemiological Problems in Neurology. A prospective study on the incidence and prognosis of Guillain–Barré syndrome in Emilia-Romagna region, Italy (1992–1993). *Neurology* 1997;48:214–21.

5. Winner SJ, Evans JG. Age-specific incidence of Guillain–Barré syndrome in Oxfordshire. *QJM* 1990;77:1297–1304.

6. Beghi E, Kurland LT, Mulder DW, Wiederholt WC. Guillain–Barré syndrome. Clinico-epidemiologic features and effect of influenza vaccine. *Arch Neurol* 1985;42:1053–7.

7. Bak P. Guillain–Barré syndrome in a Danish county. *Neurology* 1985;35:207–11.

8. Hankey GJ. Guillain–Barré syndrome in western Australia, 1980–1985. *Med J Aust* 1987;146:130–3.

9. Halls J, Bredkjaer C, Friis ML. Guillain–Barré syndrome: diagnostic criteria, epidemiology, clinical course and prognosis. *Acta Neurol Scand* 1988;78:118–22.

10. Sedano MJ, Calleja J, Canga E, Berciano J. Guillain–Barré syndrome in Cantabria, Spain. An epidemiological and clinical study. *Acta Neurol Scand* 1994;89:287–92.

11. van Koningsveld R, Van Doorn PA, Schmitz PIM, Ang CW, van der Meche FG. Mild forms of Guillain–Barré syndrome in an epidemiologic survey in the Netherlands. *Neurology* 2000;54:620–5.

12. Jacobs BC, Rothbarth PH, van der Meche FG, et al. The spectrum of antecedent infections in Guillain–Barré syndrome: a case-control study. *Neurology* 1998;51:1110–15.

13. Hahn AF. Guillain–Barré syndrome. *Lancet* 1998;352(9128):635–41.

14. Radhakrishnan K, el-Mangoush MA, Gerryo SE. Descriptive epidemiology of selected neuromuscular disorders in Benghazi, Libya. *Acta Neurol Scand* 1987;75:95–100.

15. Paolino E, Govoni V, Tola MR, Casetta I, Granieri E. Incidence of the Guillain–Barré syndrome in Ferrara, northern Italy, 1981–1987. *Neuroepidemiology* 1991;10:105–11.

16. Jiang GX, de Pedro-Cuesta J, Fredrikson S. Guillain–Barré syndrome in South-west Stockholm, 1973–1991, 1. Quality of registered hospital diagnoses and incidence. *Acta Neurol Scand* 1995;91:109–17.

17. McKhann GM, Cornblath DR, Griffin JW, et al. Acute motor axonal neuropathy: a frequent cause of acute flaccid paralysis in China. *Ann Neurol* 1993;33:333–42.

18. Winer JB, Hughes RAC, Anderson MJ, Dones JM, Kangro H, Watkins RPF. A prospective study of acute idiopathic neuropathy. II. Antecedent events. *J Neurol Neurosurg Psychiatry* 1988;51:613–18.

19. Arnason BGW. Acute inflammatory demyelinating polyradiculoneuropathies. In Dyck PJ, Thomas PK, Lambert EH, Bunge R, (Eds.). *Peripheral Neuropathy*. Philadelphia: W. B. Saunders, 1984:2050–100.

20. Kinnunen E, Farkkila M, Hovi T, Juntunen J, Weckstrom P. Incidence of Guillain–Barré syndrome during a nationwide oral poliovirus vaccine campaign. *Neurology* 1989;39:1034–6.

21. Fagius J, Osterman PO, Siden A, Wiholm BE. Guillain–Barré syndrome following zimeldine treatment. *J Neurol Neurosurg Psychiatry* 1985;48:65–9.

22. Schonberger LB, Bregman DJ, Sullivan JZ, et al. Guillain–Barré syndrome following vaccination in the national influenza immunization program, United States, 1976–1977. *Am J Epidemiol* 1979;110:105–23.

23. Raschetti R, Maggini M, Popoli P, et al. Gangliosides and Guillain–Barré syndrome. *J Clin Epidemiol* 1995;48:1399–1405.

24. Cabrera J, Griffin DE, Johnson RT. Unusual features of the Guillain–Barré syndrome after rabies vaccine prepared in suckling mouse brain. *J Neurol Sci* 1987;81:239–45.

25. Pollard JD, Selby G. Relapsing neuropathy due to tetanus toxoid. Report of a case. *J Neurol Sci* 1978;37:113–25.

26. Jiang GX, de Pedro-Cuesta J, Strigard K, Olsson T, Link H. Pregnancy and Guillain–Barré syndrome: a nationwide register cohort study. *Neuroepidemiology* 1996;15:192–200.

27. Arnason BG, Asbury AK. Idiopathic polyneuritis after surgery. *Arch Neurol* 1968;18:500–7.

28. Klingon GH. Guillain–Barré syndrome associated with cancer. *Cancer* 1965;18:157–63.

29. Kaldor J, Speed BR. Guillain–Barré syndrome and *Campylobacter jejuni*: a serological study. *BMJ* (Clin Res Ed) 1984;288(6434):1867–70.

30. Visser LH, van der Meché FGA, Meulstee J, et al. Cytomegalovirus infection and Guillain–Barré syndrome; the clinical, electrophysiologic and prognostic features. *Neurology* 1996;47:668–73.

31. Steele JC, Thanasophon S, Gladstone RM, Fleming PC. *Mycoplasma pneumoniae* as a determinant of the Guillain–Barré syndrome. *Lancet* 1969;4(7623):710–14.

32. Ropper AH. *Campylobacter* diarrhea and Guillain–Barré syndrome. *Arch Neurol* 1988;45:655–6.

33. Speed BR, Kaldor J, Watson J, et al. *Campylobacter jejuni/Escherichia coli*-associated Guillain–Barré syndrome. Immunoblot confirmation of the serological response. *Med J Aust* 1987;147:13–16.

34. Vriesendorp FJ, Mishu B, Blaser MJ, Koski CL. Serum antibodies to GM1, GD1b, peripheral nerve myelin, and *Campylobacter jejuni* in patients with Guillain–Barré syndrome and controls: correlation and prognosis. *Ann Neurol* 1993;34:130–5.

35. Mishu B, Ilyas AA, Koski CL, et al. Serologic evidence of previous *Campylobacter jejuni* infection in patients with the Guillain–Barré syndrome. *Ann Intern Med* 1993;118:947–53.

36. Rees JH, Soudain SE, Gregson NA, Hughes RAC. *Campylobacter jejuni* infection and Guillain–Barré syndrome. *N Engl J Med* 1995;333:1374–9.

37. Visser LH, van der Meché FGA, Van Doorn PA, et al. Guillain–Barré syndrome without sensory loss (acute motor neuropathy). A subgroup with specific clinical, electrodiagnostic and laboratory features. Dutch Guillain–Barré Study Group. *Brain* 1995;118:841–7.

38. Jacobs BC, Van Doorn PA, Schmitz PIM, et al. *Campylobacter jejuni* infections and anti-GM1 antibodies in Guillain–Barré syndrome. *Ann Neurol* 1996;40:181–7.

39. Oomes PG, Jacobs BC, Hazenberg MP, Banffer JR, van der Meche FG. Anti-GM1 IgG antibodies and *Campylobacter* bacteria in Guillain–Barré syndrome: evidence of molecular mimicry. *Ann Neurol* 1995;38:170–5.

40. Jacobs BC, Endtz HPh, van der Meché FGA, Hazenberg MP, Achtereekte HAM, Van Doorn

PA. Serum anti-GQ1b IgG antibodies recognize surface epitopes on *Campylobacter jejuni* from patients with Miller Fisher syndrome. *Ann Neurol* 1995;37:260–4.

41. Yuki N, Taki T, Inagaki F, et al. A bacterium lipopolysaccharide that elicits Guillain–Barré syndrome has a GM1 ganglioside-like structure. *J Exp Med* 1993;178:1771–5.

42. Jacobs BC, Endtz HP, van der Meche FG, Hazenberg MP. Humoral immune response against *Campylobacter jejuni* lipopolysaccharides in Guillain–Barré and Miller Fisher syndrome. *J Neuroimmunol* 1997;79:62–8.

43. Asbury AK, Arnason BG, Karp HR, McFarlin DE. Criteria for diagnosis of Guillain–Barré syndrome. *Ann Neurol* 1978;3:565–6.

44. Berciano J, Coria F, Monton F, Calleja J, Figols J, LaFarga M. Axonal form of Guillain–Barré syndrome: evidence for macrophage-associated demyelination. *Muscle Nerve* 1993;16:744–51.

45. Cros D, Triggs WJ. There are no neurophysiologic features characteristic of "axonal" Guillain–Barré syndrome. *Muscle Nerve* 1994;17:675–7.

46. van der Meché FGA, Meulstee J, Kleyweg RP. Axonal damage in Guillain–Barré syndrome. *Muscle Nerve* 1991;14:997–1002.

47. Fuller GN, Jacobs JM, Lewis PD, Lane RJ. Pseudoaxonal Guillain–Barré syndrome: severe demyelination mimicking axonopathy. A case with pupillary involvement. *J Neurol Neurosurg Psychiatry* 1992;55:1079–83.

48. Brown WF, Feasby TE, Hahn AF. Electrophysiological changes in the acute "axonal" form of Guillain–Barré syndrome. *Muscle Nerve* 1993;16:200–5.

49. Yuki N, Yoshino H, Sato S, Miyatake T. Acute axonal polyneuropathy associated with anti-GM1 antibodies following *Campylobacter* enteritis. *Neurology* 1990;40:1900–2.

50. Van den Berg LH, Marrink J, de Jager AEJ, et al. Anti-GM1 antibodies in patients with Guillain–Barré syndrome. *J Neurol Neurosurg Psychiatry* 1992;55:8–11.

51. Kornberg AJ, Pestronk A, Bieser K, et al. The clinical correlates of high-titer IgG anti-GM1 antibodies. *Ann Neurol* 1994;35:234–7.

52. Yuki N, Sato S, Tsuji S, Ohsawa T, Miyatake T. Frequent presence of anti-GQ1b antibody in Fisher's syndrome. *Neurology* 1993;43:414–17.

53. McKhann GM, Griffin JW, Cornblath DR, Mellits ED, Fisher RS, Quaskey SA. Plasmapheresis and Guillain–Barré syndrome: analysis of prognostic factors and the effect of plasmapheresis. *Ann Neurol* 1988;23:347–53.

54. van der Meché FGA, Schmitz PIM, Dutch Guillain–Barré Study Group. A randomized trial comparing intravenous immune globulin and plasma exchange in Guillain–Barré syndrome. *N Engl J Med* 1992;326:1123–9.

55. Ropper AH. The Guillain–Barré syndrome. *N Engl J Med* 1992;326:1130–6.

56. de Jager AEJ, Minderhoud JM. Residual signs in severe Guillain–Barré syndrome: analysis of 57 patients. *J Neurol Sci* 1991;104:151–6.

57. Ropper AH. Severe acute Guillain–Barré syndrome. *Neurology* 1986;36:429–32.

58. Gruener G, Bosch EP, Strauss RG, Klugman M, Kimura J. Prediction of early beneficial response to plasma exchange in Guillain–Barré syndrome. *Arch Neurol* 1987;44:295–8.

59. Winer JB, Hughes RAC, Osmond C. A prospective study of acute idiopathic neuropathy. I. Clinical features and their prognostic value. *J Neurol Neurosurg Psychiatry* 1988;51:605–12.

60. Miller RG, Peterson GW, Daube JR, Albers JW. Prognostic value of electrodiagnosis in Guillain–Barré syndrome. *Muscle Nerve* 1988;11:769–74.

61. Smith GD, Hughes RAC. Plasma exchange treatment and prognosis of Guillain–Barré syndrome. *QJM* 1992;85:751–60.

62. Visser LH, Schmitz PIM, Meulstee J, Van Doorn PA, van der Meché FGA. Prognostic factors of Guillain–Barré syndrome after intravenous immunoglobulin or plasma exchange. *Neurology* 1999;53:598–604.

63. The prognosis and main prognostic indicators of Guillain–Barré syndrome. A multicentre prospective study of 297 patients. The Italian Guillain–Barré Study Group. *Brain* 1996;119:2053–61.

64. Genis D, Busquets C, Manubens E, Davalos A, Baro J, Oterino A. Epidural morphine analgesia in Guillain–Barré syndrome. *J Neurol Neurosurg Psychiatry* 1989;52:999–1001.

65. The Guillain–Barré study group. Plasmapheresis and acute Guillain–Barré syndrome. *Neurology* 1985;35:1096–104.

66. French Cooperative Group on plasma exchange in Guillain–Barré Syndrome. Efficiency of plasma exchange in Guillain–Barré syndrome: role of replacement fluids. *Ann Neurol* 1987;22:753–61.

67. Randomised trial of plasma exchange, intravenous immunoglobulin, and combined treatments in Guillain–Barré syndrome. Plasma Exchange/Sandoglobulin Guillain–Barré Syndrome Trial Group. *Lancet* 1997;349(9047):225–30.

68. The Dutch Guillain–Barré Study Group. Treatment of Guillain–Barré syndrome with high-dose immune globulins combined with methylprednisolone: a pilot study. *Ann Neurol* 1994;35:749–52.

69. Brewis M, Poskanzer DC, Rolland C, Miller H. Neurological disease in an English city. *Acta Neurol Scand* 1966;42(Suppl.):1–89.

70. Chen KM, Brody JA, Kurland LT. Patterns of neurologic diseases on Guam. *Arch Neurol* 1968;19:573–8.

71. Gudmundsson KR. Prevalence and occurrence of some rare neurological diseases in Iceland. *Acta Neurol Scand* 1969;45:114–18.

72. Kennedy RH, Danielson MA, Mulder DW, Kurland LT. Guillain–Barré syndrome: a 42-year epidemiologic and clinical study. *Mayo Clin Proc* 1978;53:93–9.

73. Soffer D, Feldman S, Alter M. Epidemiology of Guillain–Barré syndrome. *Neurology* 1978;28:686–90.

74. Hogg JE, Kobrin DE, Schoenberg BS. The Guillain–Barré syndrome: epidemiologic and clinical features. *J Chronic Dis* 1979;32:227–31.

75. D'Ambrosio G, De AG, Vizioli R. Epidemiology of Guillain–Barré syndrome in Campania (south Italy). Preliminary results. *Acta Neurol* 1983;5(Napoli):245–52.

76. Kaplan JE, Poduska PJ, McIntosh GC, Hopkins RS, Ferguson SW, Schonberger LB. Guillain–Barré syndrome in Larimer county, Colorado: a high-incidence area. *Neurology* 1985;35:581–4.

77. Bahemuka M. Guillain–Barré syndrome in Kenya: a clinical review of 54 patients. *J Neurol* 1988;235:418–21.

78. Congia S, Melis M, Carboni MA. Epidemiologic and clinical features of the Guillain–Barré syndrome in Sardinia in the 1961–1980 period. *Acta Neurol* (Napoli) 1989;11:15–20.

79. Farkkila M, Kinnunen E, Weckstrom P. Survey of Guillain–Barré syndrome in southern Finland. *Neuroepidemiology* 1991;10:236–41.

80. Koobatian TJ, Birkhead GS, Schramm MM, Vogt RL. The use of hospital data for public health surveillance of Guillain–Barré syndrome. *Ann Neurol* 1991;30:618–21.

81. McLean M, Duclos P, Jacob P, Humphreys P. Incidence of Guillain–Barré syndrome in Ontario and Quebec, 1983–1989, using hospital service databases. *Epidemiology* 1994;5:443–8.

82. Matias-Guiu J, Martin R, Blanquer J, et al. Incidence of Guillain–Barré syndrome and ganglioside intake in Alcoi, Spain [letter]. *Neuroepidemiology* 1993;12:58–60.

83. Howlett WP, Vedeler CA, Nyland H, Aarli JA. Guillain–Barré syndrome in northern Tanzania: a comparison of epidemiological and clinical findings with western Norway. *Acta Neurol Scand* 1996;93:44–9.

84. Rees JH, Thompson RD, Smeeton NC, Hughes RA. Epidemiological study of Guillain–Barré syndrome in south east England. *J Neurol Neurosurg Psychiatry* 1998;64;74–7.

17

Encephalitis and meningitis

Ettore Beghi

The occurrence and clinical spectrum of infectious disorders of the central nervous system (CNS) in developed and developing countries present a temporal and geographic variability, depending on the variable distribution of the etiological agents and their vectors, different cultural attitudes towards disease control and prevention, and methodological inconsistencies of the available epidemiological studies. The latter include the use of different definitions of CNS infections, poor definition of the populations at risk, and incompleteness of diagnostic assessment. The majority of the studies are case reports, hospital series, and reports of presumed outbreaks of an infectious disease. These peculiarities and limitations must be considered when an assessment is made of the patterns of distribution and the comparability of the commonest rubrics of the CNS infections, i.e., encephalitis and meningitis.

Diagnosis

The infectious agents may provoke CNS impairment ranging from mild meningeal reactions to severe meningeal and/or parenchymal damage, which prevents clear separation between encephalitis and meningitis. With reference to standard criteria (1,2), encephalitis can be diagnosed in the presence of an acute or subacute onset of symptoms with neurological signs (clinical or laboratory) suggesting brain parenchyma involvement, in the absence of other diagnoses, including noninflammatory CNS infections. Meningitis can be defined by the presence of acute or subacute symptoms with signs of meningeal irritation and cerebrospinal fluid (CSF) pleocytosis (i.e., more than five leucocytes per mm^3), with no signs of cerebral parenchyma involvement and no evidence of other diagnoses. Bacterial meningitis can be separated from viral (or aseptic) meningitis by the presence of at least 1000 white blood cells (WBC) with $>50\%$ polymorphonucleocytes (PMNL) and/or glucose level <40 mg/dl, or less than 1000 WBC with $>50\%$ PMNL and glucose level <40 mg/dl. CSF examination is diagnostic in most cases of meningitis and encephalitis, although routine lumbar puncture can be of less value in neonates, in whom the risk of hemorrhagic tap is high and pathogens may be more frequently identified in blood cultures (3). Polymerase chain reaction (PCR) analysis can identify the etiologic agent when prior antibacterial treatment interferes with the bacterial growth (4). PCR techniques are also useful for the diagnosis of herpes simplex virus infections early in the course of encephalitis (5) and for the diagnosis of enterovirus infections (6). CSF total proteins are significantly different in patients with bacterial meningitis, in those with viral meningitis, and in those with no evidence of infection; lactate concentration is reduced and interleukin-6, interleukin-1 beta and tumor necrosis factor-alpha concentrations are elevated in bacterial meningitis compared to the other groups (7,8). Latex particle agglutination tests in the CSF are useful for the diagnosis of *Haemophilus influenzae*, *Neisseria meningitidis* and *Streptococcus pneumoniae* infection where laboratory facilities are limited (9).

Patterns of distribution and incidence rates

The patterns of distribution and the main epidemiological indexes of CNS infections are given in Table 17.1 for encephalitis and aseptic meningitis and in Table 17.2 for bacterial meningitis. These data are based on the report of endemic cases. However, epidemics are frequent for the majority of bacterial and viral infections, especially in developing countries. For any given infection, an epidemic is suspected when more than 15 cases per 100 000 per week (averaged over 2 weeks) are reported.

Almost all the studies on encephalitis and aseptic meningitis (Table 17.1) were hospital-based and some of them were limited to children and adolescents. Except for Israel and Libya, the study populations were from industrialized areas in the Northern hemisphere (six reports from Finland). The incidence of encephalitis ranged from 1 to 7.4 cases per 100 000 per year in patients of all ages and from 1 to 16.7 cases per 100 000 per year in children and adolescents. The corresponding rates for aseptic meningitis were 10.9–26.7 for children and adults combined and 27.8 in patients aged less than 14 years. Although the different rates can be largely interpreted on the basis of different study method, the incidence of encephalitis was generally lower than that of aseptic meningitis and children were at higher risk of CNS infection than adults.

The only community study on the epidemiology of encephalitis and aseptic meningitis was that of Beghi et al. (2) who examined the medical records of the Olmsted County population seen at the Mayo Clinic facilities during the period 1950–81. Using the definitions reported above, the age- and sex-adjusted incidence rate of viral encephalitis was 7.4 per 100 000. The rate was 8.6 for men and 6.3 for women. The incidence was highest in children of both sexes under age 10

Table 17.1. Patterns of distribution and incidence rates of encephalitis (E) and aseptic meningitis (AM)

Author (ref. no.)	Country	Commonest etiological agents (in decreasing order)	Source of cases (age)	Study period	No. of cases	Incidence (per 100 000 population per year)
Klemola (1965) (10)	Finland	Mumps, Adenovirus, Herpes simplex, Polio, Echo	Hospital records (all ages)	1945–63	108 (E)	2–3
Soffer (1977) (11)	Israel	—	Hospital records (all ages)	1969–70	1359 (AM)	21.6
Ponka (1982) (12)	Finland	Mumps	Hospital records (all ages)	1980	113 (AM)	26.7
					9 (E)	3.5
Beghi (1984) (2)	Minnesota, US	California, Mumps, Herpes simplex, Echo, Coxsackie	Medical records linkage (all ages)	1950–81	189 (E)	7.4
					283 (AM)	10.9
Rantakallio (1986) (13)	Finland	Mumps, Coxsackie	Hospital records EEG records (<14 yr)	1966–81	21 (E)	12.6
					46 (AM)	27.8
Radhakrishnan (1987) (14)	Libya	Herpes simplex, Rabies	Hospital records (all ages)	1983–84	5 (E)	1
					17 (AM)	3.4
Rantala (1989) (15)	Finland	Varicella, Mumps, Herpes simplex, Measles	Hospital and EEG records (<16 yr)	1973–87	95 (E)	8.8
Koskiniemi (1991) (16)	Finland	Enteroviruses, Herpes simplex Respiratory viruses, Mycoplasma	Hospital records (<16 yr) (<1 yr)	1968–87	405 (E)	1–16.7

| Ishikawa (1993) (17) | Japan | Measles, rubella, Herpes simplex | Hospital records (<16 yr) | 1990–92 | 256 (E) | 3.3 (6.6 <5 yr) (2.0 5–15 yr) |
| Koskiniemi (1997) (18) | Finland | Varicella, respiratory and enteroviruses | Hospital records (<16 yr) | 1993–94 | 175 (E) | 10.5 (18.4 <1 yr) |

Table 17.2. Patterns of distribution and incidence rates of bacterial meningitis

Author (ref. no.)	Country	Commonest etiological agents (in decreasing order)	Source of cases (age)	Study period	No. of cases	Incidence (per 100 000 population per year)
Fraser (1973) (19)	South Carolina, US	HI, SP, NM	Hospital records Death certificates Reports (all ages)	1961–71	260	5.6 (White) 18.9 (Black)
Fraser (1974) (20)	New Mexico, US	HI, SP, NM	Hospital records Death certificates (all ages)	1964–71	184	7.3
Floyd (1974) (21)	Tennessee, US	NM, HI, SP	Hospital records Death certificates Reports (all ages)	1963–71	391	7.7 (urban) 4.6 (rural)
Gilsdorf (1977) (22)	Alaska, US	HI, SP	Hospital records (all ages)	1971–74	39	94.2
Ponka (1982) (12)	Finland	HI, SP, NM	Hospital records (all ages)	1980	23	5.2
Schlech (1985) (23)	US (27 States)	HI, NM, SP	CDC reports (all ages)	1978–81	13974	2.9–4.4
Spanjaard (1985) (24)	Holland	NM, HI, SP	Hospital records Notifications Lab. records	1977–82	4150	8 22 (<5 yr)
Rantakallio (1986) (13)	Finland	NM, HI	Hospital records EEG records (<14 yr)	1966–81	55	33.3
Nicolosi (1986) (1)	Minnesota, US	HI, SP, NM	Medical records linkage (all ages)	1950–81	280	8.6
Radhakrishnan (1987) (14)	Libya	SP, NM	Hospital records (all ages)	1983–84	10	2.0
Salwen (1987) (25)	Sweden	HI, NM, SP	Hospital records (1 mo–16 yr)	1956–65	201	5.6 13.0
Rosenthal (1988) (26)	Israel	HI, SP, NM	Hospital records (<13 yr)	1981–85	100	328 (Bedouins <5 yr) 173 (Jews <5 yr)

Reference	Country	Organisms	Method	Period	Number	Incidence
Zaki (1990) (27)	Kuwait	HI, SP, NM	Hospital records	1981–87	110	3.2 (13 <12 yr)
Carter (1990) (28)	Scotland	NI, HI	Hospital records (<13 yr)	1946–61	285	16.9
				1971–86	274	17.8
Wenger (1990) (29)	US	HI, SP, NM	Lab. reports (all ages)	1986	2158	1.9–4.0
Aronson (1991) (30)	Rhode Island, US	–	Hospital records (all ages)	1976–85	667	6.9
Fortnum (1993) (31)	England	NM, HI, SP	Hospital records, Lab. records Health Authority area reports (<17 yr)	1980–89	300	16
Ishikawa (1996) (32)	Japan	HI, SP, GBS, EC	Hospital records (<16 yr)	1984–93	328	2.3 (7.2 <5 yr; 0.5 5–15 yr)
Yang (1996) (33)	China	HI, NM, SP	Hospital records (<16 yr)	1990–92		9.3 (19.2 ≤5 yr)
Schuchat (1997) (34)	US	SP, NM, GBS, LM, HI	Active population-based surveillance (all ages)	1995	248	2.4
Hussey (1997) (35)	South Africa	NM, HI, SP	Hospital records (<14 yr)	1991–92	201	34 (76 <5 yr; 257 <1 yr)

HI, *Hemophilus influenzae*; SP, *Streptococcus pneumoniae*; NM, *Neisseria meningitidis*; GBS, Group B streptococci; EC, *Escherichia coli*; LM, *Listeria monocytogenes*.

(<1 year 22.5; 1–4 years 15.2; 5–9 years 30.2). The disease had a seasonal pattern, with peak incidence in the summer months. The age- and sex-adjusted incidence of aseptic meningitis was 10.9 per 100 000 (men 13.1; women 9.6). Children aged less than 1 year of age had the highest incidence of aseptic meningitis (82.4). The incidence dropped with increasing age and was lowest in patients aged 60 + years (0.7).

Hospital records, CDC reports, and the Mayo Clinic Records Linkage System were the sources of patients in the studies on the epidemiology of bacterial meningitis (Table 17.2). Most of the data came from different states of the US and referred to patients of all ages. In children and adults the incidence of bacterial meningitis ranged from 2 to 94.2 cases per 100 000 per year, with different rates according to race (white vs. black) and living environment (urban vs. rural). Studies in children reported higher rates (2–328 per 100 000 per year). Again the wide differences in the reported rates reflect mostly a different intensity in the recruitment of patients and the use of a different study design. The study by Nicolosi et al. (1) is the only community survey in which patients with bacterial meningitis (diagnosed according to the definition given above) were traced during the period 1950–81 through their medical records. In that study, the age- and sex-adjusted incidence rate was 8.6 (men 9.4; women 7.9). The incidence was highest in the youngest age groups (<1 year 161.3; 1–4 years 32.3) and in the elderly (70 + years 14.7).

Etiology

Encephalitis and meningitis can be caused by many etiological agents. A list of the commonest causes is given in Tables 17.1 and 17.2. The different incidence and distribution of the commonest etiological agents is mostly based on the target populations (children vs. adults), the sources of cases (hospital records, laboratory records, death certificates, reports to regulatory agencies), the study design (prospective or retrospective), and the diagnostic criteria used for case acceptance. The most comprehensive sources of information on the causes of brain infection are the microbiological series. However, even in these cases, underreporting is evident, as inapparent infections can be detected using specific microbiological techniques to assess antibody prevalence rates (36).

Arboviral, enteroviral, and parainfectious encephalitides are the commonest viral infections. Arboviral infections (mosquito-borne and tick-borne) have a different geographic distribution and seasonal incidence depending on the habitat and life cycles of the vectors. Numerous outbreaks of arboviral infections, mostly equine and Japanese B encephalitides, have been reported, with variable mortality rates (37). Human enteroviruses have a worldwide distribution (38) and a life cycle which varies according to the geographical area and climate. In temperate areas enterovirus infections peak in summer and early fall. Enterovirus infections are more common in children and usually more severe in the newborn, older children, and adults. The commonest isolates are Echo and Coxsackie viruses and the most frequent neurological disorders are, in decreasing order, aseptic meningitis and encephalitis (37). Aseptic meningitis has also been reported in 1–2% of patients infected with polio virus. However, the disease has almost disappeared in developed countries since the introduction of mass immunization. Herpes simplex encephalitis has an estimated incidence of 1–4 cases per million population per year (39). In adults and children older than 2 years, over 90% of cases are caused by Herpes simplex virus type 1. The infection is more frequent among neonates and children of lower socioeconomic groups, where the prevalence of Herpes simplex antibodies is also higher (40). No epidemiological data are available on Herpes zoster encephalitis, although possible risk factors include age, immunosuppression, and disseminated cutaneous zoster. Parainfectious encephalitides have been reported to decrease significantly after the introduction of vaccination campaigns. Prior to the introduction of the vaccine, CNS involvement by mumps virus was present in up to 30% of cases (41); it then fell to 0.2% (37). The corresponding values for measles encephalitis before and after vaccination are 1:1000 and 1.5:100 000. Subacute sclerosing panencephalitis (SSPE) has been reported in almost all ethnic groups with variable incidence (0.1–7.7 cases per 100 000 per year) (37), mostly in patients with early age of measles infection, unvaccinated individuals, and among Blacks and Arabs. The incidence of varicella encephalitis, including acute cerebellar ataxia, is 1.5 per 100 000 population (2.6 per 10 000 varicella cases) (42). Although vaccines containing whole, killed organisms and live-attenuated viruses are thought to cause encephalopathies (43), epidemiological data on the CNS complications of vaccines are scanty. An excess risk of neurological complications of pertussis immunization (1:110 000 inoculations) has been documented through a case-control study (44). The incidence of encephalopathy after measles vaccination is less than one case per million doses (45). Mumps meningitis is 1:1000 vaccine recipients (46).

Hemophilus influenzae (HI), *Streptococcus pneumoniae* and *Neisseria meningitidis* are the commonest causes of bacterial meningitis in population-based and hospital-based studies (Table 17.2). HI and other bacterial meningitides are most frequent in infants and young children, patients with chronic illnesses, military recruits, and communities where crowding and poor living conditions are prevalent (47). The incidence of HI meningitis ranges from 1 to 5 per 100 000. Recently, epidemics of *Hemophilus* meningitis have been reported in several pediatric and adult communities, including day care centers (48,49). The incidence of *Hemophilus* meningitis has been shown to decrease after the introduction of vaccines.

An inverse relationship over time has been documented between the number of affected cases and the number of vaccine doses sold (50). The incidence of streptococcus meningitis is between 3 and 6 per 100 000 (51), with higher rates for children, the elderly, and people living in crowded areas. The annual incidence of *Neisseria* meningitis has been reported to vary between 1 and 3 cases per 100 000, serogroup B being the commonest etiologic agent. Outbreaks of meningococcal meningitis are still frequently reported in crowded environments.

Less frequent causes of encephalitis and meningitis include *Rickettsiae*, *Bordetella pertussis*, *Toxoplasma gondii* (ingestion of undercooked meals and contaminated water or milk), Group B streptococci, staphylococci, *Escherichia coli*, Salmonella and Proteus species, *Pseudomonas aeruginosa* and *Enterobacter aerogenes* (head trauma and surgical contamination), *Klebsiella pneumoniae* (ENT and community-acquired infections), *Pasteurella* and *Brucella* species (individuals exposed to animals and dairy products), corynebacteriacae, *Mycobacterium tuberculosis* and *Mycoplasma pneumoniae* (causing bacterial and aseptic meningitis), Lyme disease and other spirochetal CNS disorders, and *Plasmodium falciparum* (37,48).

Bacterial meningitis occurring in the newborn can be considered a separate entity as its etiology is different (48). *Escherichia coli*, *Streptococcus agalactiae*, *Klebsiella pneumoniae*, *Streptococcus* species, and *Listeria monocytogenes* are the commonest causative agents. The different etiology of neonatal meningitis reflects the mode of acquisition of the infection and immunological status of the child. The incidence of neonatal meningitis has been estimated to be 0.5–1.9 per 1000 live births, being higher in preterm neonates with low birth weight or prolonged rupture of the amniotic membranes. Other meningitides caused by bacteria, fungi, or protozoa are becoming of increasing interest because they represent opportunistic infections.

Prognosis

The large majority of patients with viral encephalitis tend to recover with minimal or no residua. The mean annual mortality rate in Olmsted County, Minnesota, has been reported to be 0.5 per 100 000, with a case fatality ratio of 4% (1,2). Fairly similar findings were reported in Finland (1–10%) (10,13,15) and in France (<5%) (52). In hospital series greater case fatality ratios have been reported, with significant variations depending on the type of infection and the recorded epidemic. In these cases, the higher mortality is mostly based on the underascertainment of milder cases. Arboviral encephalitides have been reported to carry variable case-fatality ratios (from less than 1% to 75%) with maximal rates for eastern equine encephalitis and Japanese encephalitis (37). Mortality has been reported in up to 33% of patients with Herpes simplex encephalitis (53) and in 0–3% of patients with Herpes zoster encephalitis (54). Mortality in patients with aseptic meningitis is almost nil (2).

Bacterial meningitis is generally a more severe disease, with a case-fatality ratio approximating 100% in untreated patients. When antibacterial agents came into general use, the mortality rates dropped significantly. In Olmsted County the mortality rate was 2.7 per 100 000 per year and the case-fatality ratio totalled 15% (1). Mortality varied significantly according to the etiologic agent, being maximal with *Streptococcus pneumoniae*. Case-fatality ratios fell from 82% (1935–40) to 29% (1941–49), 12% (1950–59), 14% (1960–69), 6.5% (1970–81). In the same population neonatal meningitis had a case-fatality ratio of 45% (declining from nearly 100% to 25% during the same intervals). Age and bacteremia increase a fatal outcome in patients with meningococcal disease (55).

Surviving patients may have sequelae (reported by 16% of the survivors in the Olmsted County study) (1). Sequelae are usually multiple and most frequently characterized by hearing defects (10%), mental retardation (10%), seizures (2–8%), motor (3–7%) and visual defects (2–4%) (56). Less severe complications, including headache, inability to concentrate, loss of memory, and dizziness, have been reported in 81% of patients given a questionnaire to investigate their health status (57). Factors related to the organism (*Hemophilus influenzae*, *Streptococcus pneumoniae*), the disease (longer duration of symptoms, overall disease severity, early seizures) and the host (younger or older age, neurological abnormalities at diagnosis, glucose, lactate, and cytokine levels, malnutrition) are important in determining the outcome of bacterial meningitis (48,58). Recurrent episodes of bacterial meningitis are occasionally reported, depending on anatomical congenital defects of the skull or the CNS, surgical defects, parameningeal chronic infections, impaired immune defense mechanisms, and the sequelae of head trauma. Recurring meningitis is generally caused by the same etiologic agent and is rarely fatal.

Intervention

The control of viral infections of the CNS is mostly based on prevention measures (59). Arboviral infections can be prevented by mosquito control programs and the use of inactivated or live attenuated vaccines (against equine and tick-borne encephalitides) that can be given to high-risk categories, such as laboratory workers and people living in endemic areas. The introduction of mass immunization with live attenuated viruses led to an almost complete eradication of poliomyelitis and its complications in the large industrialized countries of the temperate zones. The incidence of parainfectious childhood encephalitides (measles, SSPE, mumps, rubella) showed a remarkable decrease after the introduction of the vaccines. Mass vaccination is recommended in these cases.

The only CNS viral infection for which an effective treatment has been developed is Herpes simplex encephalitis. The currently accepted treatment is a 10-day course of acyclovir given intravenously at a dosage of 10 mg/kg every 8 hours (53,60).

Better insight into the pathophysiology of bacterial meningitis and the emergence of resistant organisms has led to significant changes in the basic principles of antimicrobial therapy (61). When the etiologic agent is still undetected, an empirical therapy of purulent meningitis must be based on the presence of predisposing factors (age, immunocompromised state, trauma, surgical intervention), as the commonest organisms tend to vary depending on the host characteristics and physical status. In general, ampicillin is the drug of first choice in the youngest children and the elderly, and third generation cephalosporins (cefotaxime or ceftriaxone), eventually associated with ampicillin, are preferred in patients aged 3 months to 50 years. Vancomycin is indicated for immunocompromised patients, head trauma, and surgery. Specific antimicrobial therapy tends also to vary according to the type of etiology. Ampicillin is the standard treatment of CNS infections caused by *Hemophilus* beta-lactamase negative strains and third generation cephalosporins are used for beta-lactamase positive strains. Benzylpenicillin or ampicillin are the standard treatment of *Neisseria* and *Streptococcus* infections. Streptococcal infections with minimal inhibitory concentration 0.1 mg/L or higher require use of third generation cephalosporins or vancomycin. Ceftazidime is the drug of choice for *Pseudomonas aeruginosa*, ampicillin (or benzylpenicillin) for *Listeria monocytogenes*, and vancomycin for staphylococcal infections.

Widespread immunization of infants with *Hemophilus influenzae* type B conjugate vaccine has been recommended (62). *Streptococcus pneumoniae* has shown increasing resistance to antibacterial agents in the last few years (63). The available polyvalent vaccine is effective in patients at higher risk, except for the elderly, the immunocompromised patients, and younger children (64). *Neisseria meningitidis* serogroup A, which was responsible of epidemics worldwide until World War II, can now be controlled by mass vaccination of selected high-risk groups (e.g., military recruits). An effective vaccine against group B meningococcus must be developed and the immunogenicity of the pneumococcal and quadrivalent meningococcal vaccines must be improved. BCG has been shown by meta-analysis to be protective against tuberculous meningitis (65). The prevention of auditory sequelae in pediatric bacterial meningitis does not seem to be affected by the antibacterial regimens (66).

Adjunctive treatment with steroids is also recommended on the basis of a recognized control of the intense inflammatory subarachnoid reaction occurring with bacterial infections. A meta-analysis of double-blind placebo-controlled trials on the use of dexamethasone in infants and children showed lower incidence of bilateral hearing loss with active treatment (67). However, the use of steroids remains controversial for the methodological inconsistencies of published trials (68).

The decision to use antibacterial agents for prophylaxis to family contacts, close neighbor contacts or children attending day-care centers is controversial (69).

Implications for clinical practice

A remarkable change in the rates of CNS infections has been noted in recent years, which may be correlated to a series of factors, including change in the type of exposure, introduction of effective preventive measures, development of bacterial strains resistant to available treatments, and new high-risk categories (elderly and immunocompromised patients). Although these notable changes may raise the interest in the epidemiology of encephalitis and meningitis, the notification rates, mostly based on passive reports, are still low (about 50%) for bacterial infections (31) and may be even lower for viral infections. In addition, the diagnosis of CNS infection is suboptimal, especially in the adult population (70). Passive notification systems are also unsatisfactory as patients who are reported do not reflect the origin of affected populations and the time to report is long. Sensitive and rapid case definition is needed for local monitoring of outbreaks and for prophylactic coverage. In addition, clear guidelines for notification and reporting are needed. Regulatory agencies, microbiologists, clinicians, and environmental health officers should cooperate more actively and review arrangements for data exchange.

Excessive prescribing of antibacterial agents tends to increase the chance of serious adverse drug reactions and the development of drug resistance. Clear guidelines for notification and reporting and a standard diagnostic, preventive, and therapeutic approach are needed to optimize the clinical approach to CNS infections, especially in countries where health care resources are limited.

REFERENCES

1. Nicolosi A, Hauser WA, Beghi E, Kurland LT. Epidemiology of central nervous system infections in Olmsted County, Minnesota, 1950–1981. *J Infect Dis* 1986;154:399–408.
2. Beghi E, Nicolosi A, Kurland LT, et al. Encephalitis and aseptic meningitis, Olmsted County, Minnesota, 1950–1981: I. Epidemiology. *Ann Neurol* 1984;16:283–94.
3. Baziomo JM, Krim G, Kremp O, et al. Retrospective analysis of 1331 samples of cerebrospinal fluid in newborn infants with suspected infection. *Arch Pediatr* 1995;2:833–9.

4. Haolin N, Knight AI, Cartwright K, Palmer WH, McFadden J. Polymerase chain reaction for diagnosis of meningococcal meningitis. *Lancet* 1992;340:1432–4.

5. Cinque P, Cleator GM, Weber T, Monteyne P, Sindic CJ, van Loon AM for the EU Concerted Action on Virus Meningitis and Encephalitis. The role of laboratory investigation in the diagnosis and management of patients with suspected herpes simplex encephalitis: a consensus report. *J Neurol Neurosurg Psychiatry* 1996;61:339–45.

6. Rotbart HA, Sawyer MH, Fast S, et al. Diagnosis of enteroviral meningitis by using PCR with a colorimetric microwell detection assay. *J Clin Microbiol* 1994;32:2590–2.

7. Hashim IA, Walsh A, Hart CA, Shenkin A. Cerebrospinal fluid interleukin-6 and its diagnostic value in the investigation of meningitis. *Ann Clin Biochem* 1995;32:289–96.

8. Lopez Cortes LF, Cruz Ruiz M, Gomez Mateos J, et al. Measurement of levels of tumor necrosis factor-alpha and interleukin-1 beta in the CSF of patients with meningitis of different etiologies: utility in the differential diagnosis. *Clin Infect Dis* 1993;16:534–9.

9. Camargos PA, Almeida MS, Cardoso I, et al. Latex particle agglutination test in the diagnosis of *Haemophilus influenzae* type B, *Streptococcus pneumoniae* and *Neisseria meningitidis* A and C meningitis in infants and children. *J Clin Epidemiol* 1995;48:1250–4.

10. Klemola E, Kaariainen L, Ollila O, et al. Studies on viral encephalitis. *Acta Med Scand* 1965;177:707–16.

11. Soffer D, Alter M, Kahana E, Yaar I. Aseptic meningitis: frequency among Israeli ethnic groups. *J Neurol* 1977;214:89–96.

12. Ponka A, Petterson T. The incidence and etiology of central nervous system infections in Helsinki in 1980. *Acta Neurol Scand* 1982;66:529–35.

13. Rantakallio P, Leskinen M, von Wendt L. Incidence and prognosis of central nervous system infections in a birth cohort of 12 000 children. *Scand J Infect Dis* 1986;18:287–94.

14. Radhakrishnan K, Maloo JC, Poddar SK, Mousa ME. Central nervous system infections in Benghazi, Libya: experience from a community-based adult medical neurology set-up. *J Trop Med Hyg* 1987;90:123–6.

15. Rantala H, Uhari M. Occurrence of childhood encephalitis: a population-based study. *Pediatr Infect Dis J* 1989;8:426–30.

16. Koskiniemi M, Rautonen J, Lehtokoski-Lehtiniemi E, Vaheri A. Epidemiology of encephalitis in children: a year survey. *Ann Neurol* 1991;29:492–7.

17. Ishikawa T, Asano Y, Morishima T, et al. Epidemiology of acute childhood encephalitis. Aichi Prefecture, Japan, 1984–90. *Brain Dev* 1993;15:192–7.

18. Koskiniemi M, Korppi M, Mustonen K, et al. Epidemiology of encephalitis in children. A prospective multicentre study. *Eur J Pediatr* 1997;156:541–5.

19. Fraser DW, Darby CP, Koehler RE, et al. Risk factors in bacterial meningitis: Charleston County, South Carolina. *J Infect Dis* 1973;127:271–7.

20. Fraser DW, Geil CC, Feldman RA. Bacterial meningitis in Bernalillo County, New Mexico: a comparison with three other American populations. *Am J Epidemiol* 1974;100:29–34.

21. Floyd RF, Federspield CF, Shaffner W. Bacterial meningitis in urban and rural Tennessee. *Am J Epidemiol* 1974;99:395–407.

22. Gilsdorf J. Bacterial meningitis in Southwestern Alaska. *Am J Epidemiol* 1977;106:388–91.

23. Schlech WF 3d, Ward JI, Band JD, Hightower A, Fraser DW, Broome CV. Bacterial meningitis in the United States, 1978 through 1981. The National Bacterial Meningitis Surveillance Study. *JAMA* 1985;253:1749–54.

24. Spanjaard L, Bol P, Ekker W, Zanen HC. The incidence of bacterial meningitis in the Netherlands – a comparison of three registration systems, 1977–1982. *J Infect* 1985;11:259–68.

25. Salwen KM, Vikerfors T, Olcen P. Increased incidence of childhood bacterial meningitis. A 25-year study in a defined population in Sweden. *Scand J Infect Dis* 1987;19:1–11.

26. Rosenthal J, Dagan R, Press J, Sofer S. Differences in the epidemiology of childhood community-acquired bacterial meningitis between two ethnic populations cohabiting in one geographic area. *Pediatr Infect Dis J* 1988;7:630–3.

27. Zaki M, Daoud AS, ElSaleh Q, West PW. Childhood bacterial meningitis in Kuwait. *J Trop Med Hyg* 1990;93:7–11.

28. Carter PE, Barclay SM, Galloway WH, Cole GF. Changes in bacterial meningitis. *Arch Dis Child* 1990;65:495–8.

29. Wenger JD, Hightower AW, Facklam RR, et al. Bacterial meningitis in the United States, 1986: report of a multistate surveillance study. *J Infect Dis* 1990;162:1316–23.

30. Aronson SM, DeBuono BA, Buechner JS. Acute bacterial meningitis in Rhode Island: a survey of the years 1976 to 1985. *R I Med J* 1991;74:33–6.

31. Fortnum HM, Davis AC. Epidemiology of bacterial meningitis. *Arch Dis Child* 1993;68:763–7.

32. Ishikawa T, Asano Y, Morishima T, et al. Epidemiology of bacterial meningitis in children. *Pediatr Neurol* 1996;14:244–50.

33. Yang Y, Leng Z, Shen X, et al. Acute bacterial meningitis in children in Hefei, China 1990–1992. *Chinese Med J* 1996;109:385–8.

34. Schuchat A, Robinson K, Wenger JD, et al. Bacterial meningitis in the United States in 1995. Active Surveillance Team. *N Engl J Med* 1997;337:970–6.

35. Hussey G, Schaaf H, Hanslo D, et al. Epidemiology of post-neonatal bacterial meningitis in Cape Town children. *South Afr Med J* 1997;87:51–6.

36. Grimstad PR, Barrett CL, Humphrey RL, Sinsko MJ. Serologic evidence for widespread infections with LaCrosse and St. Louis encephalitis viruses in the Indiana human population. *Am J Epidemiol* 1984;119:913–30.

37. Beghi E. Epidemiology of encephalitis. In Gorelick PB, Alter M (Eds.). *Handbook of Neuroepidemiology.* New York: Marcel Dekker Inc, 1994:457–90.

38. Melnick JL. Enteroviruses: polioviruses, coxsackieviruses, echoviruses and newer enteroviruses. In Fields BN, Knipe DM, Chanock RM, Melnick JL, Roizmsn B, Shopc RE (Eds.). *Virology.* New York: Raven Press, 1985:739–94.

39. Whitley RJ, Schlitt M. Encephalitis caused by herpes viruses, including B virus. In Scheld WM, Whitley RJ, Durack DT (Eds.). *Infections of the Central Nervous System.* New York: Raven Press, 1991:41–86.

40. Baker AB. Viral encephalitis. In Baker AB, Baker LH (Eds.). *Clinical Neurology.* Philadelphia: Harper & Row, 1984:1–147.

41. Gnann JW. Meningitis and encephalitis caused by mumps virus. In Scheld WM, Whitley RJ, Durack DT (Eds.). *Infections of the Central Nervous System*. New York: Raven Press, 1991:113–25.

42. Guess HA, Broughton DD, Melton LJ III, Kurland LT. Population-based studies of varicella complications. *Pediatrics* 1986;78:723–7.

43. Fenichel GM. Neurological complications of immunization. Ann Neurol 1982;12:119–28.

44. Miller DL, Ross EM, Alderslade R, Bellman MH, Rawson NS. Pertussis immunization and serious acute neurological illness in children. *BMJ* 1981;282:1595–9.

45. Centers for Disease Control. Measles prevention. *MMWR* 1987;36:409.

46. Cizman M, Mozetic M, Radescek Rakar R, et al. Aseptic meningitis after vaccination against measles and mumps. *Pediatr Infect Dis J* 1989;8:302–8.

47. Urwin G, Yuan MF, Feldman RA. Prospective study of bacterial meningitis in North East Thames region 1991–3, during introduction of *Haemophilus influenzae* vaccine. *BMJ* 1994;309:1412–14.

48. Nicolosi A. Epidemiology of bacterial meningitis and brain abscess. In Gorelick PB, Alter M (Eds.). *Handbook of Neuroepidemiology*. New York: Marcel Dekker Inc, 1994:493–529.

49. Cochi SL, Fleming DW, Hightower AW, et al. Primary invasive *Haemophilus influenzae* type B disease: a population based assessment of risk factors. *J Pediatr* 1986;108:887–96.

50. Peltola H, Kilpi T, Anttila M. Rapid disappearance of *Haemophilus influenzae* type b meningitis after routine childhood immunization with conjugate vaccines. *Lancet* 1992;340:592–4.

51. Centers for Disease Control. Recommendations of the Immunization Practices Advisory Committee (ACIP); pneumococcal polysaccharide vaccine. *MMWR* 1981;30:410–18.

52. Tardieu M. Meningites et encephalites virales aigues de l'enfant. *Pediatrie* 1987;42:675–80.

53. Skoldenberg B, Forsgren M, Alestig K, et al. Acyclovir versus vidarabine in herpes simplex encephalitis. Randomized multicentre study in consecutive Swedish patients. *Lancet* 1984;2:707–11.

54. Mazur MH, Dolin R. Herpes zoster at the NIH: a 20 year experience. *Am J Med* 1978;65:738–44.

55. Scholten RJ, Bijlmer HA, Valkenburg HA, Dankert J. Patient and strain characteristics in relation to the outcome of meningococcal disease: a multivariate analysis. *Epidemiol Infect* 1994;112:115–24.

56. Dodge PR. Sequelae of bacterial meningitis. Pediatr Infect Dis 1986;5:618–20.

57. Bohr V, Hansen B, Kjersem H, et al. Sequelae from bacterial meningitis and their relation to the clinical condition during acute illness, based on 667 questionnaire returns. Part II of a three part series. *J Infect* 1983;7:102–10.

58. Kaaresen PI, Flaegstad T. Prognostic factors in childhood bacterial meningitis. Acta Paediatr 1995;84:873–8.

59. Mangano M, Plotkin SA. Viral vaccines that protect the central nervous system. In Scheld WM, Whitley RJ, Durack DT (Eds.). *Infections of the Central Nervous System*. New York: Raven Press, 1991:233–4.

60. Whitely RJ, Alford Jr CA, Hirsch MS, et al. Vidarabine versus acyclovir therapy of herpes simplex encephalitis. *N Engl J Med* 1986;314:144–9.

61. Rockowitz J, Tunkel AR. Bacterial meningitis. Practical guidelines for management. *Drugs* 1995;50:838–53.

62. Lieberman JM, Greenberg DP, Ward JI. Prevention of bacterial meningitis. Vaccines and chemoprophylaxis. *Infect Dis Clin North Am* 1990;4:703–29.

63. Klugman KP. Pneumococcal resistance to antibiotics. Clin Microbiol Rev 1990;3:171–96.

64. Kass EH (Ed.) Assessment of the pneumococcal polysaccharide vaccine: a workshop held at the Harvard Club of Boston, Boston, Massachussetts, Oct. 6, 1990. *Rev Infect Dis* 1991;3(suppl):S1–S197.

65. Rodrigues LC, Diwan VK, Wheeler JG. Protective effect of BCG against tuberculous meningitis and miliary tuberculosis: a meta-analysis. *Int J Epidemiol* 1993;22:1154–8.

66. Yurkowski PJ, Plaisance KI. Prevention of auditory sequelae in pediatric bacterial meningitis: a meta-analysis. *Pharmacotherapy* 1993;13:494–9.

67. Geiman BJ, Smith AL. Dexamethasone and bacterial meningitis: a meta-analysis of randomized controlled trials. *West J Med* 1992;157:27–31.

68. Prasad K, Haines T. Dexamethasone treatment for acute bacterial meningitis: how strong is the evidence for routine use? *J Neurol Neurosurg Psychiatry* 1995;59:31–7.

69. Cuevas LE, Hart CA. Chemoprophylaxis of bacterial meningitis. *J Antimicrob Chemother* 1993;31(suppl B):79–91.

70. Mathiassen B, Thomsen H, Landsfeldt U. An evaluation of the accuracy of clinical diagnosis at admission in a population with epidemic meningococcal disease. *J Intern Med* 1989;226:113–16.

18

HIV infection

Ned C. Sacktor, Gerald J. Dal Pan and Justin C. McArthur

Introduction

Human immunodeficiency virus (HIV) infection has expanded to become a global pandemic which threatens health in most areas of the world, and is now the leading cause of death among some segments of the population. For example, in 1995 in the USA, AIDS surpassed cancer as the predominant cause of death in young African–American women (25–44 years) (1). From the beginning of the epidemic through to 31 December 1997, there have been 641 086 cases of AIDS and 390 692 AIDS deaths in the USA, according to the Centers for Disease Control (CDC) (2). Rates in women, children, and injecting drug users (IDUs) and infection through heterosexual contact have been rising. In the USA in 1996, African–Americans represented 41% of adults/adolescents reported with AIDS, exceeding the proportion who are Caucasians for the first time (2). On a world-wide scale, the World Health Organization (WHO) has estimated that, as of the end of 1995, 6 million AIDS cases and approximately 20 million people were alive and infected with the HIV-1 virus (3). WHO estimates that nearly 10 000 new infections occur each day.

For the first time since the beginning of the epidemic, the number of AIDS deaths in the USA declined by 13% in the first half of 1996 compared to 1995. Most of the dramatic change, however, was seen among Caucasian homosexual males, and women and minorities continued to show increases in AIDS death rates. The factors explaining this discrepancy probably reflect restricted access for these groups to medical care, and particularly to the newer combination anti-retroviral therapies.

Infection with HIV-1, a member of the lentivirus subfamily of retroviruses, produces a wide spectrum of clinical manifestations, ranging from asymptomatic infection to severe, life-threatening opportunistic infections. Within 6 weeks of infection, an acute seroconversion illness can occur. Neurological features of early infection may include meningoencephalitis, inflammatory demyelinating peripheral neuropathy, facial palsy, brachial neuritis, or radiculopathy.

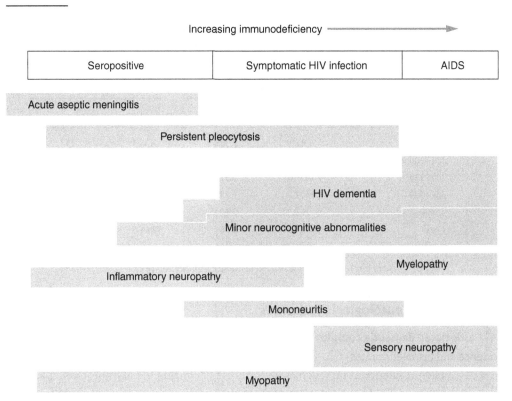

Figure 18.1 Relative timing of HIV-related neurologic disease with respect to systemic disease and relative frequency (represented by width of bar). ARC, AIDS-related complex (6).

Following acute infection, most individuals enter an asymptomatic period, in which patients are free from opportunistic infections or tumors, but functional CD4+ T cell depletion is occurring (4). Recent studies show that this is not a period of virological latency; rather viral replication occurs at a high level but is sequestered in lymphoid tissue (5). The median incubation period ranges from 8–11 years, and is increasing. Following the asymptomatic period, HIV patients progress into a symptomatic period, without profound immunosuppression (AIDS-related complex; ARC), and eventually into a period with profound immunosuppression (AIDS). Most neurologic illnesses are confined to the symptomatic stages of HIV infection (ARC or AIDS) (6) (Figure 18.1), reflecting either the effects of HIV in the central nervous system (CNS) or peripheral nervous system, or the consequence of cellular immunodeficiency.

Table 18.1. Incidence of HIV-related neurological disease per 100 person-years by CD4 + cell count: Multicenter AIDS Cohort Study (1988–1992)

CD4 + cell count	Dementia		Neuropathy	
	PY	IR	PY	IR
≤ 100	818.9	7.34	826.3	7.75
101–200	690.2	3.04	699.3	3.43
201–350	1370.4	1.31	1385.2	0.72
351–500	1427.7	1.75	1445.2	0.76
> 500	263.3	0.46	2648.6	0.49
Total	6944.5	1.96	7004.6	1.74

PY, person years free of specific disease; IR, incidence rate per 100 person years. From (9).

HIV-associated neurological syndromes

HIV-1 associated dementia complex (HIV dementia)

Incidence and prevalence rates

The prevalence of HIV dementia is only 0.4% during the asymptomatic phase of infection (7). In patients with AIDS, dementia develops in 15–20%. Data from the Multicenter AIDS Cohort Study (MACS), a cohort of homosexual men, has shown that HIV dementia occurs at an annual incidence of 7% after the development of AIDS (8). Incidence rates are higher in those with lower CD4 + counts (Table 18.1) (9). HIV dementia has now become an important cause of dementia in adults younger than age 60.

Diagnosis

HIV dementia is characterized by cognitive symptoms (e.g., memory loss, poor concentration, mental slowing), behavioral symptoms (e.g., apathy, depression), and motor dysfunction (e.g., unsteady gait, poor coordination, tremor).

Potential risk factors for dementia include low CD4 + count, anemia, low body mass index, older age, the presence of more constitutional symptoms before AIDS (8), injection drug use (10), and female sex (11).

Children are also affected by a progressive encephalopathy with loss of milestones. The estimated frequency of the progressive encephalopathy is 30% in children with AIDS (12) with a typical survival of 6 to 24 months. In children, progressive dementia occurs more commonly than CNS opportunistic infections (13,14).

More subtle forms of cognitive impairment termed minor cognitive/motor disorder (MC/MD) exist in 20% of symptomatic HIV-seropositive patients (15,16). The risk for progression to dementia and prognostic impact of MC/MD is unclear. However, several studies (17,18) have independently shown that the presence of cognitive impairment (MC/MD or dementia) in HIV infection is predictive of poor survival.

The diagnosis of HIV dementia is established by a history of a progressive cognitive or behavioral decline with apathy, memory loss, or slowed mental processing and by appropriate ancillary studies. Neuropsychological assessment shows progressive deterioration on serial testing in at least two areas including motor speed, frontal/executive functioning, and memory. Imaging studies in HIV dementia reveal diffuse cerebral atrophy with ill-defined white matter hyperintensities on magnetic resonance imaging. Imaging studies are also performed to exclude any central nervous system opportunistic processes. Cerebrospinal fluid analysis is also useful to exclude cryptococcal meningitis or neurosyphilis.

Prognosis

The progression of HIV dementia is variable. Some patients have a relatively rapid progression over 3–6 months, whereas a third may have a slow/stable course over years. Low CD4 + count, injection drug use, and prominent psychomotor slowing may be associated with more rapid progression of neurological deficits (15).

Intervention

Antiretroviral treatment may improve some of the cognitive deficits associated with HIV dementia. Portegies et al. (19) observed a dramatic fall in the point-prevalence of HIV dementia from 53% before the introduction of zidovudine to about 10% after zidovudine (used in high doses of 1200–1500 mg/day) was made available in Amsterdam (19). This finding has not been confirmed in other studies, but most of these have not used the high doses of zidovudine administered in the 1980s. (Lower doses are now used because of myelotoxicity at higher doses of zidovudine.) The impact of combination antiretroviral medication therapy and protease inhibitors on the epidemiology of HIV dementia remains to be determined. In a study of temporal trends in neurological diseases from the Multicenter AIDS Cohort Study (MACS) between 1988 and 1992, there was no change in incidence of HIV dementia after adjustment for CD4 + counts, with no major protective effect of regular doses of zidovudine on the development of HIV dementia (8) (Figure 18.2). Recent observations since January 1996 (when highly active antiretroviral medications including protease inhibitors came into use) show conflicting results on the incidence of HIV dementia. In the Frankfurt AIDS Cohort Study, the incidence of HIV dementia has decreased (20). The CDC reported an increase in reported cases of HIV dementia, whereas the MACS

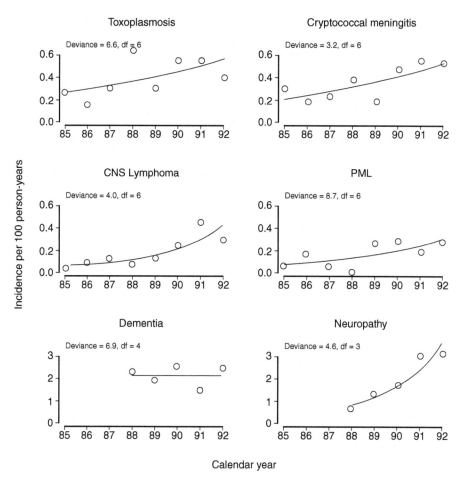

Figure 18.2 Incidence of HIV-related neurologic diseases in the Multicenter AIDS Cohort Study, 1985–1992. Open circles represent observed data; solid lines represent expected incidence based on Poisson regression models, unadjusted for level of immunosuppression. PML, progressive multifocal leukoencephalopathy (9).

reported a decrease in cases (Figure 18.3). The decrease in incidence in the MACS may represent less active surveillance for dementia in the MACS. These observations need to be confirmed over a longer period.

Epidemiology of other HIV-associated neurological syndromes

Myelopathies

HIV-1 associated vacuolar myelopathy (HIV myelopathy) is characterized by a vacuolar degeneration affecting predominantly the thoracic spinal cord. Symptoms include a slowly progressive spastic paraparesis, with bowel and bladder

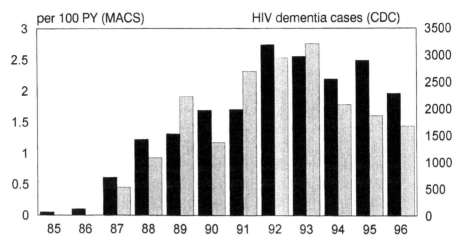

Figure 18.3 Incidence of HIV dementia in the Multicenter AIDS Cohort Study (MACS) and USA (CDC). Solid bar and left axis represent incidence in the MACS per 100 person-years (PY). Hatched bar and right axis represent HIV dementia as a percentage of AIDS indicator illnesses.

involvement occurring late in the course. Its prevalence from autopsy series ranges from 22–55% (21–22), with clinical expression in only 10% or less. HIV myelopathy is often accompanied by dementia. Myelopathies due to other infections (syphilis, HTLV-1 virus, herpes group viruses, cytomegalovirus (CMV), mycobacteria, toxoplasmosis) or neoplastic causes (lymphoma) have been reported (23–28), although their frequency is relatively low.

HIV-related neuromuscular disorders

A variety of peripheral nervous system disorders can complicate HIV infection (29–33). During the asymptomatic period of infection, acute and chronic inflammatory demyelinating polyneuropathies can occur in 1% or less of patients (34). A multiple mononeuropathy also may complicate HIV infection in 0.5–3.0% of patients (35,36), usually when other constitutional symptoms are present, but before the development of AIDS-indicator illnesses.

The most common neuropathy is a predominantly sensory peripheral neuropathy (HIV neuropathy) which usually occurs in the later stages of HIV infection (30). Symptoms include severe pain in the feet, which can impair walking markedly. Estimates of the prevalence of symptomatic neuropathy vary from 13% in a clinical referral population (30) to 35% in hospitalized AIDS patients (37). Using clinical and electrophysiologic criteria, Levy et al. (36) found a prevalence of neuropathy of 89% with 42% of the neuropathy cases being symptomatic (36). There has been an increasing incidence of HIV neuropathy (Figure 18.3), probably reflecting increasing survival with severe immunosuppression and the cumulative effects of neurotoxic drugs (38).

A toxic neuropathy associated with the antiretroviral agents, didanosine (ddI) (39), zalcitabine (ddC) (40), and stavudine (d4T) can occur in 13, 34, and 15–20 of patients respectively. The symptoms of HIV-associated sensory neuropathy and the toxic neuropathy are identical. This neurotoxic effect is a major factor limiting the use of these antiretroviral agents.

Myopathy in HIV-seropositive patients can be related to HIV infection itself or to the myotoxic effects of zidovudine treatment (41). Myopathy can occur at any stage of HIV infection. The frequencies of these disorders are not well established. In a study comparing zidovudine to placebo the incidence of a composite diagnosis of myopathy was 3% in the zidovudine treated group compared to 0.4% in the placebo group (42). Autopsy studies have found that about 25% of persons who have died of AIDS have muscle pathology attributable to HIV myopathy.

Epidemiology of HIV-associated neurological opportunistic infections

Opportunistic infections and neoplasms of the CNS are common in association with HIV infection, and usually do not develop until the CD4 + count is below 200, reflecting the underlying immunodeficiency. Patients may have multiple concurrent opportunistic processes, or opportunistic processes may coexist with HIV-related neurological disorders. An AIDS patient who develops an opportunistic infection will need lifelong maintenance therapy.

Cryptococcal meningitis

Cryptococcus neoformans, a ubiquitous encapsulated yeast, causes neurological disease in about 10% of AIDS patients (43). It is the most common CNS opportunistic infection in AIDS patients. Symptoms include fever, headache, photophobia, and an altered mental status. In up to 5% of patients, it may be the first recognized opportunistic infection. In 1997, 1168 cases of extrapulmonary cryptococcosis (the vast majority being cryptococcal meningitis) were reported to the CDC, accounting for 5% of all initial AIDS-indicator opportunistic infections in the USA. Assay of the CSF cryptococcal antigen is nearly 100% sensitive and specific and can be performed rapidly (44). As primary and secondary prophylaxis with antifungal agents such as fluconazole become more widespread, the rates of cryptococcal meningitis in AIDS patients may decline.

Central nervous system toxoplasmosis

Toxoplasma gondii, an obligate intracellular protozoan, can cause multifocal cerebral abscesses. Symptoms include fever, hemiparesis, confusion, seizure, ataxia, and other focal neurological abnormalities. Clinical CNS toxoplasmosis is the result of reactivation of a latent infection. Grant et al. estimated that the 3-year probability of ever developing CNS toxoplasmosis was 28% for HIV-infected patients also seropositive for antibodies to *Toxoplasma gondii* (45). There is wide variation in the prevalence of latent infection among different populations, reflecting differences in dietary and other sociocultural factors. In 1997, 1073 cases of CNS toxoplasmosis were reported to the CDC, accounting for 4% of all initial AIDS-indicator conditions in the USA. Current prophylactic regimens directed toward primary prevention of *Pneumocystis carinii* pneumonia, including trimethoprim/sulfamethoxazole and dapsone, also are effective in reducing the incidence of CNS toxoplasmosis (9,46–48). In the era of combination therapy, the incidence of CNS toxoplasmosis has decreased (20).

Primary CNS lymphoma

Up to 3% of AIDS patients develop primary CNS lymphoma (PCNSL), making AIDS the most common disease associated with this tumor. About one-half of these tumors are clinically silent and detected only at autopsy. Almost all PCNSL are B cell-derived (49). The typical presentation is one of slowly progressive neurological deterioration with headache, mental change, seizures, and focal deficits (49). Treatment with radiotherapy with or without chemotherapy is only modestly effective, increasing median survival from 1–2 months in untreated cases to 3–6 months (50). The majority of PCNSL cases occur when the CD4 + count is less than 50 cells/mm³ (51). In 1997, 170 cases of PCNSL were reported to the CDC, accounting for 1% of all initial AIDS-indicator conditions in the USA. These figures underestimate the true burden of PCNSL, as this condition is often seen after other AIDS-indicator illnesses have developed, i.e., is a secondary condition. As the use of primary antimicrobial prophylaxis decreases the frequency of CNS toxoplasmosis and as more individuals are surviving longer periods in immunosuppressed states due to the use of antiretroviral agents, PCNSL may become an increasingly important cause of mass lesions in HIV-infected patients.

Progressive multifocal leukoencephalopathy

Progressive multifocal leucoencephalopathy (PML), a complication in 2–4% of AIDS cases, is a demyelinating CNS disorder caused by infection of oligodendrocytes and astrocytes with a reactivated virus called the JC virus, a member of the Papovaviridae. Primary infection with the JC virus, although usually clinically silent, is common in childhood and early adulthood, with 80–90% of the general population infected by middle adulthood. Common presenting symptoms are cognitive dysfunction, weakness, and visual loss. CSF JC virus polymerase chain reaction (PCR) is positive in 30–60% of cases (52). In 1997, 213 cases of PML were reported to the CDC, accounting for 1% of all AIDS-indicator conditions in the USA. Survival after PML generally is poor, with a median survival of about 4 months, although survival of up to 30 months has been reported (53).

Cytomegalovirus infection

Cytomegalovirus (CMV) is a common pathogen in the advanced stages of AIDS, producing disease when the CD4+ count is usually less than 100 cells/mm^3. CMV-induced disease represents reactivation of latent infection. In the general population, the seroprevalence of antibodies to CMV is about 50% (54). In HIV-seropositive homosexual men, however, the seroprevalence of anti-CMV antibodies is closer to 100% (55). CMV retinitis, a common manifestation of CMV-induced disease and a main cause of visual loss and blindness, occurs in 15–28% of AIDS patients (56,57), although the introduction of protease inhibitors may be decreasing the incidence of CMV disease.

CMV encephalitis presents with acute or subacute confusion, disorientation, and memory loss, and tends to have a more rapid progression than HIV dementia. CSF CMV PCR is positive in 30–100% of cases. CMV encephalitis has been reported in up to 2% of AIDS patients (35,58), although it may be misdiagnosed for HIV dementia, and this figure may underrepresent the true frequency (59). Autopsy studies reveal evidence of CMV infection in 10–50% of brains from AIDS patients (60–63).

CMV polyradiculitis is characterized by the subacute onset of a flaccid paraparesis, sacral pain, paresthesias, and sphincter dysfunction (64,65). CSF findings include a polymorphonuclear pleocytosis and hypoglycorrhachia. In about 50% of cases of polyradiculitis, CSF viral cultures yield CMV, and CMV PCR is usually positive. Polyradiculitis occurs in about 2% of AIDS patients (31,34,35,66).

With the introduction of highly active antiretroviral therapy, CMV-induced disease has become less common.

Implications of highly active antiretroviral therapies for clinical practice

Combination antiretroviral medication therapies including protease inhibitors and the ability to monitor disease progression through plasma viral load measurement are having a significant impact on the epidemiology of systemic HIV infection. Their influence on the epidemiology of HIV-associated neurological conditions is unclear. With the use of combination antiretroviral regimens and increased use of prophylactic regimens to prevent opportunistic infections, HIV-infected persons are having increased survival. With suppression of the virus in the systemic compartment, neurological disease could decrease as well. Recent data in the Multicenter AIDS Cohort Study suggests that in the era of highly active antiretroviral therapy, the incidence of HIV dementia, cryptococcal meningitis, CNS toxoplasmosis, and primary CNS lymphoma may be decreasing (67). However, subjects in this cohort maintain excellent adherence to complicated antiretroviral regimens. In patients with poor adherence, the CNS may act as a reservoir for the development of neurovirulent strains, and HIV-associated neurological disease could increase. In the future, an increasing proportion of care for patients with HIV or AIDS may be related to neurological conditions.

REFERENCES

1. Centers for Disease Control and Prevention. HIV/AIDS Surveillance Report 1995;7:1–39.
2. Centers for Disease Control and Prevention. US HIV and AIDS cases reported through December 1997. *HIV/AIDS Surveillance Report* 1997;8:1–43.
3. Mertens TE, Low-Beer D. HIV and AIDS: where is the epidemic going? *Bull WHO* 1996;74:121–9.
4. Phillips AN, Lee CA, Elford J, et al. Serial CD4 lymphocyte counts and development of AIDS. *Lancet* 1991;337:389–92.
5. Ho DD, Neumann AU, Perelson AS, Chen W, Leonard JM, Markowitz M. Rapid turnover of plasma virions and CD4 lymphocytes in HIV-1 infection. *Nature* 1995;373:123–6.
6. Johnson RT, McArthur JC, Narayan O. The neurobiology of human immunodeficiency virus infections. *FASEB J* 1988;2:2970–81.
7. Bartholomew C, Saxinger WC, Clark JW, et al. Transmission of HTLV-I and HIV among homosexual men in Trinidad. *JAMA* 1987;257:2604–8.
8. McArthur JC, Hoover DR, Bacellar H, et al. Dementia in AIDS patients: incidence and risk factors. *Neurology* 1993;43:2245–52.
9. Bacellar H, Munoz A, Miller EN, et al. Temporal trends in the incidence of HIV-1 related neurologic diseases: Multicenter AIDS Cohort Study, 1985–1992. *Neurology* 1994;44:1892–1900.
10. Janssen RS, Nwanyanwu OC, Selik RM, Stehr-Green JK. Epidemiology of human immunodeficiency virus encephalopathy in the United States. *Neurology* 1992; 42:1472–6.
11. Chiesi A, Seeber AC, Dally LG, Floridia M, Rezza G, Vella S. AIDS dementia complex in the Italian National AIDS Registry: temporal trends (1987–1993) and differential incidence according to mode of transmission of HIV-1 infection. *J Neurol Sci* 1996;144:107–13.
12. Belman AL, Diamond G, Dickson D, et al. Pediatric acquired immunodeficiency syndrome. Neurologic syndromes [published erratum appears in *Am J Dis Child* 1988 May;142(5):507]. *Am J Dis Child.* 1988;142:29–35.
13. Epstein LG, Sharer LR, Joshi VV, Fojas MM, Koenigsberger MR, Oleske JM. Progressive encephalopathy in children with acquired immune deficiency syndrome. *Ann Neurol* 1985;17:488–96.
14. Mintz M, Epstein LG, Koenigsberger MR. Neurological manifestations of acquired immunodeficiency syndrome in children. *Int Pediatrics* 1989;4:161–71.

15. Bouwman FH, Skolasky R, Hes D, et al. Variable progression of HIV-associated dementia. *Neurology* 1998;50:1814–20.

16. Janssen RS, Cornblath DR, Epstein LG, McArthur J, Price RW. Human immunodeficiency virus (HIV) infection and the nervous system: report from the American Academy of Neurology AIDS Task Force. *Neurology* 1989;39:119–22.

17. Sacktor NC, Bacellar H, Hoover DR, et al. Psychomotor slowing in HIV infection. A predictor of dementia, AIDS, and death. *J Neurovirol* 1996;2:404–10.

18. Mayeux R, Stern Y, Tang MX, et al. Mortality risks in gay men with human immunodeficiency virus infection and cognitive impairment. *Neurology* 1993;43:176–82.

19. Portegies P, de Gans J, Lange JM, et al. Declining incidence of AIDS dementia complex after introduction of zidovudine treatment [published erratum appears in *BMJ* 1989 Nov 4;299(6708):1141]. *BMJ* 1989;299:819–21.

20. Brodt HR, Kamp BS, Gute P, Knupp B, Staszewski S, Helm EB. Changing incidence of AIDS-defining illnesses in the era of antiretroviral combination therapy. *AIDS* 1997;11:1731–8.

21. Artigas J, Grosse G, Niedobitek F. Vacuolar myelopathy in AIDS. A morphological analysis. *Pathol Res Pract* 1990;186:228–37.

22. Dal Pan GJ, Glass JD, McArthur JC. Clinicopathological correlations of HIV-1-associated vacuolar myelopathy: an autopsy-based case-control study. *Neurology* 1994;44:2159–64.

23. Berger JR. Spinal cord syphilis associated with human immunodeficiency virus infection: a treatable myelopathy. *Am J Med* 1992;92:101–3.

24. Britton CB, Mesa-Tejada R, Fenoglio CM, Hays AP, Garvey GG, Miller JR. A new complication of AIDS: thoracic myelitis caused by herpes simplex virus. *Neurology* 1985;35:1071–4.

25. Herskovitz S, Siegel SE, Schneider AT, Nelson SJ, Goodrich JT, Lantos G . Spinal cord toxoplasmosis in AIDS. *Neurology* 1989;39:1552–3.

26. McArthur JC, Griffin JW, Cornblath DR, et al. Steroid-responsive myeloneuropathy in a man dually infected with HIV-1 and HTLV-I. *Neurology* 1990;40:938–44.

27. Tucker T, Dix RD, Katzen C, Davis RL, Schmidley JW. Cytomegalovirus and herpes simplex virus ascending myelitis in a patient with acquired immune deficiency syndrome. *Ann Neurol* 1985;18:74–9.

28. Woolsey RM, Chambers TJ, Chung HD, McGarry JD. Mycobacterial meningomyelitis associated with human immunodeficiency virus infection [see comments]. *Arch Neurol* 1988;45:691–3.

29. Cornblath DR. Treatment of the neuromuscular complications of human immunodeficiency virus infection. *Ann Neurol* 1988;23:S88–S91.

30. Cornblath DR, McArthur JC. Predominantly sensory neuropathy in patients with AIDS and AIDS-related complex. *Neurology* 1988;38:794–6.

31. Miller RG, Storey JR, Greco CM. Ganciclovir in the treatment of progressive AIDS-related polyradiculopathy. *Neurology* 1990;40:569–74.

32. Parry GJ. Peripheral neuropathies associated with human immunodeficiency virus infection. *Ann Neurol* 1988;23:S49–S53.

33. Simpson DM, Wolfe DE. Neuromuscular complications of HIV infection and its treatment. *AIDS* 1991;5:917–26.

34. Fuller GN, Jacobs JM, Guiloff RJ. Nature and incidence of peripheral nerve syndromes in HIV infection. *J Neurol Neurosurg Psychiatry* 1993;56:372–81.

35. Guiloff RJ, Fuller GN, Roberts A, et al. Nature, incidence and prognosis of neurological involvement in the acquired immunodeficiency syndrome in central London. *Postgrad Med J* 1988;64:919–25.

36. Levy RM, Bredesen DE, Rosenblum ML. Neurological manifestations of the acquired immunodeficiency syndrome (AIDS): experience at UCSF and review of the literature. *J Neurosurg* 1985;62:475–95.

37. So YT, Holtzman DM, Abrams DI, Olney RK. Peripheral neuropathy associated with acquired immunodeficiency syndrome. Prevalence and clinical features from a population-based survey. *Arch Neurol* 1988;45:945–8.

38. Dal Pan GJ, Nance-Sproson TE, Cohen BA, Lopez OL, Miller EN, Guccione M. HIV-associated predominantly sensory neuropathy: risk factors and survival characteristics in the Multicenter AIDS Cohort Study (MACS). Neuroscience of HIV Infection: Basic and Clinical Frontiers, Vancouver, BC, Aug 2–5 1994.

39. Yarchoan R, Pluda JM, Thomas RV, et al. Long-term toxicity/activity profile of 2′,3′-dideoxyinosine in AIDS and AIDS-related complex. *Lancet* 1990;336:526–9.

40. Blum AS, Dal Pan GJ, Feinberg J, et al. Low dose zalcitabine (ddC)-related toxic neuropathy: frequency, natural history, and risk factors. *Neurology* 1996;46:999–1003.

41. Manji H, Harrison MJG, Round JM, et al. Muscle disease, HIV and zidovudine: the spectrum of muscle disease in HIV-infected individuals treated with zidovudine. *J Neurol* 1993;240:479–88.

42. Simpson DM, Slasor P, Dafni U, Berger J, Fischl MA, Hall C. Analysis of myopathy in a placebo-controlled zidovudine trial. *Muscle Nerve* 1997;2:382–5.

43. Larsen RA, Leal MA, Chan LS. Fluconazole compared with amphotericin B plus flucytosine for cryptococcal meningitis in AIDS. A randomized trial. *Ann Intern Med* 1990;113:183–97.

44. Bartlett JG. *Medical Management of HIV Infection*. Glenview, IL : Physicians & Scientists Publishing Co., 1996.

45. Grant IH, Gold JWM, Rosenblum M, Niedzwiecki D, Armstrong D. *Toxoplasma gondii* serology in HIV-infected patients: the development of central nervous system toxoplasmosis in AIDS. *AIDS* 1990;4:519–21.

46. Carr A, Tindall B, Brew BJ, et al. Low-dose trimethoprim-sulfamethoxazole prophylaxis for toxoplasmic encephalitis in patients with AIDS. *Ann Intern Med* 1992;117:106–11.

47. Girard PM, Landman R, Gaudebout C, et al. Dapsone pyrimethamine compared with aerosolized pentamidine as primary prophylaxis against pneumocystis-carinii pneumonia and toxoplasmosis in HIV infection. *N Engl J Med* 1993;328:1415–520.

48. Hardy WD, Feinberg J, Finkelstein DM, et al. A controlled trial of trimethoprim sulfamethoxazole or aerosolized pentamidine for secondary prophylaxis of pneumocystis-carinii pneumonia in patients with the acquired immunodeficiency syndrome – AIDS Clinical Trial Group Protocol 021. *N Engl J Med* 1992;327:1842–8.

49. Rosenblum ML, Levy RM, Bredesen DE, So YT, Wara W, Ziegler JL. Primary central nervous system lymphomas in patients with AIDS. *Ann Neurol* 1988;23:S13–S16.

50. Baumgartner JE, Rachlin JR, Beckstead JH, et al. Primary central nervous system lymph-

omas: natural history and response to radiation therapy in 55 patients with acquired immunodeficiency syndrome. *J Neurosurg* 1990;73:206–11.

51. Levine AM, Sullivan-Halley J, Pike MC, et al. Human immunodeficiency virus-related lymphoma – prognostic factors predictive of survival. *Cancer* 1991;68:2466–72.

52. Cinque P, Scarpellini P, Vago L, Linde A, Lazzarin A. Diagnosis of central nervous system complications in HIV-infected patients: cerebrospinal fluid analysis by the polymerase chain reaction. *AIDS* 1997;11:1–17.

53. Berger JR, Kaszovitz B, Post MJ, Dickinson G. Progressive multifocal leukoencephalopathy associated with human immunodeficiency virus infection. A review of the literature with a report of sixteen cases. *Ann Intern Med* 1987;107:78–87.

54. Drew WL. Cytomegalovirus infection in patients with AIDS. *J Infect Dis* 1988;158:449–56.

55. Leach CT, Cherry JD, English PA, et al. The relationship between T-cell levels and CMV infection in asymptomatic HIV-1 antibody-positive homosexual men. *J Acquir Immune Defic Syndr Hum Retrovirol* 1993;6:407–13.

56. Cheong I, Flegg PJ, Brettle RP, et al. Cytomegalovirus disease in AIDS: the Edinburgh experience. *Int J STD AIDS* 1992;3:324–8.

57. Jabs DA, Green WR, Fox R, Polk BF, Bartlett JG. Ocular manifestations of acquired immunodeficiency syndrome. *Ophthalmology* 1989;96:1092–9.

58. Degans J, Portegies P. Neurological complications of infections with human immunodeficiency virus type 1. A review of literature and 241 cases. *Clin Neurol Neurosurg* 1989;91:199–219.

59. Holland NR, Power C, Mathews VP, Glass JD, Forman M, McArthur JC. CMV encephalitis in acquired immunodeficiency syndrome (AIDS). *Neurology* 1994;44:507–14.

60. Budka H, Costanzi G, Cristina S, et al. Brain pathology induced by infection with the human immunodeficiency virus (HIV). A histological, immunocytochemical, and electron microscopical study of 100 autopsy cases. *Acta Neuropathol.(Berl.)* 1987;75:185–98.

61. Kure K, Llena JF, Lyman WD, et al. Human immunodeficiency virus-1 infection of the nervous system: an autopsy study of 268 adult, pediatric, and fetal brains. *Hum Pathol* 1991;22:700–10.

62. Petito CK, Cho ES, Lemann W, Navia BA, Price RW. Neuropathology of acquired immunodeficiency syndrome (AIDS): an autopsy review. *J Neuropathol Exp Neurol* 1986;45:635–46.

63. Wiley CA, Nelson JA. Role of human immunodeficiency virus and cytomegalovirus in AIDS encephalitis. *Am J Pathol* 1988;133:73–81.

64. Mahieux F, Gray F, Fenelon G, et al. Acute myeloradiculitis due to cytomegalovirus as the initial manifestation of AIDS. *J Neurol Neurosurg Psychiatry* 1989;52:270–4.

65. Miller RG, Kiprov DD, Parry G, Bredesen DE. Peripheral nervous system dysfunction in acquired immunodeficiency syndrome. In Rosenblum ML, Levy RM, Bredesen DE (Eds.). *AIDS and the Nervous System.* New York: Raven Press, 1987:65–78.

66. Leger JM, Bouche P, Bolgert F, et al. The spectrum of polyneuropathies in patients infected with HIV. *J Neurol Neurosurg Psychiatry* 1989;52:1369–74.

67. Sacktor N, Lyles RH, Skolasky, R, et al. HIV-associated neurologic incidence changes: Multicenter AIDS Cohort Study, 1990–1998, *Neurology* 2001;56:257–60.

19

Prion diseases

Esther A. Croes and Cornelia M. van Duijn

Introduction

Prion disorders form a group of transmissible spongiform encephalopathies that may afflict humans and other mammalians (1–3). They are transmissible within and between species by inoculation of infected tissue in the brain or administration to the blood, and, to a lesser extent, by ingestion of infected material. The most conspicuous feature at microscopic brain examination consists of spongiform changes due to cell loss. The clinical outcome of the encephalopathy consists mainly of dementia, behavioural changes, and cerebellar disorders. Human prion disorders include Creutzfeldt–Jakob disease (CJD), Gerstmann–Sträussler–Scheinker syndrome (GSS), fatal familial insomnia (FFI) and kuru. Prion disorders occur in inherited, acquired, and sporadic forms.

Despite their rare occurrence, the unique infectious and inheritable etiology of these dementias make them not only highly interesting scientifically but also important with regard to public health. The causative agent is thought to be a "prion," which is an acronym for proteinaceous infectious particle (1). Unlike the "traditional" infectious agents such as bacteria and viruses, the prion contains little or no nucleic acid (1) and shows an unusual resistance to traditional disinfectants, preservatives and ionizing radiation, which signifies its potential hazards. This resistance was dramatically illustrated by the outbreak of a bovine spongiform encephalopathy (BSE) epidemic in the UK during the 1980s, for which a change in decontamination procedure of ovine and bovine material for animal feeding was held responsible. In this chapter the etiology, diagnosis, occurrence, and prognosis of human prion disorders will be reviewed. The emphasis will be on CJD, by far the most common and complex prion disorder in humans.

Etiology

The pathogenesis of prion disorders remains an issue of ongoing debate. The normal, or cellular, prion protein (PrP^C) is situated in all body cells, but mainly in the brain and spinal cord. Its function is unknown. There is growing evidence pointing to an abnormal isoform of the prion protein (indicated as PrP^{Sc}) as the transmissible factor (4). PrP^{Sc} is thought to be derived from the normal host protein PrP^{C} through a conformational change (1,4,5). A plausible model proposed is that PrP^{Sc} may act as a template for the conversion of normal host PrP^{C} into PrP^{Sc} (1,4,5). Since PrP^{Sc} is not degradable, this abnormal isoform accumulates and forms aggregates in varying parts of the brain, where it blocks the normal function.

In relation to etiologic subtypes, the three classical forms distinguished in prion diseases are the inherited, acquired, and sporadic forms. Inherited forms of human prion disease constitute up to 5–10% of CJD and virtually all GSS and FFI cases (1–3,6,7). Familial CJD, GSS, and FFI are all caused by mutations in the prion protein gene (PRNP) (1–3,6,7). Not all patients with a dominant PRNP mutation have a family history of prion disease (7), suggesting there is incomplete penetrance of the disease. It is important to realize that the clinical presentation of the disease may differ considerably between mutation carriers from a single family; carriers may present with various neurodegenerative and neuropsychiatric illnesses (8). In addition to dominant mutations in PRNP a milder genetic variation (or polymorphism) in the gene has been implicated in the susceptibility for the acquired, sporadic, and variant form (1–3,9). This concerns the codon 129 polymorphism. In the caucasian population 39% of healthy individuals are homozygous for methionine, 51% heterozygous and 12% homozygous for valine (9). Subjects homozygous for methionine at this codon are at significantly increased risk for acquired and sporadic CJD compared to heterozygotes, whereas homozygotes for valine are at an increased risk for early-onset acquired and sporadic CJD (9). Other genetic or nongenetic risk factors may further underlie the disease. The apolipoprotein E gene, the predominant genetic risk factor for the most common cause of dementia, Alzheimer's disease (10), has been studied in relation to CJD. Although some studies found evidence for an association, a relation to CJD was not confirmed in other investigations (11,12).

In addition to the causes of the disease, prion diseases may be transmitted from man to man. The classical example is kuru, in which the disease has been transmitted through cannibalistic rituals. Iatrogenic transmission of CJD has occurred through dura mater transplantation (13), neurosurgery and electro-encephalographic electrode implantation (14–16), corneal transplantation (17), and administration of human growth (18–20) and gonadotrophin (21) hormone.

In the large majority of patients CJD occurs sporadically. Studies on risk factors for sporadic CJD have yielded controversial results (22–28). An increased risk of CJD has been shown for subjects with a history of infection (22,25), surgery of the head (23,24), and trauma to the head or body (23,24) in some studies but not in others (27). A retrospective case-control study found a significant association between the development of sporadic CJD after surgical procedures (29). The risk increased with the number of surgical treatments, to a maximum of three procedures with an odds ratio of 2.3 (95% confidence interval 1.34–3.41). None of these findings were supported in a joint analysis of five European studies (28,30). Although experimental research indicates that the possibility of transmission through blood products cannot be excluded (31,32), up until now there has been no epidemiological or clinical evidence for transmission of sporadic CJD from man to man through blood transfusion (27,28,33). Findings of studies on dietary transmission, through the consumption of (organ) meat (22,25,28), milk products (28), and exposure to animals (23,26,28) in sporadic CJD have not yielded consistent results (27). The strongest evidence for transmission of spongiform encephalopathies from animal to man through food is found for a form of CJD indicated as variant CJD (vCJD) (34). vCJD was discovered in the UK following the BSE epidemic. Experimental studies strongly suggest that vCJD is linked to the occurrence of an epidemic of BSE (35–37). At present of major concern is the spread of vCJD. Although the number of BSE cases is reduced, there are still affected animals entering the human food chain in the UK and elsewhere.

Diagnosis

Prion disorders are characterized pathologically by the triad of spongy degeneration, neuronal loss, and astrocyte proliferation. In all prion disorders accumulation of the abnormal protease-resistant isoform of the prion protein (PrP^{Sc}) is found in the brain (1). Clinically, classical CJD usually presents between 60 and 70 years of age with a rapidly progressive dementia and end-stage myoclonus. Further, cerebellar ataxia, extrapyramidal features, cortical blindness, and pyramidal signs are frequently present. Characteristic EEG changes consist of generalized periodic sharp wave activity occurring at 1–2 Hz. The diagnostic criteria for possible, probable, and definite classical CJD are listed in Table 19.1. These criteria are based upon Masters' diagnostic criteria (38). The most recent alteration in these criteria concerns the 14-3-3 protein test in cerebrospinal fluid. The 14-3-3 protein reflects a rapid neurodegeneration. When this test is applied to patients with a diagnosis of possible CJD sensitivity and specificity may reach 95% (39). This is much higher than the reported sensitivity and specificity for the EEG (67 and 86% respectively) (40). New developments may be anticipated with regard to the use of magnetic resonance imaging (MRI) in the diagnosis of CJD. There is evidence for an increased signal in the putamen and caudate nucleus, especially on T2-weighted images and proton density scans, in sporadic CJD patients (41). Further, it has been suggested that diffusion-weighted MRI shows changes with

Table 19.1. Diagnostic criteria for classical CJD

I.	rapidly progressive dementia
II.	A. myoclonus
	B. visual or cerebellar problems
	C. pyramidal or extrapyramidal features
	D. akinetic mutism
III.	typical EEG
IV.	positive 14-3-3 protein test

Definite: neuropathological or immunohistochemical confirmation.
Probable: I + 2 of II + III or *possible* + IV.
Possible: I + 2 of II + duration < 2 years.

Table 19.2. Diagnostic criteria for vCJD

I.	A. Progressive neuropsychiatric disorder
	B. Duration of illness > 6 months
	C. Routine investigations do not suggest an alternative diagnosis
	D. No history of potential iatrogenic exposure

Clinical features

II.	A. Early psychiatric symptoms
	B. Persistent painful sensory symptoms
	C. Ataxia
	D. Myoclonus or chorea or dystonia
	E. Dementia

Investigations

III.	A. EEG does not show the typical appearance of classical CJD or no EEG performed
	B. Bilateral pulvinar high signal on MRI scan
IV.	Positive tonsil biopsy

Definite: IA + neuropathological confirmation of vCJD.
Probable: I + 4 of II + IIIA + IIIB or I + IV.
Possible: I and 4 of II + IIIA.

high intensity in the cerebral cortex (42). However, sensitivity and specificity of the current assessment of the MRI are lower than those of the 14-3-3 protein test, and are comparable to that of the EEG (43).

The clinical presentation of classical CJD is highly variable and may depend on the etiology. A distinct clinical picture is seen for vCJD, which is related to BSE (34). The diagnostic criteria are listed in Table 19.2. These patients present at an unusually early age (mean 29 years) with behavioral and psychiatric disturbances and ataxia, rather than dementia (34). Early psychiatric symptoms in vCJD include depression, anxiety, apathy, withdrawal, and delusions. Persistent painful sensory symptoms are also often present, including both frank pain and unpleasant dysesthesia. In a later stage of vCJD dementia and other neurological disorders appear as in the classical form of CJD. The typical EEG abnormalities for classical CJD are absent (34). The 14-3-3 protein test has a sensitivity of only 50% in vCJD patients. Findings on brain MRI-scan, tonsil biopsy and pathology also differ from those in classical CJD. In vCJD, on MRI-scanning a bilateral high signal is seen in the thalamus, especially the pulvinar (44). In tonsil biopsy samples accumulation of the pathogenic protein can be shown (45). Neuropathology shows extensive plaque formation, surrounded by vacuoles (florid plaques), and an unusual pattern of prion staining throughout the cerebrum and cerebellum (34).

For all prion disorders, DNA diagnostics may be used to support the diagnosis. Several dominant mutations in the PRNP gene are known to lead to CJD. In patients with possible CJD from families in which prion disease or dementia segregates as an autosomal dominant disorder, screening of the PRNP gene may elucidate the diagnosis. GSS and FFI are also typically autosomal dominant disorders (6,46,47). The clinical presentation of patients with each of the PRNP mutations known to date may be extremely diverse, ranging from cerebellar disorders or dementia to progressive insomnia and autonomic, endocrine, and motor dysfunction (46,47).

Incidence

Prion diseases are rare among humans. The most common prion disease, CJD, is reported worldwide with a mortality of around one death per million persons (7,38,48,49). Increased frequencies have been found in isolated populations in Slovakia and in Libyan Israelis, in both cases due to an increased frequency of mutations in the PRNP gene (50–52). Most incidence studies have been based on nationwide retrospective searches; therefore the interpretation of the findings is hampered by differences in case-ascertainment and diagnosis. This problem was largely overcome in the European Union, when in 1993 a collaborative study was started in order to monitor the incidence of CJD in Belgium, France, Germany, Italy, the Netherlands, Slovakia, and the UK according to a common protocol (7). The registers aimed to ascertain all patients diagnosed in those countries with definite or probable CJD. In 2000, the reported mortality varied from 0.64 to 1.72 deaths per million (53). From 1993, there has been a modest increase in mortality, which can be attributed to better case ascertainment due to the inclusion of the

14-3-3 protein test in the diagnostic criteria (54,55). Further, this rise may be explained by an increased awareness among neurologists since the recognition of vCJD. Of all CJD patients, 5–10% are classified as familial and up to 5% as iatrogenic, with the remainder being sporadic (7). These percentages may vary between countries. Iatrogenic CJD is mainly attributed to growth hormone treatment, particularly in the UK and France. Transmission by dura mater transplantation is seen mainly in Japan, but is clearly on the rise in other countries. Up until 2000, vCJD has been diagnosed in 91 patients, of whom 88 are inhabitants of the UK, two of France and one of Ireland. From 1995 to 2000 a statistically significant rise in mortality of 33% per year was seen (56). At present it is not possible to predict the size of the epidemic of vCJD in the UK and elsewhere. Predictions range from 100 to more than 100 000 patients (57).

The other classical prion disorders, GSS, FFI, and kuru, are far more rare than CJD. The exact incidence of GSS and FFI is unknown, but estimated to be between 1 and 10 per 100 million (3). Although an epidemic of kuru occurred in the beginning of the twentieth century in the Fore speaking tribes in Papua New Guinea, the disease has virtually disappeared after cessation of ritual cannibalism (58).

Prognosis and intervention

Effective therapy is not available for any of the prion disorders known to date. Within months after diagnosis of CJD, there is a progressive deterioration of the clinical condition to akinetic mutism. The median survival is estimated to be 5 to 6 months (1,2,7). The duration of disease is found to be longer in familial and genetically determined CJD patients (2,46). In vCJD the median duration between onset of symptoms and death is 14 months (34). With regard to the other prion disorders, the course of disease in kuru patients is also devastating, in most cases leading to death within a year (46). The median duration of illness in GSS patients is estimated to be between 4 and 5 years (46).

In the absence of effective therapy, intervention is limited to prevention of prion disorders. The iatrogenic transmission of CJD through human growth hormone has led to a ban on this product after the development of an analogous synthetic compound. The epidemic of CJD patients due to transmission via dura mater transplants has called for preventive measurements in the processing of dura mater.

Of major concern is whether subclinical forms of BSE in animals other than cows, which are used for human consumption, exist and if so, can be transmitted to humans (59). Another point of concern is the possible transmission of prion disorders through medicinal products from animal to man or from man to man.

In BSE and vCJD, infectivity of nonneuronal material is higher compared to classical CJD; in particular lymphoreticular tissue is infective (45). Because of the long incubation period and absence of a screening method for blood donors, man-to-man transmission may occur. In the UK preventive measures have been taken such as the withdrawal from blood banks of blood and blood products from vCJD patients, collection of plasma from outside the UK, and leukodepletion of erythrocyte and thrombocyte concentrate. However, the risk of accidental transmission of vCJD may also be increased during other medical procedures. In particular surgical procedures involving lymphoreticular tissue, e.g. appendectomy or tonsillectomy, might convey a risk of transmission.

Implications

Prion diseases are rare disorders with a unique pathogenesis. Major progress has been achieved in unraveling the genetic etiology. The work on the molecular genetics of these disorders has not only elucidated the pathophysiology, but has also led to the recognition that an unexpectedly wide disease spectrum is associated with various PRNP mutations. PRNP testing may be used as a diagnostic test. However, results may have major implications for relatives, and because of psychological and socio-economic implications testing may be restricted to patients with a clearly positive family history of neuropsychiatric disorders (60). The diagnosis of sporadic CJD has been further improved by the introduction of the 14-3-3 protein test and MRI scanning of the brain.

With regard to the etiology of prion disorders, little is known of risk factors for sporadic CJD. The major challenges in CJD research in Europe will be related to the BSE epidemic. Possible transmission of vCJD through other animals and medicinal products remains an issue of great concern. An important issue to tackle in future research of risk factors is the exposure assessment. Putative models for the transmission from cow to man includes nutrition, medication, and animal exposure. None of these exposures are easily quantified in epidemiologic research. To assess exposure to BSE-infected tissue specifically is particularly difficult. Up until now it has been impossible to trace the products of BSE cows in food or medication. An important point for clinical research concerns the variability of disease expression. As signified by vCJD, disease expression may be atypical. An important question to be answered by neurologists in the near future is whether patients without the methionine-methionine genotype at codon 129 of the PRNP gene will develop vCJD, and what their clinical phenotype will be. The twentieth century has shown that prion diseases are unpredictable.

Prion disorders are rare disorders. However, they are highly relevant because of the potential of iatrogenic transmission. The possibility of transmission of any form of CJD in particular through blood products and surgical procedures remains an issue of concern from a clinical point of view. In the light of iatrogenic transmission, early diagnosis, preferably preclinically, is important for surgery, blood transfusion, and organ-donation policies. This concerns in particular vCJD. Although most patients have been found in the UK, the present spread of contagious diseases through tourism and professional exchange between countries demands close monitoring.

Acknowledgement

This work is supported by grants of the Netherlands Organization for Scientific Research (NWO), the Dutch Ministry of Health (VWS) and the Netherlands Institute for Health Sciences (NIHES).

REFERENCES

1. Prusiner SB. Prions and neurodegenerative diseases. *N Engl J Med* 1987;317:1571–81.
2. Brown P, Cathala F, Raubertas RF, Gajdusek D, Castaigne P. The epidemiology of Creutzfeldt–Jakob disease: conclusion of a 15-year investigation in France and review of the world literature. *Neurology* 1987;37:895–904.
3. Prusiner SB, Hsiao KK. Human prion diseases. *Ann Neurol* 1994;35:385–95.
4. Pan KM, Baldwin M, Nguyen J, et al. Conversion of α-helices into β-sheets features in the formation of the scrapie prion protein. *Proc Natl Acad Sci USA* 1993;90:10962–6.
5. Prusiner SB, Scott M, Foster D, et al. Transgenetic studies implicate interaction between homologous PrP isoforms in scrapie prion replication. *Cell* 1990;63:673–86.
6. Collinge J, Harding AE, Owen F, et al. Diagnosis of Gerstmann–Straussler syndrome in familial dementia with prion protein gene analysis. *Lancet* 1989;2:15–17.
7. Will RG, Alpérovitch A, Poser S, et al. Creutzfeldt-Jakob disease in Europe 1993–1995. Descriptive epidemiology. *Ann Neurol* 1998;43:763–7.
8. Collinge J, Brown J, Hardy J, et al. Inherited prion disease with 144 base pair gene insertion. II. Clinical and pathological features. *Brain* 1992;115:687–710.
9. Collinge J, Palmer MS, Dryden AJ. Genetic predisposition to iatrogenic Creutzfeldt–Jakob disease. *Lancet* 1991;337:1441–2.
10. Strittmatter WJ, Saunders AM, Schmechel D, et al. Apolipoprotein E: high avidity binding to beta-amyloid and increased frequency of type 4 allele in late-onset familial Alzheimer's disease. *Proc Natl Acad Sci USA* 1993;90:1977–81.
11. Amouyel P, Vidal O, Launay JM, Laplanche JL. The apolipoprotein E alleles as major susceptibility factors for Creutzfeldt–Jakob disease. The French Research Group on Epidemiology of Human Spongiform Encephalopathies. *Lancet* 1994;344:1315–18.
12. Saunders AM, Schmader K, Breitner JCS, et al. Apolipoprotein E ε4 allele distributions in

late-onset Alzheimer's disease and in other amyloid-forming diseases. *Lancet* 1993;342:710–11.

13. Thadani V, Penar PL, Partington J, et al. Creutzfeldt–Jakob disease probably acquired from a cadaveric dura mater graft. *J Neurosurg* 1988;69:766–9.

14. Masters CL, Richardson EP Jr. Subacute spongiform encephalopathy Creutzfeldt–Jakob disease: the nature and progression of spongiform change. *Brain* 1978;101:333–44.

15. Will RG, Matthews WB. Evidence for case-to-case transmission of Creutzfeldt–Jakob disease. *J Neurol Neurosurg Psychiatry* 1982;45:235–44.

16. Bernouilli C, Siegfried J, Baumgartner G, et al. Danger of accidental person to person transmission of Creutzfeldt–Jakob disease by surgery. *Lancet* 1977;1:478–9.

17. Duffy P, Wolf J, Collins G, et al. Possible person to person transmission of Creutzfeldt–Jakob disease. *N Engl J Med* 1974;290:692–3.

18. Powell-Jackson J, Weller R, Kennedy P, et al. Creutzfeldt–Jakob disease following human growth hormone administration. *Lancet* 1985;2:244–6.

19. Gibbs C, Joy A, Heffner R, et al. Clinical and pathological features and laboratory confirmation of Creutzfeldt–Jakob disease in a recipient of pituitary-derived human growth hormone. *N Engl J Med* 1985;313:734–9.

20. Brown P, Gajdusek DG, Gibbs CJ, Asher DM. Potential epidemic of Creutzfeldt–Jakob disease from human growth hormone therapy. *N Engl J Med* 1985;313:728–31.

21. Cochius JI, Mack K, Burns RJ, Alderman CP, Blumbergs PC. Creutzfeldt–Jakob disease in a recipient of human pituitary gonadotrophin. *Austr NZ J Med* 1990;20:592–3.

22. Bobowick AR, Brody JA, Matthews MR, Roos R, Gajdusek DC. Creutzfeldt–Jakob disease: a case-control study. *Am J Epidemiol* 1973;98:381–94.

23. Kondo K, Kuroiwa Y. A case-control study of Creutzfeldt–Jakob disease: association with physical injuries. *Ann Neurol* 1982;11:377–81.

24. Davanipour Z, Alter M, Sobel E, et al. Creutzfeldt–Jakob disease: possible medical risk factors. *Neurology* 1985;35:1483–6.

25. Davanipour Z, Alter M, Sobel E, et al. A case-control study of Creutzfeldt–Jakob disease: dietary risk factors. *Am J Epidemiol* 1985;98:381–94.

26. Harries-Jones R, Knight R, Will RG, et al. Creutzfeldt–Jakob disease in England and Wales, 1980–1984: a case-control study of potential risk factors. *J Neurol Neurosurg Psychiatr* 1988;51:1113–19.

27. Wientjens DPWM, Davanipour Z, Hofman, Kondo K, Matthews WB, Will RG, van Duijn CM. Risk factors for Creutzfeldt–Jakob disease: a re-analyisis of case-control studies. *Neurology* 1996;46:1287–91.

28. Van Duijn CM, Delasnerie-Lauprêtre N, Zerr I, et al. Risk factors for Creutzfeldt–Jakob disease: the EU collaborative studies. *Lancet* 1998;351:1081–85.

29. Collins S, Law MG, Fletcher A, et al. Surgical treatment and risk of sporadic Creutzfeldt–Jakob disease: a case-control study. *Lancet* 1999;353:693–7.

30. Zerr I, Brandel JP, Masullo C, et al. European Surveillance on Creutzfeldt–Jakob disease: a case-control study for medical risk factors. *J Clin Epidemiol* 2000;53:747–54.

31. Manuelidis E, Kim JH, Mericangas J, Manuelidis L. Transmission to animals of Creutzfeldt–Jakob disease from human blood. *Lancet* 1985;ii:896–7.

32. Tateishi J. Transmission of Creutzfeldt–Jakob disease from human blood and urine into mice. *Lancet* 1985;ii:1074.

33. Wilson K, Code C, Ricketts MN. Risk of acquiring Creutzfeldt–Jakob disease from blood transfusions: systematic review of case-control studies. *BMJ* 2000;321:17–19.

34. Will RG, Zeidler M, Stewart GE, et al. Diagnosis of new variant Creutzfeldt–Jakob disease. *Ann Neurol* 2000;47:575–82.

35. Collinge J, Sidle KCL, Mead J, et al. Molecular analysis of prion strain variation and the aetiology of "new variant" CJD. *Nature* 1996;383:685–90.

36. Bruce ME, Will RG, Ironside JW, et al. Transmission to mice indicates that "new variant" CJD is caused by the BSE agent. *Nature* 1997;389:498–501.

37. Hill AF, Desbruslais M, Joiner S, et al. The same prion strain causes vCJD and BSE. *Nature* 1997;389:448–50.

38. Masters CL, Harris JO, Gajdusek DC, et al. Creutzfeldt–Jakob disease: patterns of worldwide occurrence and the significance of familial and sporadic clustering. *Ann Neurol* 1979;5:177–88.

39. Zerr I, Bodemer M, Gefeller O, et al. Detection of 14-3-3 protein in the cerebrospinal fluid supports the diagnosis of Creutzfeldt–Jakob disease. *Ann Neurol* 1998;43:32–40.

40. Steinhoff BJ, Racker S, Herrendorf G, et al. Accuracy and reliability of periodic sharp wave complexes in Creutzfeldt–Jakob disease. *Arch Neurol* 1996;53:162–6.

41. Finkenstaedt M, Szudra A, Zerr I, et al. MR imaging of Creutzfeldt–Jakob disease. *Radiology* 1996;199:793–8.

42. Demaerel P, Heiner L, Robberecht W, et al. Diffusion weighted MRI in sporadic Creutzfeldt–Jakob disease. *Neurology* 1999;52:205–8.

43. Poser S, Mollenhauer B, Krauss A, et al. How to improve the clinical diagnosis of Creutzfeldt–Jakob disease. *Brain* 1999;122:2345–51.

44. Sellar RJ, Will W, Zeidler M. MR imaging of new variant Creutzfeldt–Jakob disease. *Neuroradiology* 1997;39:S53.

45. Hill AF, Butterworth RJ, Joiner S, et al. Investigation of variant Creutzfeldt–Jakob disease and other human prion diseases with tonsil biopsy samples. *Lancet* 1999;353:183–9.

46. Prusiner SB. Genetic and infectious prion diseases. *Arch Neurol* 1993;50:1129–53.

47. Medori R, Tritschler H-J, LeBlanc A, et al. Fatal familial insomnia, a prion disease with a mutation at codon 178 of the prion protein gene. *N Engl J Med* 1992;326:444–9.

48. Sadatoshi T, Kuroiwa Y. Creutzfeldt–Jakob disease in Japan. *Neurology* 1983;33:1503–6.

49. Holman RC, Khan AS, Kent J, Strine TW, Schonberger LB. Epidemiology of Creutzfeldt–Jakob disease in the United States, 1979–1990: an analysis of national mortality data. *Neuroepidemiology* 1995;14:174–81.

50. Mitrová E. Epidemiological analysis of Creutzfeldt–Jakob disease in Slovakia (1972–1985). In Court L (Ed.). *Virus non conventionnels du système nerveux central.* Paris: Masson 1988:19–29.

51. Kahana E, Alter M, Braham J, Sofer D. Creutzfeldt–Jakob disease: focus among Libyan Jews in Israel. *Science* 1974;183:90–1.

52. Neugat RH, Neugat AI, Kahana E, et al. Creutzfeldt–Jakob disease: familial clustering among Libyan-born Israelis. *Neurology* 1979;29:225–31.

53. www.eurocjd.ed.ac.uk

54. Cohen CH. Does improvement in case ascertainment explain the increase in sporadic Creutzfeldt–Jakob disease since 1970 in the United Kingdom? *Am J Epidemiol* 2000;152:474–9.

55. Brandel JP, Delasnerie-Laupretre N, Laplanche JL, et al. Diagnosis of Creutzfeldt–Jakob disease: effect of clinical criteria on incidence estimates. *Neurology* 2000;54:1095–9.

56. Andrews NJ, Farrington CP, Cousens SN, et al. Incidence of variant Creutzfeldt–Jakob disease in the UK. *Lancet* 2000;356:481–2.

57. Ghani AC, Ferguson NM, Donnely CA, et al. Predicted vCJD mortality in Great Britain. *Nature* 2000;406:583–4.

58. Gajdusek DC. Unconventional viruses and the origin and disappearance of kuru. *Science* 1977;197:943–60.

59. Hill AF, Joiner S, Linehan J, et al. Species-barrier-independent prion replication in apparently resistant species. *PNAS* 2000;97:10248–53.

60. Croes EA, Dermaut B, van der Cammen TJM, et al. Genetic testing should not be advocated as a diagnostic tool in familial forms of dementia. *Am J Hum Genet* 2000;67:1033–5.

20

Neoplastic disease

John F. Annegers

Introduction

This chapter will highlight current issues in the epidemiology of brain tumors. The areas of interest are the classification of brain tumors in epidemiologic studies, the spatial and temporal occurrence of brain tumors, and risk factors for brain tumors. More thorough reviews of the literature are available for adults (1) and for children (2).

Classification of central nervous system neoplasia

The classification of intracranial tumors for epidemiologic studies is plagued by large variations in inclusion and exclusion criteria. A reasonable, working classification system is essential, however, for descriptive epidemiology and etiologic studies. There are several axes of classification of central nervous system neoplasia. There are anatomic location, histology, site of origin, and means of ascertainment.

The term "intracranial tumor" is generally used to refer to neoplasia of the nervous system and anatomic proximate tumors of the pituitary gland and craniopharyngeal duct (3). The major histological types of intracranial neoplasia are presented in Table 20.1. Because of the distinct occurrence, prognosis, and known or suspected etiologic factors for each type of neoplasia, there is little justification to combine all intracranial neoplasia. However, since most mortality and incidence data include all primary central nervous system (CNS) tumors, much of the descriptive epidemiology compares the rates of all primary central nervous neoplasia. Pituitary tumors, craniopharyngioma, and neurilemmoma, although often included as intracranial tumors, will not be addressed in this chapter.

Metastatic tumors of the brain may be derived from many primary sites and are of clinical significance because of seizures and other neurologic symptoms. The most common primary sites are the lungs in males and breast in females. Since the epidemiologic interest in metastatic tumors rests in the primary site, this chapter will be restricted to primary intracranial neoplasia.

Table 20.1. Primary intracranial tumors

Tumors of neuroglial cells (gliomas)
    Astrocytic series
    Astrocytoma (Grades I and II)
    Glioblastoma (Grades III and IV)
    Oligodendroglioma
    Ependymoma
Medulloblastoma
Tumors of mesodermal tissues
    Meningioma
Tumors of cranial nerve roots
    Neurilemmoma
Tumors of blood vessels
    Hemangioma
Pituitary tumors (Adenomas)
Craniopharyngioma
Pinealoma

Adapted from (3).

Besides the anatomic, histologic, and site of origin axes of classification, brain tumors may also be considered by their means of ascertainment. That is symptomatic versus incidental diagnosis. The prevalence of incidental autopsy findings of gliomas in routine CNS autopsies was 0.5% in the population over 65 years of age and the prevalence was over 1% for meningiomas in autopsies on individuals over age 55 (4). Since the detection of incidental brain tumors at autopsy is a function of mortality rates and the frequency of CNS autopsies, comparisons should be based on prevalence at autopsy rather than including incidental autopsy cases in incidence rate computations.

Spatial and temporal patterns of incidence and mortality

The incidence rates from different countries are presented in Figure 20.1. The highest rates are reported from the Scandinavian countries and Israel, while the remainder of Europe and the Americas report intermediate rates, and Japan and China report the lowest rates (5). The differences, however, are more likely explained by variations in ascertainment and classification rather than real differences in rates. The Israeli rates include benign tumors while the Danish registry also includes tumors found incidentally at autopsy.

The geographic patterns of brain tumor incidence and mortality rates are relatively stable as is found in many other neurologic diseases such as amyotrophic

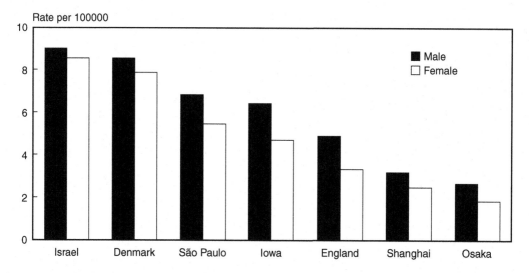

Figure 20.1 Brain and central nervous system cancer incidence circa 1980. Age standardized to WHO standard distribution. Source: Cancer in Five Continents 1987.

lateral sclerosis (ALS) and idiopathic epilepsy. This is in contrast to the large variations found for most malignant neoplasia of other sites and suggests that there are no environmental risk factors that will explain more than a small proportion of primary brain tumors.

Mortality and incidence rates of primary malignant CNS tumors have increased over the past few decades (see Figures 20.2 and 20.3). The increased rates have occurred almost exclusively among the elderly in the United States (6–8), Canada (9), and most European countries (10). In Norway, the incidence of intracranial neoplasms in 1983–92 compared to 1963–72 increased 1.26-fold for those under 55 years of age, 1.76-fold for age 55–74 and 3.35-fold for over age 75 (10). Birth cohort analyses from Connecticut (12) and Canada (13) point to a secular change rather than a unique birth cohort experience.

The secular trends of brain tumors are due, at least in part, to the introduction of computerized axial tomography (CAT) in the mid-1970s. However, since the increased mortality rates predate the widespread use of CAT in the late 1970s and the increase is not confined to lower grade tumors (13), additional factors must be involved. Several suggestions have been offered for the introduction of new risk factor(s) for brain tumors. However, the factor(s) would have to differentially bias the incidence by age. The failure of etiologic studies to detect risk factors in general, or risk factors that have a strong interaction with age, does not support this contention.

An innovative explanation was suggested by Riggs (14), who noted that the

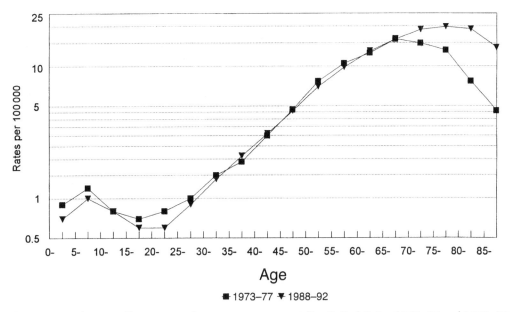

Figure 20.2 Primary malignant central nervous system mortality, United States 1973–77 and 1988–92. Source: SEER Program.

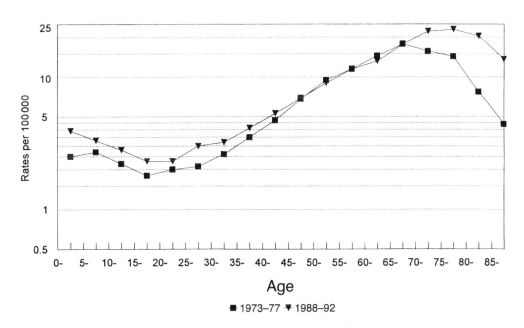

Figure 20.3 Primary malignant central nervous system incidence, United States, 1973–77 and 1988–92. Source: SEER Program.

increasing mortality rates from brain tumors have paralleled the decreasing mortality rates from ischemic heart disease and cerebrovascular disease since the mid-1960s in the United States. If these new survivors to the elderly population are also much more susceptible to brain tumors, then mortality from brain tumors would increase, especially in the oldest age groups. However, this explanation would also require strong comorbidity between cardiovascular disease and malignant brain tumors and a birth cohort effect, which has not been shown.

The secular trends are most likely the result of three factors: (1) the availability of CAT beginning in the mid-1970s; (2) changes in attitude toward medical care among the elderly; and (3) support programs such as Medicare that facilitate the use of diagnostic procedures (15). The concurrent rise of ALS mortality among the elderly suggests a role for factors 2 and 3 since there has been no comparable advance in diagnostic technology but there is a similar, although of lesser magnitude, upward shift in the age-specific ALS mortality rates.

Risk factors

Due to relative rarity, heterogeneity, and uniform occurrence, the search for environmental causes of brain tumors has not been rewarding. Most risk factors proposed by clinical or epidemiologic investigations have not withstood the tests of replication, dose response, and consistency.

Trauma

Traumatic brain injury has long been considered a risk factor for intracranial neoplasia, especially meningioma. This impression is based on case reports, and some case-control studies have reported a modest association for meningioma and glioma (16–18). It is possible that more complete recall of head trauma episodes by cases is a bias in case-control studies of head trauma and brain tumors. In a case-control study of 540 children with primary brain tumors and 801 controls the risk of brain tumor among children with a previous head injury that resulted in medical attention was slightly elevated: odds ratio (OR) 1.4 (1.0–1.9) (19). Other case-control studies of fatal brain cancer (20) and incident astrocytomas (21) have failed to find an association. In a cohort of 2953 traumatic brain injuries there was no increase of astrocytoma or meningioma, although only a few cases were expected (22). Thus, if there is an association between brain trauma and brain cancer, it is weak, less than 1.5.

Radiation

The survivors of the atomic bombing of Hiroshima and Nagasaki have demonstrated the increased risks of leukemia and other cancers from radiation exposure.

These cohorts, however, do not show increased mortality rates from CNS tumors (23).

A number of case reports of meningioma have been presented for therapeutic radiation for tinea capita and vascular nevi (24). In a cohort of 10 804 children irradiated for ringworm of the scalp and an equal number of unexposed children the relative risk (RR) was 9.5 (3.5–25.7) for meningioma (25). The incidence of glioma was also elevated, but not significantly, with a RR of 2.6 (0.8–8.6). An increasing relative risk with dose provides additional support for an etiologic role of radiation exposure (25).

The studies of Preston-Martin show a weak but suggestive association with the number of full-mouth dental X-rays for men and women for meningiomas and gliomas (18,26). Other case-control studies have failed to show an association between diagnostic radiographic exposure and brain tumors in Germany (27), Australia (28), and the United States (29).

N-Nitroso compounds – diet

An association between consumption of cured meats and meningioma was interpreted as a possible role of nitrite exposure (30). However, these findings have not been confirmed by other case-control studies (20,28,29,31).

Occupational

Clusters of brain tumors among synthetic rubber workers (32) and petrochemical workers (33) initially suggested an etiologic link. However, they were not confirmed by large industry-specific cohort studies in rubber workers (34), or petrochemical employees (35). A pooled analysis of the worldwide petroleum industry employees reported 210 observed brain cancer deaths and 209.7 expected (35).

The most convincing occupational exposure associated with brain tumor is vinyl chloride exposure before 1973. A proportionate mortality ratio (PMR) of 4.17 was found among vinyl chloride workers in the United States (36). A small but consistently increased standardized mortality ratio (SMR) was reported in studies of workers involved in the manufacture of vinyl chloride (37,38). The SMR for men exposed in the United States for brain cancer mortality was 1.8 (1.14–2.71) (38). Although a differential diagnosis explanation might be raised, it was unnecessary to presume such a difference to resolve the issue of increased incidence of brain tumors in occupations such as petrochemical employees. The identification of the modest increased mortality of brain tumors associated with vinyl chloride, perhaps 1.5-fold, probably occurred only because the far stronger association with angiosarcoma of the liver prompted studies of the exposed population worldwide.

Farming and pesticides

Many studies have reported an association between brain cancer and farming occupations (39–41). These findings suggest a possible effect of exposure to herbicides, insecticides, or fungicides. The initial studies of heavily exposed cohorts of pesticides applicators reported a nonsignificantly elevated SMR of 2.5 (42). However, large cohort studies from various countries have consistently reported SMRs of close to 1.0 (43–45).

Epilepsy and anticonvulsants

Brain tumor cases have a higher prevalence of a history of epilepsy and anticonvulsant drug use than controls. Carpenter (46) found that four of 65 brain tumor cases compared to two of 249 controls had a history of epilepsy, OR 5.7 (1.0–32.1). Gold (47) reported an increased risk of brain tumors in children exposed to barbiturates when they combined prenatal and childhood exposures. The authors noted that the use of medications began many years prior to the diagnosis of brain tumor and suggested that the association was etiologic rather than the expression of an underlying association of seizures with brain tumors.

Two cohort studies (48,49) show a very high rate of brain cancer after the diagnosis of epilepsy. In both studies, the authors interpreted the finding of a decreasing standardized incidence ratio (SIR) with duration from seizure diagnosis 0–4 years SIR = 47.4; 5–9 years SIR = 11.8; and 10 + years SIR = 5.9 (49) as evidence that undetected brain tumors were the cause of the seizures rather than evidence of an etiologic role for the anticonvulsants. The association with in utero barbiturate exposure has not been replicated. A case-control study of 86 cases and 172 controls found an OR of 0.96 (0.47–1.94) for in utero barbiturate exposure (50).

Electromagnetic fields

Among deaths in white males over 20 years of age in Washington State from 1950 through 1982, there was a small but significantly elevated PMR of 1.23 for workers employed in occupations with exposure to electromagnetic fields (51). A case-control study reported an OR of 2.3 (1.3–4.2) for electrical and electronic workers (52). However, a case-control study of all types of brain tumors found an OR of 1.0 for occupations thought to involve electromagnetic fields (53). Stratification by histologic type resulted in a nonsignificant OR of 1.7 (0.7–4.4) for gliomas but also a protective effect for meningioma with an OR of 0.3 (0.03–3.2).

Cohort studies do not show an increased incidence of brain tumors for occupations involving exposure to electromagnetic fields. In a large Swedish cohort, the SMR for brain tumors was 0.9 (0.7–1.3) for electrical/electronic engineers and technicians, 0.9 (0.7–1.2) for electricians, and 1.1 (0.7–1.8) for linemen (53). No association was found between brain tumor risk and radio frequency radiation among Norwegian electrical workers identified in the 1960 census and followed through 1985 (54). In that study 119 brain tumors were observed compared to 109 expected or an SMR of 1.09 (0.9–1.4). Thus, if there is an effect of electromagnetic fields on the incidence of brain tumors, it is too small to measure in conventional epidemiologic studies.

Diagnosis

The most common presenting symptoms in patients with glioblastoma are seizure and headache followed by mental confusions and hemiparesis. The tumors are then usually demonstrated by MRI (55). However, especially for low grade astrocytomas and in the elderly, many tumors are recognized as the result of an MRI for other indications or incidental findings at autopsy.

Prognosis

The prognosis for malignant brain tumors is poor. The SEER program of the National Cancer Institute presents 5-year relative survival data for persons with a diagnosis of invasive brain and other nervous system cancer (7). These are virtually all glioblastoma. The relative survival calculation removes the effect of other causes of death adjusting for age and sex. For all cases diagnosed in 1986–91, the relative survival was 28.9%. Although this represents a significant improvement over the relative survival of 22.3% for cases diagnosed in 1974–76, it is probably explained, at least in part, by earlier diagnosis. The most important prognostic factor is the age at diagnosis. The relative survival is 56.7% under age 44, 20.7% for 45–54, 8.7% for 55–64, 5.4% for 65–74 and only 2.9% for over 75 years of age.

Implications for practice

The onset of seizure in people aged 35–64 must first be evaluated for benign or malignant brain tumor. Only very rarely can the etiology of a brain tumor be reasonably attributed to a specific cause. Unlike most cancer sites where well-defined risk factors have been established, brain tumors are like many other neurologic diseases where high-risk populations cannot be defined by established risk factors. The association with family history is not particularly useful since due to the low incidence of brain tumors, the increased risk in relatives is a very low absolute risk.

REFERENCES

1. Inskip PD, Linet MS, Heineman EF. Etiology of brain tumors in adults. *Epidemiol Rev* 1995;17:382–414.
2. Kuijten RR, Bunin GR. Risk factors for childhood brain tumors. *Cancer Epidem Biomarkers Prev* 1993;2:277–88.
3. Schoenberg BS, Christine BW, Whisnant JP. The descriptive epidemiology of primary intracranial neoplasms: the Connecticut experience. *Am J Epidemiol* 1976;104:499–510.
4. Annegers JF, Schoenberg BS, Okazaki H, Kurland LT. Epidemiologic study of primary intracranial neoplasms. *Arch Neurol* 1981;38:217–19.
5. IARC. Cancer Incidence in Five Continents. Age-standardized incidence rates, four-digit rubrics, and age-standardized and cumulative incidence rates, three-digit rubrics. *IARC Sci Publ* 1992;871–1011.
6. Horm JW, Asire AJ, Young Jr. JL, Pollack ES (Eds.) SEER Program: cancer incidence and mortality in the United States, 1973–81. National Cancer Institute. *NIH Pub. No. 85-1837.* Bethesda, MD (rev) 1984.
7. Kosary CL, Ries LAG, Miller BA, Hankey BF, Harras A, Edwards BK (Eds.) SEER cancer statistics review, 1973–1992: tables and graphs, National Cancer Institute. *NIH Pub. No. 96-2789.* Bethesda, MD, 1995.
8. Greig NH, Ries LG, Yancik R, Rapoport SI. Increasing annual incidence of primary malignant brain tumors in the elderly. *J Natl Cancer Inst* 1990;82:1621–4.
9. Mao Y, Desmeules M, Semenciw RM, Hill G, Gaudette L, Wigle DT. Increasing brain cancer rates in Canada. *Can Med Assoc J* 1991;145:1583–91.
10. Boyle P, Maisonneuve P, Saracci R, Muir CS. Is the increased incidence of primary malignant brain tumors in the elderly real? [editorial; comment] [see comments]. *J Natl Cancer Inst* 1990;82:1594–6.
11. Helseth A. The incidence of primary central nervous system neoplasms before and after computerized tomography availability. *J Neurosurg* 1995;83:999–1003.
12. Polednak AP. Time trends in incidence of brain and central nervous system cancers in Connecticut. *J Natl Cancer Inst* 1991;83:1679–81.
13. Werner MH, Phuphanich S, Lyman GH. The increasing incidence of malignant gliomas and primary central nervous system lymphoma in the elderly. *Cancer* 1995;76:1634–42.
14. Riggs JE. Rising primary malignant brain tumor mortality in the elderly. A manifestation of differential survival. *Arch Neurol* 1995;52:571–5.
15. Modan B, Wagener DK, Feldman JJ, Rosenberg HM, Feinleib M. Increased mortality from brain tumors: a combined outcome of diagnostic technology and change of attitude toward the elderly. *Am J Epidemiol* 1992;135:1349–57.
16. Hochberg F, Toniolo P, Cole P. Head trauma and seizures as risk factors of glioblastoma. *Neurology* 1984;34:1511–14.
17. Preston-Martin S, Yu MC, Henderson BE, Roberts C. Risk factors for meningiomas in men in Los Angeles County. *J Natl Cancer Inst* 1983;70:863–6.
18. Preston-Martin S, Paganini-Hill A, Henderson BE, Pike MC, Wood C. Case-control study

of intracranial meningiomas in women in Los Angeles County, California. *J Natl Cancer Inst* 1980;65:67–73.

19. Gurney JG, Preston-Martin S, McDaniel AM, Mueller BA, Holly EA. Head injury as a risk factor for brain tumors in children: results from a multicenter case-control study. *Epidemiology* 1996;7:485–9.

20. Carpenter AV, Flanders WD, Rome EL, Cole P, Fry SA. Brain cancer and nonoccupational risk factors: a case-control study among workers at two nuclear facilities. *Am J Public Health* 1987;77:1180–2.

21. Ahlbom A, Navier IL, Norell S, Olin R, Spannare B. Nonoccupational risk indicators for astrocytomas in adults. *Am J Epidemiol* 1986;124:334–7.

22. Annegers JF, Laws ER Jr, Kurland LT, Grabow JD. Head trauma and subsequent brain tumors. *Neurosurgery* 1979;4:203–6.

23. Preston DL, Kato H, Kopecky K, Fujita S. Studies of the mortality of A-bomb survivors. 8. Cancer mortality, 1950–1982. *Radiat Res* 1987;111:151–78.

24. Spallone A, Gagliardi FM, Vagnozzi R. Intracranial meningiomas related to external cranial irradiation. *Surg Neurol* 1979;12:153–9.

25. Ron E, Modan B, Boice JD, et al. Tumors of the brain and nervous system after radiotherapy in childhood. *N Engl J Med* 1988;319:1033–9.

26. Preston-Martin S, Mack W, Henderson BE. Risk factors for gliomas and meningiomas in males in Los Angeles County. *Cancer Res* 1989;49:6137–43.

27. Schlehofer B, Blettner M, Becker N, Martinsohn C, Wahrendorf J. Medical risk factors and the development of brain tumors. *Cancer* 1992;69:2541–7.

28. Ryan P, Lee MW, North B, McMichael AJ. Risk factors for tumors of the brain and meninges: results from the Adelaide Adult Brain Tumor Study. *Int J Cancer* 1992;51:20–7.

29. Hochberg F, Toniolo P, Cole P, Salcman M. Nonoccupational risk indicators of glioblastoma in adults [published erratum appears in *J Neurooncol* 1990 Aug;9(1):90]. *J Neurooncol* 1990;8:55–60.

30. Preston-Martin S, Yu MC, Benton B, Henderson BE. N-Nitroso compounds and childhood brain tumors: a case-control study. *Cancer Res* 1982;42:5240–5.

31. Giles GG, McNeil JJ, Donnan G, et al. Dietary factors and the risk of glioma in adults: results of a case-control study in Melbourne, Australia. *Int J Cancer* 1994;59:357–62.

32. Mancuso TF, Ciocco A, el-Attar AA. An epidemiological approach to the rubber industry. A study based on departmental experience. *J Occup Med* 1968;10:213–32.

33. Alexander V, Leffingwell SS, Lloyd JW, Waxweiler RJ, Miller RL. Brain cancer in petrochemical workers: a case series report. *Am J Ind Med* 1980;1:115–23.

34. Englund A, Ekman G, Zabrielski L. Occupational categories among brain tumor cases recorded in the cancer registry in Sweden. *Ann NY Acad Sci* 1982;381:188–96.

35. Wong O, Raabe GK. Critical review of cancer epidemiology in petroleum industry employees, with a quantitative meta-analysis by cancer site [see comments]. *Am J Ind Med* 1989;15:283–310.

36. Monson RR, Peters JM, Johnson MN. Proportional mortality among vinyl-chloride workers. *Lancet* 1974;2:397–8.

37. Simonato L, L'Abbe KA, Andersen A, et al. A collaborative study of cancer incidence and mortality among vinyl chloride workers. *Scand J Work Environ Health* 1991;17:159–69.

38. Wong O, Whorton MD, Foliart DE, Ragland D. An industry-wide epidemiologic study of vinyl chloride workers, 1942–1982. *Am J Ind Med* 1991;20:317–34.

39. Reif JS, Pearce N, Fraser J. Occupational risks for brain cancer: a New Zealand Cancer Registry-based study. *J Occup Med* 1989;31:863–7.

40. Musicco M, Sant M, Molinari S, Filippini G, Gatta G, Berrino F. A case-control study of brain gliomas and occupational exposure to chemical carcinogens: the risk to farmers. *Am J Epidemiol* 1988;128:778–85.

41. Heineman EF, Gao YT, Dosemeci M, McLaughlin JK. Occupational risk factors for brain tumors among women in Shanghai, China. *J Occup Environ Med* 1995;37:288–93.

42. Blair A, Grauman DJ, Lubin JH, Fraumeni JF Jr. Lung cancer and other causes of death among licensed pesticide applicators. *J Natl Cancer Inst* 1983;71:31–7.

43. Corrao G, Calleri M, Carle F, Russo R, Bosia S, Piccioni P. Cancer risk in a cohort of licensed pesticide users. *Scand J Work Environ Health* 1989;15:203–9.

44. Wiklund K, Dich J, Holm LE, Eklund G. Risk of cancer in pesticide applicators in Swedish agriculture. *Br J Ind Med* 1989;46:809–14.

45. Bohnen NI, Kurland LT. Brain tumor and exposure to pesticides in humans: a review of the epidemiologic data. *J Neurol Sciences* 1995;132:110–21.

46. Carpenter AV, Flanders WD, Frome EL, Cole P, Fry SA. Brain cancer and nonoccupational risk factors: a case-control study among workers at two nuclear facilities. *Am J Public Health* 1987;77:1180–2.

47. Gold E, Gordis L, Tonascia J, Szklo M. Risk factors for brain tumors in children. *Am J Epidemiol* 1979;109:309–19.

48. Clemmesen J, Hjalgrim-Jensen S. Brain tumors in children exposed to barbiturates [letter]. *J Natl Cancer Inst* 1981;66:215.

49. Shirts SB, Annegers JF, Hauser WA, Kurland LT. Cancer incidence in a cohort of patients with seizure disorders. *J Natl Cancer Inst* 1986;77:83–7.

50. Goldhaber MK, Selby JV, Hiatt RA, Quesenberry CP. Exposure to barbiturates in utero and during childhood risk of intracranial and spinal cord tumors. *Cancer Res* 1990;50:4600–3.

51. Milham S Jr. Mortality in workers exposed to electromagnetic fields. *Environ Health Perspect* 1985;62:297–300.

52. Thomas TL, Stolley PD, Stemhagen A, et al. Brain tumor mortality risk among men with electrical and electronics jobs: a case-control study. *J Natl Cancer Inst* 1987;79:233–8.

53. Mack W, Preston-Martin S, Peters JM. Astrocytoma risk related to job exposure to electric and magnetic fields. *Bioelectromagnetics* 1991;12:57–66.

54. Tornqvist S, Knave B, Ahlbom A, Persson T. Incidence of leukaemia and brain tumours in some "electrical occupations." *Br J Ind Med* 1991;48:597–603.

55. Kaba SE, Kyritsis AP. Recognition and management of gliomas. *Drugs* 1997;53:235–44.

21

Cerebral palsy

Karin B. Nelson

Introduction

Understanding of the etiology of cerebral palsy has changed markedly over the past two decades, as epidemiologic studies have supplanted anecdote and uncontrolled case series. Unfortunately, there has been no parallel progress in reducing the rate of occurrence of cerebral palsy over a similar period, despite striking improvements in both obstetric and neonatal care (1,2).

Cerebral palsy (CP) is a group of chronic motor disorders of central nervous system origin, characterized by aberrant control of movement or posture, beginning early in life and not due to recognized progressive disease. Major malformations of the CNS are usually excluded. In studies of etiology disorders arising after the first month of life are also excluded. The term cerebral palsy thus denotes a chronic, usually congenital, motor disorder. "Cerebral palsy" is not an etiologic diagnosis but indicates developmental motor disability; the term is thus analogous to "mental retardation," a term denoting chronic, usually congenital, cognitive disability.

CP may be categorized into its clinical subtypes (spastic quadriplegia, diplegia, hemiplegia; dyskinetic or ataxic forms, and mixed), by severity, and may be further grouped according to whether or not etiology is considered known through neuroimaging, chromosomal, metabolic, or other evidence.

Prevalence

Studies of the prevalence of CP, although they differ by date, age of ascertainment, and exclusions, are reasonably comparable in different developed countries, with an overall prevalence of 1.4 to 2.3 per thousand (3–6). For disabling congenital CP, an American population-based study observed a prevalence at three years of 1.23 per thousand survivors (7). As discussed below, the rate of CP among very premature livebirths is much higher than among term infants (8), and appears to have risen markedly, apparently due to the dramatically increased survival of very preterm babies.

Etiology

The old hypothesis that birth asphyxia is the major cause of CP and other developmental disabilities is not sustained by research in defined populations (2,9,10). Abnormalities of birth and clinical evidence suggestive of birth asphyxia are present in a nontrivial proportion of normal people; such events occur in a higher proportion of those with CP but do not account for most CP (11,12). Because there are no specific and generally available means to recognize asphyxia during birth and other factors (notably exposure to infection or inflammation or thrombo-embolic event) that may produce similar findings, an impression of the presence of birth asphyxia may involve serious misattribution of cause. The hypothesis that birth asphyxia is a major cause of CP has not led to the development of therapies producing a net decrease in CP.

Known risk factors for CP in very low birthweight (VLBW) infants differ somewhat from those in term babies, so these will be outlined separately.

VLBW infants

Both low birthweight and short gestation are important risk factors for CP. Risk is greatest in the youngest or smallest babies. An infant born weighing less than 1500 g had 100 times the risk of moderate or severe CP as compared with an infant born weighing 3000 to 3500 g, the most common birthweight group (7). In VLBW infants, fixed anatomical lesions and syndromic entities explain relatively few cases (5,13). With increased survival of VLBW infants in recent decades, this group now contributes a larger proportion of CP, and a greater absolute number of cases, than in the past (6).

Some but not all factors related to risk that a child will be born too early or too small are also related to risk of CP *among* VLBW children. For example, a family history of premature birth, twinning, and maternal smoking are all related to risk of low birthweight, but while VLBW children of families with a history of preterm birth are at higher risk of CP than other VLBW children, data are not consistent in indicating that a low birthweight child who was a twin or triplet, or born to a smoker, is at higher risk than another child of similar birthweight who was a singleton or born to a nonsmoker. In VLBW infants, maternal preeclampsia is associated with *lower* risk of CP (14,15); possible reasons for this have been discussed elsewhere (16). Some observational studies have noted that exposure to magnesium sulfate, administered for maternal preeclampsia or in an attempt to stop preterm labor, was associated with a lower rate in CP in VLBW infants

(14,17,18), while others have not (19–21). This question is now being examined in randomized trials.

Maternal reproductive tract infection is an important cause of preterm birth (22,23). Some investigators have observed such infection to be related to neonatal ultrasonographic findings which are in turn associated with high risk of CP and with risk of CP itself; these observations, not entirely consistent from study to study, have been subjected to recent meta-analysis (24).

Other risk factors for CP in VLBW infants include short interbirth interval, birth in a hospital lacking specialized personnel and equipment for cases of premature or ill newborns, and birth within a short time of the mother's admission to the hospital, associated with a 49-fold increase in risk of CP in a population-based study (13).

Neonatal hypothyroxinemia or maternal thyroid disease have been linked with increase in risk of CP or mental handicap (25,26). A randomized trial of administration of thyroxine in VLBW infants, administered before testing of individual infants, was not associated with lower risk of CP (27).

Conditions that can lead to primary compromise of oxygen supply, such as placental abruption or cord prolapse, are not more frequent in VLBW infants with CP than in VLBW infants without CP, nor are abnormalities on electronic fetal heart rate monitoring more frequent (13,15). Most VLBW children with CP were not acidotic soon after birth. Although cerebral ischemia has been thought to play a role in CP in VLBW infants, it has not been shown that ischemia, when present, is often related to primary disorders of oxygen supply rather than to infectious or other etiologies.

A number of illnesses and neuroimaging abnormalities in the neonate, especially echolucensies on early ultrasonography, are associated with increased risk of CP. These are presumably consequences of earlier-acting but usually unidentified causal factors.

Term infants

Although at much lower individual risk than children born VLBW, babies of normal birthweight contribute more than half of CP. Intracranial and extracranial malformations are more common in children with CP than in the general population (9,10). In infants born at term, brain malformations or prenatal destructive lesions observed on neuroimaging, or congenital nonbacterial infections, are relatively more common than in smaller infants (5,28).

Multiple births constitute a much smaller percentage of infants of normal birthweight than of smaller babies, but it is in normal birthweight infants that being a twin is associated with heightened risk of CP (29,31). An important factor in that risk is death of a cotwin, associated with a 100-fold greater likelihood of CP in the survivor (29,30,32).

Potentially asphyxiating obstetrical conditions such as abruptio placentae, cord prolapse, and tight nuchal cord occur with higher frequency in term children with CP than in term controls, but account for only a minority – perhaps in the neighborhood of 10% – of CP in term babies (2,9,12,33). Asphyxiating conditions are most strongly related to the spastic quadriplegic subtype of CP, especially when accompanied by dyskinesia. Spastic quadriplegia with dyskinesia is not specific to asphyxia, however. Specific abnormal fetal heart rate patterns on electronic monitoring in labor are more frequent in children with CP, but unfortunately the high prevalence of such abnormalities, 32–79% in some series (34,35) and the low prevalence of birth asphyxia-related CP in this term and near-term group (about 1 in 15 000 births), combined with lack of proven efficacy of interventions, makes electronic fetal monitoring a poor indicator for management decisions in labor aimed at the prevention of CP (36).

Exposure to maternal infection is a risk factor for CP in babies of normal birthweight (37,9,28), and is a common antecedent of low Apgar scores and other signs of early depression in the infant, even when the infant is not known to be infected. Other reported risk factors for CP in term or normal birthweight babies include maternal hyperthyroidism, seizures, or mental retardation, atypical menstrual cycles, bleeding in pregnancy, severe proteinuria (9), and early age at menarche (38). Unlike VLBW infants, babies born at term to women with preeclampsia may be at increased risk of CP (34). In industrialized countries, physical trauma at birth is no longer an important etiologic factor in brain injury; its role and that of malnutrition, iodine deficiency, and neonatal hypothermia in developing countries are not known.

Since the initial description by Silver et al. in 1992 (39), a number of case reports and a few controlled studies, of which some have included perinatal strokes, indicate that antiphospholipid antibodies, the factor V Leiden mutation and other abnormalities of coagulation can be associated with CP, especially with hemiplegic CP (40–42). Perhaps at least in part because of the association of these conditions with placental vascular pathology, there is relatively often a history of pregnancy complications, fetal growth retardation, low Apgar scores, low pH, and neonatal seizures in affected infants (43,44).

A range of neonatal signs and illnesses have been observed more frequently in children with CP than in controls, but the antecedents of these signs and illnesses are seldom identified.

Middlesized infants

Few studies have addressed the etiology of CP in infants born weighing 1501 to 2499 g. This is likely to be an etiologically heterogeneous group in which growth retardation and syndromic entities may be important.

Diagnosis

The diagnosis of CP rests on identification of abnormalities of tone, reflexes, and posture, as assessed after the first year of life and preferably not before age 3 years; earlier diagnostic assessments are unstable, especially in children born prematurely. Deviation from normal motor development is often the first clue to the presence of CP, and is an indication that careful evaluation is needed. Allen and Alexander (45) have discussed motor milestones on sequential examinations as an important screening procedure for CP, to be followed by detailed neurologic examination.

Spastic hemiplegia is recognized by hypertonus and pathologic reflexes predominating unilaterally, with arm usually more affected than leg; limb asymmetries are common. Spastic quadriplegia affects all four limbs, the upper extremities usually more severely than the lower, often with bulbar signs; spastic diplegia is spastic involvement dominantly of the legs, although upper extremities may also be involved to a lesser extent; ataxic or dyskinetic disorders may occur alone or with spasticity.

Prognosis

In VLBW neonates, physical examination is a relatively poor guide to identification of those who, if they survive, will experience neurologic disability. The best predictor of CP in these infants is information on neonatal cranial ultrasonography, especially evidence of echolucencies. In term infants, on the other hand, the best predictor of long-term neurologic abnormality is serious encephalopathy in the newborn period.

In very young children, especially those born prematurely, early motor abnormalities of mild or moderate degree tend to improve and disappear later (46,47), so that it is unusual that a child thought to have mild CP at one year of age still demonstrates CP by school age. Three years is perhaps a reasonable age at which to assess motor performance for prognostic purposes, although some improvement may occur after that time, and athetosis may first become manifest at about that age.

Mildly or moderately severely disabled children with CP have a survival rate to age 20 years little different from unaffected children, but only about half of severely disabled children survive to age 20 years (48). Severe to profound mental retardation, bilaterality of involvement, and presence of other associated neurologic disabilities including epilepsy are associated with more limited life expectancy (48–51). With good medical care, even seriously affected persons often outlive their parents, so long-term planning is important.

The employability of persons with CP is chiefly a function of their intellectual capability and severity of motor disability. Despite early and aggressive treatment and good family and technical support, economic independence is not common except in mildly affected persons.

Intervention

The goals of intervention in CP are to improve function, prevent deformities and discomfort, and make care easier. Physical therapy is likely to be the mainstay of management even if other modalities are also employed, and has an important role both before and after surgical procedures. Training of parents or caregivers in the establishment of a home program is an important supplement to professional therapists. Physical medicine or orthopedic consultants may recommend assistive devices such as leg braces, crutches, chairs, or communication aids.

Antispasmodic agents can be administered orally to lessen spasticity, with care not to interfere with strength or balance. Baclofen, a muscle relaxant and antispasmodic, can be administered orally or intrathecally via an implanted pump. Disadvantages include the sedative effects of high oral doses and the potential complications and costs of surgical implantation. Botulinum toxin has been employed for relief of spasticity (52), the effects of each injection lasting for months.

Surgical procedures are chiefly for the lower limb, where muscles are larger and fewer and requirements for fine motor performance less critical. Tenotomies, neurectomies, osteotomy, and arthrodeses to stabilize joints are among the available interventions. A relatively newer procedure for the reduction of spasticity in the lower limbs is selective dorsal rhizotomy, which involves selective surgical destruction of dorsal root fibers identified by intraoperative electrical stimulation to be associated with aberrant electrical activity (53). This procedure is not free of complications. Careful preoperative assessment and pre- and postoperative physical therapy are important to optimize outcome. Assessment of these medical and surgical therapies is a continuing process.

Implications for clinical practice

Because physical findings suggestive of CP in the first year of life, especially those of mild degree, may subsequently resolve, it is important not to label mild or moderately involved infants too early. Even in children whose mild motor signs resolve there may be deficits in other areas of neurologic function, however, so caution is also needed with respect to excessive reassurance of parents whose children are younger than about 3 years.

It is important, in considering the etiology of CP and in discussing this with families, to remember that low Apgar scores, neonatal seizures, need for ventilatory support and neonatal seizures, alone or together, are nonspecific and may be due to factors other than birth asphyxia. A history suggestive of in utero exposure to infection or autoimmune disorder, or finding abnormalities of coagulation factors such as the factor V Leiden mutation, may offer hints as to etiology in some children with CP.

Support and counseling of families and prevention of secondary complications are major realistic goals in the treatment of children with CP. Families may need aid in arranging respite care and in long-term planning. Assessment of the affected person will be required for contractures, hip instability, scoliosis, problems with nutrition or swallowing, sensory defects, educational disabilities, and seizure disorders. Older persons with CP, now surviving in larger numbers, may experience falls, infections, pain, depression, and social isolation.

Implications for research

The etiology of CP is still poorly understood. Births of VLBW infants are concentrated in specialized facilities or infants are transferred early to such facilities, and much of what we know about etiology and prognosis of CP in VLBW infants has come from followup studies from such centers. In term or near-term infants, in whom the prevalence of CP is relatively low but who contribute a majority of CP, however, births are scattered and prospective studies are probably not feasible. Only a narrow range of hypotheses have yet been tested with regard to the etiology of CP in infants of normal birthweight. Further progress in understanding the etiology of CP in children born at or near term would be accelerated by population-based investigations, of which only a few contemporary examples are available.

REFERENCES

1. Colver AF, Gibson M, Hey EN, Jarvis SN, Mackie PC, Richmond S. Increasing rates of cerebral palsy across the severity spectrum in north-east England 1964–1993. *Arch Dis Child Fetal Neonatal Ed* 2000;83:F7–F12.
2. Stanley FJ, Watson L. The cerebral palsies in Western Australia; trends, 1968–1981. *Am J Obstet Gynecol* 1988;158:89–93.

3. Murphy CC, Yeargin-Allsopp M, Decoufle P, Drews CD. Prevalence of cerebral palsy among ten-year-old children in metropolitan Atlanta, 1985 through 1987. *J Pediatr* 1993;123:S13–9.

4. Takeshita K, Ando Y, Ohtani K, Takashima S. Cerebral palsy in Tottori, Japan. *Neuroepidemiology* 1989;8:184–92.

5. Hagberg B, Hagberg G, Olow I, et al. The changing panorama of cerebral palsy in Sweden. VII. Prevalence and origin in the birth year period 1987–1990. *Acta Paediatr Scand* 1996;85:954–60.

6. Pharoah P, Cooke T, Johnson M, et al. Epidemiology of cerebral palsy in England and Scotland 1984–9. *Arch Dis Child Fetal Neonatal Ed* 1998;79:F21–5.

7. Cummins SK, Nelson KB, Grether JK. Cerebral palsy in four northern California counties, births 1983 through 1985. *J Pediatr* 1993;123:230–7.

8. Lorenz JM, Wooliever DE, Jetton JR, Paneth N. A quantitative review of mortality and developmental disability in extremely premature newborns. *Arch Pediatr Adolesc Med* 1998;152:425–35.

9. Nelson KB, Ellenberg JH. Antecedents of cerebral palsy, multivariate analysis of risk. *N Engl J Med* 1986;315:81–6.

10. Torfs CP, van den Berg G, Oechsli FW, Cummins S. Prenatal and perinatal factors in the etiology of cerebral palsy. *J Pediatr* 1990;116:615–9.

11. Nelson KB, Ellenberg JH. Obstetric complications as risk factors for cerebral palsy or seizure disorders. *JAMA* 1984;251:1843–8.

12. Yudkin PL, Johnson A, Clover LM, Murphy KW. Assessing the contribution of birth asphyxia to cerebral palsy in term singletons. *Paediatr Perinat Epidemiol* 1995;9:156–70.

13. Grether JK, Nelson KB, Emery ES III, Cummins SK. Prenatal and perinatal factors and cerebral palsy in very low birth weight infants. *J Pediatr* 1996;128:407–14.

14. Nelson KB, Grether JK. Can magnesium sulfate reduce the risk of cerebral palsy in very low birthweight infants? *Pediatrics* 1995;95:263–9.

15. Murphy DJ, Sellers S, MacKenzie IA, Yudkin PL, Johnson AM. Case-control study of antenatal and intrapartum risk factors for cerebral palsy in very preterm singleton babies. *Lancet* 1995;346:1449–54.

16. Nelson KB. Magnesium sulfate and risk of cerebral palsy in very low-birthweight infants. *JAMA* 1996;276:1843–4.

17. Schendel DE, Berg CJ, Yeargin-Allsopp M, Boyle CA, Decoufle P. Prenatal magnesium sulfate exposure and the risk for cerebral palsy or mental retardation among very low-birth-weight children aged 3 to 5 years. *JAMA* 1996;276:1805–10.

18. Matsuda Y, Kouno S, Hiroyama Y, et al. Intrauterine infection, magnesium sulfate exposure and cerebral palsy in infants born between 26 and 30 weeks of gestation. *Eur J Obstet Gynecol Reprod Biol* 2000;91:159–64.

19. Paneth N, Jetton J, Pinto B, Martin J, Susser M. Magnesium sulfate in labor and risk of neonatal brain lesions and cerebral palsy in low birthweight infants. *Pediatrics* 1997;99(Electronic suppl.):e1.

20. Wilson-Costello D, Borawski E, Friedman H, Redline R, Fanaroff AA, Hack M. Perinatal

correlates of cerebral palsy and other neurologic impairment among low birth weight children. *Pediatrics* 1998;102:315–22.

21. Grether JK, Hoogstrate J, Walsh-Greene E, Nelson KB. Magnesium sulfate for tocolysis and risk of spastic cerebral palsy in premature children born to women without preeclampsia. *Am J Obstet Gynecol* 2000;183:717–25.

22. Goldenberg RL, Rouse DJ. Prevention of premature birth. *N Engl J Med* 1998;339:313–20.

23. Mazor M, Chaim W, Maymon E, Hershkowitz R, Romero R. The role of antibiotic therapy in the prevention of prematurity. *Clin Perinatol* 1998;25:659–85.

24. Wu YW, Colford JM Jr. Chorioamnionitis as a risk factor for cerebral palsy: a meta-analysis. *JAMA* 2000;284:1417–24.

25. Reuss ML, Paneth N, Pinto-Martin JA, Lorenz JM, Susser M. The relation of transient hypothyroxinemia in preterm infants to neurologic development at two years of age. *N Engl J Med* 1996;334:821–7.

26. den Ouden AL, Kok JH, Verkerk PH, Brand R, Verloove B, Vanhorick SP. The relation between neonatal thyroxine levels and neurodevelopmental outcome at age 5 and 9 years in a national cohort of very preterm and/or very low birth weight infants. *Pediatr Research* 1996;39:142–5.

27. van Wassenaer AG, Kok JH, de Vijlder JJM, et al. Effects of thyroxine supplementation on neurologic development in infants born at less than 30 weeks' gestation. *N Engl J Med* 1997;336:21–6.

28. Grether JK, Nelson KB. Maternal infection and cerebral palsy in infants of normal birth weight. *JAMA* 1997;278:207–11.

29. Grether JK, Nelson KB, Cummins SK. Twinning and cerebral palsy in four northern California counties, births 1983 through 1985. *Pediatrics* 1993;92:854–8.

30. Petterson B, Nelson KB, Watson L, Stanley F. Twins, triplets, and cerebral palsy in births in Western Australia in the 1980s. *BMJ* 1993;301:39–43.

31. Pharoah PO, Cooke T. Cerebral palsy and multiple births. *Arch Dis Child Fetal Neonatal Ed* 1996;75:F174–7.

32. Pharoah PO, Adi Y. Consequences of in utero death in a twin pregnancy. *Lancet* 2000;355:1597–602.

33. Nelson KB, Grether JK. Potentially asphyxiating conditions and spastic cerebral palsy in infants of normal birth weight. *Am J Obstet Gynecol* 1998;179:507–13.

34. Gaffney G, Sellers S, Flavell V, Squier M, Johnson A. Case-control study of intrapartum care, cerebral palsy, and perinatal death. *BMJ* 1994;308:743–50.

35. Umstad MP, Permezel M, Pepperell RJ. Intrapartum cardiotocography and the expert witness. *Austral NZ J Obstetr Gynecol* 1994;34:20–3.

36. Nelson KB, Dambrosia JM, Ting TY, Grether JK. Uncertain value of electronic fetal monitoring in predicting cerebral palsy. *N Engl J Med* 1996;3334:613–8.

37. Eastman NJ, Deleon M. The etiology of cerebral palsy. *Am J Obstet Gynecol* 1955;69:950–61.

38. Petridou E, Koussouri M, Toupadaki N, et al. Risk factors for cerebral palsy: a case-control study in Greece. *Scand J Soc Med* 1996;1:14–26.

39. Silver RK, MacGregor SN, Pasternak JF, Neely SE. Fetal stroke associated with elevated maternal anticardiolipin antibodies. *Obstet Gynecol* 1992;80:497–9.

40. Thorarensen O, Ryan S, Hunter J, Younkin DP. Factor V Leiden mutation: an unrecognized cause of hemiplegic cerebral palsy, neonatal stroke, and placental thrombosis. *Ann Neurol* 1997;42:372–5.

41. Debus O, Koch HG, Kurlemann G, et al. Factor V Leiden and genetic defects of thrombophilia in childhood porencephaly. *Arch Dis Child Fetal Neonatal Ed* 1998;78:F121–4.

42. Golomb MR, Domi T, Mayank S, deVeber GA. Children with presumed prenatal or perinatal arterial ischemic stroke have frequent coagulation abnormalities and persistent neurological deficits [abstract]. *Ann Neurol* 2000;48:526.

43. Arias F, Romero R, Joist H, Kraus FT. Thrombophilia: a mechanism of disease in women with adverse pregnancy outcome and thrombotic lesions in the placenta. *J Matern Fetal Med* 1998;7:277–86.

44. Nelson KB, Dambrosia JM, Grether JK, Phillips TM. Neonatal cytokines and coagulation factors in children with cerebral palsy. *Ann Neurol* 1998;44:665–75.

45. Allen MC, Alexander GR. Using motor milestones as a multistep process to screen preterm infants for cerebral palsy. *Develop Med Child Neurol* 1997;39:12–16.

46. Nelson KB, Ellenberg JH. Children who "outgrew" cerebral palsy. *Pediatrics* 1982;69:529–36.

47. Roth SC, Baudin J, Pezzani B, Goldsmith M, Townsend J, Reynolds EOR, Stewart AL. Relation between neurodevelopmental status of very preterm infants at one and eight years. *Develop Med Child Neurol* 1994;36:1049–62.

48. Hutton JL, Cooke T, Pharoah POD. Life expectancy in children with cerebral palsy. *BMJ* 1994;309:431–5.

49. Crichton JU, MacKinnon M, White CP. The life expectancy of persons with cerebral palsy. *Develop Med Child Neurol* 1995;37:567–76.

50. Strauss D, Shavelle R. Life expectancy of adults with cerebral palsy. *Dev Med Child Neurol* 1998;40:369–75.

51. Williams K, Alberman E. Survival in cerebral palsy: the role of severity and diagnostic labels. *Dev Med Child Neurol* 1998;40:376–9.

52. Davis EC, Barnes MP. Botulin toxin and spasticity. *J Neurol Neurosurg Psychiatry* 2000;69:143–7.

53. Graubert C, Song KM, McLaughlin JF, Bjornson KF. Changes in gait at 1 year post-selective dorsal rhizotomy: results of a prospective randomized study. *J Pediatr Orthop* 2000;20:496–500.

22

Migraine

Ann I. Scher, Richard B. Lipton and Walter F. Stewart

Epidemiology

Migraine headache is an extremely common and temporarily disabling headache disorder. One recent population-based survey reported that 19% of women and 8% of men had suffered at least one attack of migraine in the previous year (1). However, only a minority of active migraineurs have seen a physician within the last year for headache (2–4). As a consequence, clinic-based studies are prone to significant selection bias. Population-based studies, which actively screen participants for migraine whether or not they consult physicians, provide more representative samples for research.

A large number of population-based prevalence studies of migraine have been published and summarized elsewhere (5–8). Prevalence has been shown to vary by race, age, gender, and survey methodology (below). A recent meta-analysis suggests that much of the variability in estimates of migraine prevalence is due to the variability of case definitions and sociodemographic profiles of the study subjects (9). Studies using the IHS criteria showed more consistent results (9). Table 22.1 presents the results from recent population-based studies that: (1) used IHS criteria and (2) were based on representative populations.

Age

Most studies on migraine prevalence have reported variation by age and gender. Prevalence is generally highest between the ages of 25 and 55, often with a peak in the late 30s and early 40s (10–13). Figure 22.1 (from the American Migraine Study) illustrates this pattern. The strong nonlinear association of age with prevalence accounts for some of the variability in prevalence estimates among studies, due to differing age distributions in the study populations.

Gender

A number of studies have reported the prevalence of migraine to be the same or greater in boys prior to puberty; three studies (Table 22.1) (14–16) based on

Table 22.1. Gender-specific prevalence estimates of migraine from 21 population-based studies using IHS diagnostic criteria

Author (year, ref. no)	Country	Source	Method	Sample size	Time frame	Age (years)	Migraine prevalence (%) Female	Male	Total	Comments
Abu-Arefeh (1994) (14)	Scotland	School	Clinical interview	1754	1 year	5–15	11.5	9.7	10.6	Prevalence is higher in boys prior to age 12 (1.14 : 1). After age 12, more common in girls (2.0 : 1)
Alders (1996) (100)	Malaysia	Community	Face-to-face	595	1 year	5+	11.3	6.7	9.0	
Arregui (1991) (101)	Peru	Community	Clinical interview	2257	All	12.2	4.5	8.4		
Barea (1996) (15)	Brazil	School	Clinical interview	538	1 year	10–18	10.3	9.6	9.9	2–48 hour duration allowed
Breslau (1993) (87)	US	Community	Face-to-face/ Telephone	1007	1 year	21–30	12.9	3.4	9.2	
Cruz (1985) (102)	Ecuador	Community	Clinical interview	2723	Lifetime	All	7.9	5.6	6.9	Community endemic for cysticercosis
Göbel (1994) (24)	Germany	Community	Mail SAQ	4061	Lifetime	18+	15.0	7.0	11.0	
Haimanot (1995) (10)	Ethiopia	Community	Face-to-face/ clinical interview	15 000	1 year	20+	4.2	1.7	3.0	
Henry (1992) (11)	France	Community	Face-to-face	4204	1 year	15+	11.9	4.0	8.1	
Abdul (1997) (103)	Saudi Arabia	Community	Face-to-face	5891	Lifetime	15+			8.0	
Jaillard (1997) (104)	Peru	Community	Clinical interview	3246	1 year	15+	7.8	2.3	5.3	
Merikangas (1993) (105)	Switzerland	Community	Clinical interview	379	1 year	28–29	32.6	16.1	24.5	Weighted prevalence
Michel (1996) (96)	France	Community	Mail SAQ	9411	3 months	18+	18.0	8.0	13.0	
O'Brien (1994) (25)	Canada	Community	Telephone	2922	1 year	18+	21.9	7.4	15.2	
Raieli (1995) (16)	Italy	School	Clinical interview	1445	1 year	11–14	3.3	2.7	3.0	

Study	Country	Setting	Method	N	Period	Age				Comments
Rasmussen (1991) (106)	Denmark	Community	Clinical interview	740	1 year	25–64	15.0	6.0	10.0	
Russell (1995) (107)	Denmark	Community	Clinical interview	3471	Lifetime	40	23.7	11.7	17.7	
Sakai (1997) (12)	Japan	Community	Mail SAQ	4029	1 year	15+	12.9	3.6	8.4	Female: Male prevalence ratio = 3.6. Regional differences
Stewart (1992) (20)	US	Community	Mail SAQ	20 468	1 year	12–80	17.6	5.7	12.0	
Stewart (1996) (1)	US	Community	Telephone	12 328	1 year	18–65	19.0	8.2	14.7	Racial differences
Wong (1995) (13)	Hong Kong	Community	Telephone	7356	1 year	15+	1.5	0.6	1.0	

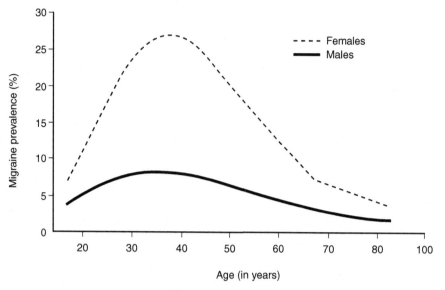

Figure 22.1 Age- and sex-specific prevalence of migraine. (Reprinted with permission from Lipton RB, Stewart WF. Migraine in the United States: Epidemiology and health care use. Neurology 1993:43[Suppl.3]:6.)

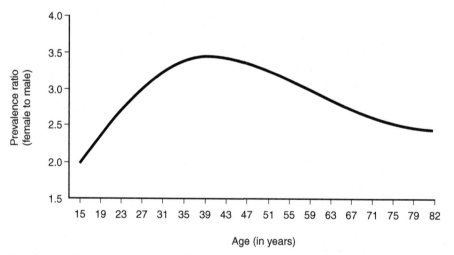

Figure 22.2 Female-to-male prevalence ratio of migraine by age. (Reprinted with permission from Lipton RB, Stewart W. Migraine in the United States: Epidemiology and health care use. Neurology 1993;43[Suppl.3]:6).

pediatric or adolescent populations show almost equal prevalence rates in boys and girls. After adolescence, prevalence ratios range between 2.0 and 3.6 (Table 22.1). This female preponderance continues throughout life, although to a less marked degree after age 40 or so. Figure 22.2 from the American Migraine Study, illustrates how this prevalence rate ratio varies by age, with a low at age 15, a peak at around age 40, and declines thereafter.

Socioeconomic status

Migraine was once considered to be a disease of the affluent. Bille found no support for this idea in a study of school children (17,18). Studies using intelligence testing and occupation as SES measures also failed to find an association between migraine prevalence and social class or intelligence (19).

As noted earlier, migraine prevalence is inversely related to household income in US population-based studies (1,20,21). Similar results were found in data from the National Health Interview Survey (NHIS) (22). In that study, although migraine prevalence was higher in low vs. middle income groups, prevalence was highest in the high income groups. However, this study relied on self-reported migraine diagnosis (which would be higher in those with higher income). Non-US studies have generally not supported the association of low SES (as measured by education, occupation, or income) with headache prevalence (14,23–25). This lack of association outside the US may be influenced by international differences in patterns of medical consulting behavior and access to health care.

Race

The American Migraine Study showed that migraine prevalence was lower in African–Americans than Asians (20). An independent US study found that prevalence was higher in caucasians than African–Americans, with the lowest prevalence in Asian–Americans (1). There have been relatively few post-IHS surveys of African or Asian populations, but a community-based Ethiopian survey (10) (Table 22.1) found a relatively low prevalence of migraine (4.2% female, 1.7% male). Studies from Hong Kong (1.5%) (13) and Japan also report a relatively low prevalence of migraine (12.9% female, 3.6% male) (12).

Incidence

There have been few population-based studies that have attempted to define age-specific migraine incidence prospectively. In one prospective study designed to determine whether those with major depression or anxiety disorders were more prone to develop migraine, Breslau et al. (26) followed a group of 21–30-year-olds who were members of a large managed-care organization in south-east Michigan. Of the 848 subjects at risk for incident migraine, 71 subsequently met criteria for migraine during the 5-year follow-up period, corresponding to an incidence rate of 17 per 1000/person years (24 female, 6 male). This excellent study is limited primarily by the narrow age range of the samples; incidence below the age of 21 could only be estimated.

In two population-based cross-sectional studies, incidence rates were estimated based on participants' recalled age of onset. In a Danish population-based study in which 1000 participants underwent a clinical interview, Rasmussen (7) estimated the (age-adjusted) incidence of migraine at 3.7 per 1000 person years (5.8 female, 1.6 male). This study did not have adequate power to assess age-specific incidence. Reported rates represent the average of young adults with high rates and older adults with very low rates. In another population-based telephone survey of 10 000, Stewart et al. (27) calculated age-specific incidence rates after correcting for telescoping, that is, the tendency to recall past events as happening more recently than they did. The peak age of onset was found to be at ages 5–10 for males and 12–13 for females for migraine with aura and 10–11 for males and 14–17 for females for migraine without aura. Peak incidence rates for migraine with aura were 6.6/1000 person years for males and 14.1/1000 person years for females and 10.1/1000 person years for males and 18.9/1000 person years for migraine without aura.

Stang et al. (28) used the linked medical records system in Olmstead County, Minnesota to identify new cases of migraine and establish the type and age of onset. Compared to the population-based study of Stewart et al. (27) they found lower rates of incidence and later incidence peaks. These findings may be explained by the low consultation rates of those with migraine and the possibility that medical consultation may occur well after the onset of symptoms.

Etiology

Familial aggregation of migraine has long been recognized and genetic studies have generally supported a role for both genetic and environmental risk factors in the etiology of migraine (29). This section reviews the recent evidence for genetic factors in migraine (30,31).

Twin studies

Clinic-based twin studies have consistently shown that monozygotic (MZ) twins are more concordant for migraine than dizygotic (DZ) twins, supporting a role for genetic factors in migraine etiology (31). Three recent studies conducted in population-based twin registries also support a genetic basis for migraine. These studies were conducted in Australia (32), Finland (33), and Sweden (34). Two studies (Australia and Sweden) used the IHS criteria, one did not. Direct interviews of both twins were used only in the Australian study.

In the Australian study, Merikangas and coworkers evaluated 5844 twins ranging in age from 19–91 by direct interview. Proband-wise concordance for female same-sex twins was 0.44 for MZ twins and 0.24 for the DZ twins. In males, the MZ concordance rate was 0.31 and the DZ concordance rate was 0.18. In all three studies, about half of the variation in migraine prevalence was attributable to genetic factors. These data also demonstrate that nongenetic factors must play a role as the MZ concordance rate was well below 1.0. Thus, the twin studies support the importance of genetic as well as environmental risk factors for migraine.

Familial aggregation

A number of studies have examined the risk of migraine among relatives of migraine probands and nonmigrainous controls (30,31). All of the family studies demonstrate an increased family risk of migraine among the relatives of migraine probands. In the early studies, relative risks ranged from 1.5 to 19.3 (30). Variation in the family relative risk in the early studies is accounted for, at least in part, by a number of methodological differences among these studies. First, diagnostic criteria were variable and often poorly specified. Second, in many studies, migraine probands were identified from specialty care centers. Since seeking medical care for migraine is strongly associated with disability (35,36) and disability is associated with familial aggregation (37), clinic-based studies are likely to overestimate familial aggregation. Third, in many studies, family history is obtained from the index case, not by direct interview of the relatives. Since probands with migraine are more likely to report migraine in their relatives than persons without migraine, this method also leads to overestimation of familial aggregation (38).

Two recent population-based migraine family studies avoid many of the limitations of earlier studies. Both of these studies show an increased risk of migraine in the relatives of those with migraine. The studies differ, however, in whether the excess risk is specific to the type of migraine in the proband. In the first study, Russell and Olesen (39) identified 378 probands with and without aura from the general population based on IHS criteria. First-degree relatives and spouses were directly interviewed by telephone to determine migraine status. First degree relatives of probands who had migraine with aura had a four-fold increased risk of migraine with aura. The relatives of probands who had migraine without aura had a 1.9-fold increased risk of migraine without aura – thus, suggesting that the transmission of migraine type within families has a degree of specificity. Interestingly, the spouses of probands with migraine without aura had a 1.5-fold increased risk of migraine without aura, suggesting the influence of either shared environmental factors or assortative mating.

Stewart et al. (37) interviewed 511 first-degree family members of 73 clinically confirmed probands with migraine and 72 matched controls without migraine. Overall, the risk of migraine was 50% higher in the relatives of the migraineurs than the nonmigraineurs. Migraine risk was particularly elevated (RR = 2.2) in the relatives of those with disabling migraine. In contrast to the study of Russell and

Olesen (39), no specificity in transmission was found. That is, the type of migraine in the proband (with aura vs. without aura) did not differentially affect the risk of migraine in relatives. Nor was the risk to relatives specific to the type of migraine in the proband, i.e., an increased risk of both types of migraine was found in family members independent of the type of migraine in the proband. This study also showed that the age of onset of migraine in the proband did not affect the risk to relatives, in contrast to the pattern seen in other disorders with a genetic basis.

Segregation analysis

The evidence from segregation analysis does not provide consistent evidence for any single mode of inheritance (40–44). The inconsistent results may reflect the genetic heterogeneity of migraine. Some families show apparent autosomal dominant transmissions while others show autosomal recessive transmission with incomplete penetrance.

Linkage studies

Linkage studies of familial hemiplegic migraine (FHM) have been an area of interest and progress. The original report of linkage of FHM to a location on chromosome 19 (45) has been confirmed in many unrelated families (46,47). However, some families with FHM did not show linkage to chromosome 19 (46,47). Thus, even this relatively stereotyped autosomal dominant disorder is genetically heterogeneous. Linkage markers for some of the nonchromosome 19 FHM families have been tentatively identified on chromosome 1 (48). The Dutch group has identified a specific pathogenic gene on chromosome 19 that codes for a calcium channel protein subunit (49). It is possible that the gene or genes involved in nonchromosome 19 FHM may code for functionally related proteins.

The relationship between this chromosome 19 locus and the more common types of migraine is not clear. One group found an association between the chromosome 19 marker and both migraine with and without aura in an affected sib-pair study of 28 families (50). Another group did not find an association in a small number of families (51). Perhaps the chromosome 19 marker is also associated with more common types of migraine but the population-attributable risk must be low. This work raises the intriguing possibility that migraine, like a number of other episodic neurologic diseases, may be an ion channelopathy.

The heterogeneity of FHM underscores the likely heterogeneity of the more common types of migraine. Future work should take heterogeneity into account by looking for families with pathogenic genes which interact with each other and with environmental factors to determine migraine risk. Population-based strategies are important for defining the attributable risk for pathogenic genes and for assessing gene–environment interactions.

Diagnosis

Diagnosis of migraine is complicated by the episodic and heterogeneous nature of the illness. Attacks vary in frequency, pain intensity, duration, and associated headache features (5). Characterization of attacks is further complicated by the fact that migraineurs often have more than one headache type and may have trouble recalling which symptoms were associated with each headache type. Even when recalled perfectly, the poor demarcation among the primary headache disorders complicates the classification of individual headache attacks which may have features that defy classification. In fact, there is some controversy as to whether migraine and tension-type headache represent distinct diseases (52,53) or are opposite ends of a continuum of severity (54–56).

To improve the classification of the headache disorders, the International Headache Society (IHS), based on expert consensus, published a classification system for a broad range of headache disorders. This system represented an enormous improvement over the past systems. Rather than using the traditional nomenclature, these guidelines provided simpler, more informative terms. In addition, the criteria were much more explicit, indicating which features were required to diagnose particular headache disorders (57). The advent of these criteria has facilitated epidemiologic research by providing standardized operational definitions of migraine. These criteria have been subjected to field testing and have been found to be comprehensive when tested in a population-based sample (58). In subspecialty clinics, however, it is difficult to classify many patients. This is primarily due to the large number of clinic patients that have chronic daily headaches evolving from migraine (59–62). Despite their limitations, the IHS criteria represent an enormous advance in headache classification.

Selection and referral bias has also substantially influenced the study of migraine. Most studies of headache are based on patients in primary or specialty care settings. However, only a minority of headache sufferers ever consult physicians, and fewer still consult neurologists or headache specialists (2–4). In clinic-based studies, factors that contributed to seeking specialty care may be mistaken for attributes of the disease. For example, several clinic-based studies reported an association between migraine and high socioeconomic status (SES). In US population-based studies, however, the inverse was found to be true – that is, low SES was associated with migraine (1,20). Thus, at least in the US, migraine is a disease of high SES in the clinic but not in the community.

Recall of headache onset (first lifetime attack) is prone to a systematic bias known as "telescoping"; events in the past are assigned a time too close to the present (17,63,64). The net effect is a distortion of age-specific incidence measurements. In addition, patients may also not reliably recall headache characteristics from the remote past – recalling only their most severe or most dramatic attacks.

Prognosis

There are relatively few longitudinal studies on the natural history of migraine. Bille followed a migrainous cohort for up to 40 years (17,18,65); although 62% were free of migraine as young adults, only 46% were migraine-free after 40 years. An additional 22% who were not migraine free reported past remissions. Thus, migraine is often a condition of very long duration. Hockaday also reported long-term remissions (66). Fry (67) and Waters (19,54), in other longitudinal studies, noted the tendency for attacks to decrease in frequency and severity as patients aged.

Clinic-based studies have reported on a subgroup of migraineurs who, after years of episodic migraine, experience increasing attack frequency often coupled with decreasing attack severity to the point that daily or near-daily headaches may occur (68–70). This syndrome has been variously called chronic daily headache evolving from migraine, transformed migraine, drug-induced headache, and malignant migraine. In clinics, 46–87% of such patients are found to be overusing acute headache medication (60,61,71–73).

Although medication overuse has been hypothesized to be the mechanism by which daily headaches are perpetuated through a rebound cycle (69), rebound headache has only been demonstrated for caffeine in a placebo-controlled trial. Drug withdrawal alone has been reported to have a success rate of about 60% (74,75). Since many clinic patients with this condition are not overusing medication, however, there may be a subgroup of migraine sufferers with a progressive condition (60,61,71–73).

The prevalence of daily headache evolving from migraine in the general population has not been well studied. Estimates of the prevalence of chronic tension-type headache (the only IHS diagnostic category for frequent headache) mostly range from 1–3% (7,10,13,24,76–78). Two population-based surveys reported a prevalence of about 1–2% for frequent headache associated with migraine (based on proposed criteria for Transformed Migraine) (62,77,78).

Implications for clinical practice

A number of conditions are more likely to occur in individuals with migraine than in the general population. Population-based studies demonstrate that migraine is comorbid with depression, anxiety disorders, and manic depressive illness (79–88) as well as epilepsy (89–92). In addition, migraine is associated with stroke in women below the age of 45 (93,94). The existence of comorbidity creates a need for heightened diagnostic vigilance; detecting migraine implies an array of other disorders are more likely. If comorbid illnesses are identified, treatment plans should reflect the concomitant diagnoses (95).

Most studies of health care utilization have shown that most migraineurs are not receiving medical care for their headaches and usually treat their headaches with over-the-counter medication. The percentage of migraineurs who report ever having consulted a physician for headache ranges from 15–60% (4,7,12,96), with higher consultation rates in women than in men. Of these migraine sufferers who have sought medical care, less than 15% have ever consulted neurologists and fewer than 2% consult headache specialists (4). Most migraineurs take medication for attacks though the majority take over-the-counter medication to the exclusion of prescription drugs (97). High levels of pain, disability, and work-loss mandate aggressive treatment for disabled migraine sufferers (12,96,98,99).

Conclusion

Migraine is a very common disorder, with highest prevalence during the peak productive years – between the ages of 25 and 55. The prevalence is greater in females than males after puberty, but the sex ratio varies with age. In the United States, migraine prevalence is higher in those with lower incomes, possibly because migraine interferes with work and schooling.

Family and twin studies support a role for genetic factors in migraine, but inheritance is likely to be complex and multifactorial. Though FHM is sometimes related to mutations on a calcium channel gene, specific mechanisms and gene–environment interactions for more common forms of migraine remain to be elucidated.

The impact of headache disorders on individuals and society is large and provides an important target for public health interventions. Despite the widespread disability produced by migraine and the increasing availability of effective treatment, the disorder remains undertreated and underdiagnosed.

REFERENCES

1. Stewart WF, Lipton RB, Liberman J. Variation in migraine prevalence by race. *Neurology* 1996;47:52–9.
2. Lipton RB, Stewart WF, Simon D. Medical consultation for migraine: results from the American Migraine Study. *Headache* 1998;38:87–96.
3. Stang PE, Osterhaus JT, Celentano DD. Migraine. Patterns of healthcare use. *Neurology* 1994;44:S47–S55.

4. Linet MS, Stewart WF, Celentano DD, Ziegler D, Sprecher M. An epidemiologic study of headache among adolescents and young adults. *JAMA* 1989;261:2211–16.

5. Stewart WF, Shechter A, Lipton RB. Migraine heterogeneity. Disability, pain intensity, and attack frequency and duration. *Neurology* 1994;44:S24–S39.

6. Stewart WF, Shechter A, Rasmussen BK. Migraine prevalence. A review of population-based studies [see comments]. *Neurology* 1994;44:S17–S23.

7. Rasmussen BK. Epidemiology of headache. *Cephalalgia* 1995;15:45–68.

8. Lipton RB, Stewart WF. Prevalence and impact of migraine. Neurol Clin 1997;15:1–13.

9. Stewart WF, Simon D, Shechter A, Lipton RB. Population variation in migraine prevalence: a meta-analysis. *J Clin Epidemiol* 1995;48:269–80.

10. Tekle Haimanot R., Seraw B, Forsgren L, Ekbom K, Ekstedt J. Migraine, chronic tension-type headache, and cluster headache in an Ethiopian rural community [see comments]. *Cephalalgia* 1995;15:482–8.

11. Henry P, Michel P, Brochet B, Dartigues JF, Tison S, Salamon R. A nationwide survey of migraine in France: prevalence and clinical features in adults. GRIM [see comments]. *Cephalalgia* 1992;12:229–37.

12. Sakai F, Igarashi H. Prevalence of migraine in Japan: a nationwide survey. *Cephalalgia* 1997;17:15–22.

13. Wong TW, Wong KS, Yu TS, Kay R. Prevalence of migraine and other headaches in Hong Kong. *Neuroepidemiology* 1995;14:82–91.

14. Abu-Arefeh I, Russell G. Prevalence of headache and migraine in schoolchildren. *BMJ* 1994;309:765–9.

15. Barea LM, Tannhauser M, Rotta NT. An epidemiologic study of headache among children and adolescents of southern Brazil. *Cephalalgia* 1996;16:545–9.

16. Raieli V, Raimondo D, Cammalleri R, Camarda R. Migraine headaches in adolescents: a student population-based study in Monreale. Cephalalgia 1995;15:5–12.

17. Bille B. Migraine in schoolchildren. *Acta Paediatr Scand Suppl* 1962;51:1–151.

18. Bille B. Migraine in children: prevalence, clinical features, and a 30-year follow-up. In: Ferrari MD, Lataste X. (Xavier) (Eds.). *Migraine and other Headaches*. Carnforth, UK: Parthenon Publishing, 1989.

19. Waters WE. Migraine: intelligence, social class, and familial prevalence. *BMJ* 1971;2:77–81.

20. Stewart WF, Lipton RB, Celentano DD, Reed ML. Prevalence of migraine headache in the United States. Relation to age, income, race, and other sociodemographic factors. *JAMA* 1992;267:64–9.

21. Kryst S, Scherl E. A population-based survey of the social and personal impact of headache. *Headache* 1994;34:344–50.

22. Stang PE, Osterhaus JT. Impact of migraine in the United States: data from the National Health Interview Survey. *Headache* 1993;33:29–35.

23. Rasmussen BK. Migraine and tension-type headache in a general population: psychosocial factors. In *J Epidemiol* 1992;21:1138–43.

24. Gobel H, Petersen-Braun M, Soyka D. The epidemiology of headache in Germany: a nationwide survey of a representative sample on the basis of the headache classification of the International Headache Society [see comments]. *Cephalalgia* 1994;14:97–106.

25. O'Brien B, Goeree R, Streiner D. Prevalence of migraine headache in Canada: a population-based survey. *Int J Epidemiol* 1994;23:1020–6.

26. Breslau N, Chilcoat HD, Andreski P. Further evidence on the link between migraine and neuroticism. *Neurology* 1996;47:663–7.

27. Stewart WF, Linet MS, Celentano DD, Van NM, Ziegler D. Age- and sex-specific incidence rates of migraine with and without visual aura. *Am J Epidemiol* 1991;134:1111–20.

28. Stang PE, Yanagihara PA, Swanson JW, et al. Incidence of migraine headache: a population-based study in Olmsted County, Minnesota. *Neurology* 1992;42:1657–62.

29. Ziegler DK. Genetics of migraine. In Vinken PJ, Rose FC (Eds.). *Headache.* Amsterdam: Elsevier Science Publishers, 1986:28–30.

30. Merikangas KR. Genetic epidemiology of migraine. In Sandler M, Collins GM (Eds.). *Migraine: a Spectrum of Ideas.* Oxford: Oxford University Press, 1990:40–7.

31. Merikangas KR. Genetics of migraine and other headache. *Curr Opin Neurol* 1996;9:202–5.

32. Merikangas KR, Tierney C, Martin NG, Heath AC, Risch NJ. Genetics of migraine in the Australian Twin Registry. In Rose FC (Ed.). *New Advances in Headache Research 4.* London: Smith-Gordon, 1994:27–8.

33. Honkasalo ML, Kaprio J, Winter T, Heikkila K, Sillanpaa M, Koskenvuo M. Migraine and concomitant symptoms among 8167 adult twin pairs. *Headache* 1995;35:70–8.

34. Larsson B, Bille B, Pedersen NL. Genetic influence in headaches: a Swedish twin study. *Headache* 1995;35:513–19.

35. Linet MS, Celentano DD, Stewart WF. Headache characteristics associated with physician consultation: a population-based survey. *Am J Prevent Med* 1991;7:40–6.

36. Lipton RB, Stewart WF, Celentano DD, Reed ML. Undiagnosed migraine headaches. A comparison of symptom-based and reported physician diagnosis. *Archiv Intern Med* 1992;152:1273–8.

37. Stewart WF, Staffa J, Lipton RB, Ottman R. Familial risk of migraine: a population-based study. *Ann Neurol* 1997;41:166–72.

38. Ottman R, Hong S, Lipton RB. Validity of family history data on severe headache and migraine. *Neurology* 1993;43:1954–60.

39. Russell MB, Olesen J. Increased familial risk and evidence of genetic factor in migraine [see comments]. *BMJ* 1995;311:541–4.

40. Devoto M, Lozito A, Staffa G, D'Alessandro R, Sacquegna T, Romeo G. Segregation analysis of migraine in 128 families. *Cephalalgia* 1986;6:101–5.

41. Russell MB, Iselius L, Olesen J. Inheritance of migraine investigated by complex segregation analysis. *Hum Genet* 1995;96:726–30.

42. D'Amico D, Leone M, Macciardi F, Valentini S, Bussone G. Genetic transmission of migraine without aura: a study of 68 families. *Ital J Neurol Sci* 1991;12:581–4.

43. Mochi M, Sangiorgi S, Cortelli P, et al. Testing models for genetic determination in migraine [see comments]. *Cephalalgia* 1993;13:389–94.

44. Ulrich V, Russell MB, Ostergaard S, Olesen J. Analysis of 31 families with an apparently autosomal-dominant transmission of migraine with aura in the nuclear family. *Am J Med Genet* 1997;74:395–7.

45. Joutel A, Bousser MG, Biousse V, et al. A gene for familial hemiplegic migraine maps to chromosome 19. *Nat Genet* 1993;5:40–5.

46. Joutel A, Ducros A, Vahedi K, et al. Genetic heterogeneity of familial hemiplegic migraine. *Am J Hum Genet* 1994;55:1166–72.

47. Ophoff RA, van ER, Sandkuijl LA, et al. Genetic heterogeneity of familial hemiplegic migraine. *Genomics* 1994;22:21–6.

48. Ducros A, Joutel A, Vahedi K, et al. Familial hemiplegic migraine: mapping of the second gene and evidence for a third locus. *Cephalalgia* 1997;17:232(Abstract).

49. Ophoff RA, Terwindt GM, Vergouwe MN, et al. Familial hemiplegic migraine and episodic ataxia type–2 are caused by mutations in the Ca2 + channel gene CACNL1A4. *Cell* 1996;87:543–52.

50. May A, Ophoff RA, Terwindt GM, et al. Familial hemiplegic migraine locus on 19p13 is involved in the common forms of migraine with and without aura. *Hum Genet* 1995;96:604–8.

51. Hovatta I, Kallela M, Farkkila M, Peltonen L. Familial migraine: exclusion of the susceptibility gene from the reported locus of familial hemiplegic migraine on 19p. *Genomics* 1994;23:707–9.

52. Rasmussen BK, Jensen R, Schroll M, Olesen J. Interrelations between migraine and tension-type headache in the general population [see comments]. *Archiv Neurol* 1992;49:914–18.

53. Ulrich V, Russell MB, Jensen R, Olesen J. A comparison of tension-type headache in migraineurs and in non-migraineurs: a population-based study. *Pain* 1996;67:501–6.

54. Waters WE. *Headache.* Littleton, MA: PSG Publishing Co., 1986.

55. Featherstone HJ. Migraine and muscle contraction headaches: a continuum. *Headache* 1985;25:194–8.

56. Raskin N. *Headache.* 2nd edition. New York: Churchill Livingstone, 1988.

57. Headache Classification Committee of the International Headache Society. Classification and diagnostic criteria for headache disorders, cranial neuralgias and facial pain. *Cephalalgia* 1988;8Suppl7:1–96.

58. Rasmussen BK, Jensen R, Olesen J. A population-based analysis of the diagnostic criteria of the International Headache Society. *Cephalalgia* 1991;11:129–34.

59. Solomon S, Lipton RB, Newman LC. Evaluation of chronic daily headache – comparison to criteria for chronic tension-type headache. *Cephalalgia* 1992;12:365–8.

60. Sandrini G, Manzoni GC, Zanferrari C, Nappi G. An epidemiological approach to the nosography of chronic daily headache. *Cephalalgia* 1993;13 Suppl 12:72–7.

61. Mathew NT. Transformed migraine. *Cephalalgia* 1993;13 Suppl 12:78–83.

62. Silberstein SD, Lipton RB, Sliwinski M. Classification of daily and near-daily headaches: field trial of revised IHS criteria. *Neurology* 1996;47:871–5.

63. Brown NR, Rips LJ, Shevell SK. The subjective dates of natural events in very-long-term memory. *Cognit Psychol* 1985;17:139–77.

64. Vahlquist B. Migraine in children. *Int Arch Allergy Immunol* 1955;7:348–55.

65. Bille B. A 40-year follow-up of school children with migraine. Cephalalgia 1997;17:488–91.

66. Hockaday JM Definitions, clinical features, and diagnosis of childhood migraine. In Hockaday JM (Ed.). *Migraine in Childhood and other Non-epileptic Paroxysmal Disorders.* Boston: Butterworths, 1988:5.

67. Fry J. *Profiles of Disease: A Study in the Natural History of Common Diseases.* Edinburgh: E. & S. Livingstone, 1966.

68. Mathew NT, Reuveni U, Perez F. Transformed or evolutive migraine. *Headache* 1987;27:102–6.

69. Mathew NT, Stubits E, Nigam MP. Transformation of episodic migraine into daily headache: analysis of factors. *Headache* 1982;22:66–8.

70. Siberstein SD, Lipton RB, Solomon S, Mathew NT. Classification of daily and near-daily headaches: proposed revisions to the IHS criteria. *Headache* 1994;34:1–7.

71. Manzoni GC, Granella F, Sandrini G, Cavallini A, Zanferrari C, Nappi G. Classification of chronic daily headache by International Headache Society criteria: limits and new proposals. *Cephalalgia* 1995;15:37–43.

72. Solomon S, Lipton RB, Newman LC. Clinical features of chronic daily headache. *Headache* 1992;32:325–9.

73. von Korff M, Galer BS, Stang P. Chronic use of symptomatic headache medications. *Pain* 1995;62:179–86.

74. Diener HC, Dichgans J, Scholz E, Geiselhart S, Gerber WD, Bille A. Analgesic-induced chronic headache: long-term results of withdrawal therapy. *J Neurol* 1989;236:9–14.

75. Andersson PG. Ergotamine headache. *Headache* 1975;15:118–21.

76. Lavados PM, Tenham E. Epidemiology of tension type headache in Santiago, Chile: a prevalence study. Personal Communication.

77. Scher AI, Stewart WF, Liberman J, Lipton RB. Wolff Award 1998. Prevalence of frequent headache in a population sample. *Headache* 1998;38:497–506.

78. Castillo J, Munoz P, Guitera V, Pascual J. Epidemiology of chronic daily headache in the general population. American Association for the Study of Headache. 40th Annual Scientific Meeting. *Headache* 1998;6:151.

79. Breslau N, Davis GC, Andreski P. Migraine, psychiatric disorders, and suicide attempts: an epidemiologic study of young adults. *Psychiatry Res* 1991;37:11–23.

80. Silberstein SD, Lipton RB, Breslau N. Migraine: association with personality characteristics and psychopathology. *Cephalalgia* 1995;15:358–69.

81. Merikangas KR, Angst J, Isler H. Migraine and psychopathology. Results of the Zurich cohort study of young adults. *Archiv Gen Psychiatry* 1990;47:849–53.

82. Stewart WF, Linet MS, Celentano DD. Migraine headaches and panic attacks. *Psychosom Med* 1989;51:559–69.

83. Stewart WF, Shechter A, Liberman J. Physician consultation for headache pain and history of panic: results from a population-based study. *Am J Med* 1992;92:35S–40S.

84. Merikangas KR, Stevens DE, Angst J. Headache and personality: results of a community sample of young adults. 18th Collegium Internationale Neuro-Psychopharmacologicum Congress: Migraine: The interface between neurology and psychiatry (1991, Nice, France). *J Psychiatr Res* 1993;27:187–96.

85. Breslau N. Migraine, suicidal ideation, and suicide attempts. Neurology 1992;42:392–5.

86. Breslau N, Davis GC. Migraine, major depression and panic disorder: a prospective epidemiologic study of young adults [see comments]. *Cephalalgia* 1992;12:85–90.

87. Breslau N, Davis GC. Migraine, physical health and psychiatric disorder: a prospective epidemiologic study in young adults. *J Psychiatr Res* 1993;27:211–21.

88. Breslau N, Davis GC, Schultz LR, Peterson EL. Joint 1994 Wolff Award Presentation. Migraine and major depression: a longitudinal study. *Headache* 1994;34:387–93.

89. Andermann E, Andermann FA. Migraine-epilepsy relationships: epidemiological and genetic aspects. In Andermann F, Lugaresi E (Eds.). *Migraine and Epilepsy.* Boston: Butterworths, 1987:281.

90. Lipton RB, Ottman R, Ehrenberg BL, Hauser WA. Comorbidity of migraine: the connection between migraine and epilepsy. *Neurology* 1994;44:S28–S32.

91. Ottman R, Lipton RB. Comorbidity of migraine and epilepsy. *Neurology* 1994;44:2105–10.

92. Ottman R, Lipton RB. Is the comorbidity of epilepsy and migraine due to a shared genetic susceptibility? *Neurology* 1996;47:918–24.

93. Tzourio C, Iglesias S, Hubert JB, et al. Migraine and risk of ischaemic stroke: a case-control study [see comments]. *BMJ* 1993;307:289–92.

94. Tzourio C, Tehindrazanarivelo A, Iglesias S, et al. Case-control study of migraine and risk of ischaemic stroke in young women. *BMJ* 1995;310:830–3.

95. Lipton RB, Silberstein SD. Why study the comorbidity of migraine? *Neurology* 1994;44:S4–S5.

96. Michel P, Pariente P, Duru G, et al. MIG ACCESS: a population-based, nationwide, comparative survey of access to care in migraine in France [published erratum appears in *Cephalalgia* 1996 May;16(3):213]. *Cephalalgia* 1996;16:50–5.

97. Celentano DD, Stewart WF, Lipton RB, Reed ML. Medication use and disability among migraineurs: a national probability sample survey. *Headache* 1992;32:223–8.

98. Lipton RB, Amatniek JC, Ferrari MD, Gross M. Migraine. Identifying and removing barriers to care. *Neurology* 1994;44:S63–S68.

99. Lipton RB. Disability assessment as a basis for stratified care. *Cephalalgia* 1998;18:40–6.

100. Alders EE, Hentzen A, Tan CT. A community-based prevalence study on headache in Malaysia. *Headache* 1996;36:379–84.

101. Arregui A, Cabrera J, Leon-Velarde F, Paredes S, Viscarra D, Arbaiza D. High prevalence of migraine in a high-altitude population. *Neurology* 1991;41:1668–9.

102. Sachs H, Sevilla F, Barberis P, Bolis L, Schoenberg B, Cruz M. Headache in the rural village of Quiroga, Ecuador. *Headache* 1985;25:190–3.

103. Abdul JM, Ogunniyi A. Sociodemographic factors and primary headache syndromes in a Saudi community. *Neuroepidemiology* 1997;16:48–52.

104. Jaillard AS, Mazetti P, Kala E. Prevalence of migraine and headache in a high-altitude town of Peru: a population-based study. *Headache* 1997;37:95–101.

105. Merikangas KR, Whitaker AE, Angst J. Validation of diagnostic criteria for migraine in the Zurich longitudinal cohort study. *Cephalalgia* 1993;13 Suppl 12:47–53.

106. Rasmussen BK, Jensen R, Schroll M, Olesen J. Epidemiology of headache in a general population – a prevalence study. *J Clin Epidemiol* 1991;44:1147–57.

107. Russell MB, Rasmussen BK, Thorvaldsen P, Olesen J. Prevalence and sex-ratio of the subtypes of migraine. *Int J Epidemiol* 1995;24:612–18.

Index

Printed in the United States
by Baker & Taylor Publisher Services